Abandoning The Predator Diet

A Comprehensive Guide to Navigate the Modern Health Crisis

Dr. Hamid Muhyidheen

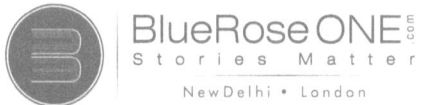

BLUEROSE PUBLISHERS
India | U.K.

Copyright © Dr. Hamid Muhyidheen 2025

All rights reserved by author. No part of this publication may be reproduced, stored in a retrieval system or transmitted in any form or by any means, electronic, mechanical, photocopying, recording or otherwise, without the prior permission of the author. Although every precaution has been taken to verify the accuracy of the information contained herein, the publisher assumes no responsibility for any errors or omissions. No liability is assumed for damages that may result from the use of information contained within.

BlueRose Publishers takes no responsibility for any damages, losses, or liabilities that may arise from the use or misuse of the information, products, or services provided in this publication.

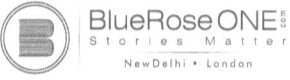

For permissions requests or inquiries regarding this publication,
please contact:

BLUEROSE PUBLISHERS
www.BlueRoseONE.com
info@bluerosepublishers.com
+91 8882 898 898
+4407342408967

ISBN: 978-93-7018-696-5

Typesetting: Sagar

First Edition: May 2025

Dedicated

To the pillars of my existence, my dear Father and Mother, with their boundless love, unwavering support, and prayers, guiding me through life's trials with wisdom at length.

Every step I take, is to make them proud.

"The Illiterate Of The 21st Century,

Will Not Be Those Who Cannot Read Or Write,

But Those Who Cannot Learn,

Unlearn,

And Relearn."

- Alvin *Eugene* Toffler

Acknowledgements

"The More Grateful I Am, The More Beauty I See" – Mary Davis

My name, **"Hamid"** means, *"One Who is Grateful."*
I have no idea if it is by the virtue of my name or not, but ever since I can remember, I have always been exceedingly grateful for everything in my life. First and foremost to The Almighty, for giving me this wonderful adventure called life, and showering me with an abundance of blessings that words could never fully capture.

Throughout my life, I have always considered myself lucky, it has always been as though, all the luck in the world is always by my side. Even through hardships and extremes, I have always had the unwavering support of my parents, grandmother, my better half, siblings and their families, relatives, friends, colleagues and mentors, who inspire and guide me, to focus my energy for a life of service.

Neither words nor actions, would never be enough to express the gratitude to my father, **Mr. Moideen. N.K**, and my mother **Mrs. Jameela. K,** without whose tireless support, prayers and love, I would never be able to take the bold steps in my life and career, which have helped me achieve more than I expected, and have given me so much satisfaction and happiness.
My eldest sister **Mrs. Majida**, her husband **Mr. Shahid Ali**, and their children **Mr. Razeen** and **Ms. Zara**, my brother **Mr. Aslam,** his wife **Mrs. Rahmath**, and their children **Mr. Azyan**, **Mr. Rayhan** and **Ms. Aliya,** my elder sister **Mrs. Najiya** and her husband **Mr. Junaise**, and their children **Ms. Ahlam** and **Mr. Aylan**, my younger sister **Mrs. Hadiya** and her husband **Mr. Khaleel**, and their children **Ms. Haleema**, **Ms. Afreen**, and **Ms. Aqsa,** my younger sister **Ms. Fadiya**, and my brother **Mr. Avvab**, have been an irreplaceable part during all my steps, and their love and support is more than I can ask for.
Even though I would like to write individually of how much each of them mean to me, as you can see, if I were to do so, my acknowledgement section would well exceed my page limit.

Words cannot articulate my gratitude to my better half, **Dr. Irfana. M**, whose unwavering support has been my constant. Your words of encouragement, even during the most challenging moments, have fuelled my determination to move forward. Thank you for your patience, understanding, and for always being there through the thick and thin.

I am indebted to **Dr. Praveen Jacob**, who is first and foremost, a wonderful human being, with whom I share a heartfelt kinship. You have been such a huge support, pushed me in the right direction, and provided me with all that I need, for this wonderful art of treating patients. His academic accomplishments, career achievements and contributions to the medical fraternity, as well as to the community as a whole, are so vast and excessive, that if I were to try and mention them all, then this book would seem as though it was about him.
So I will stop here, just mentioning my undying gratitude to you dear sir.

I am filled with gratitude to **Dr. Nagarajan** sir, who took me under his care, since my first day of college. He somehow felt that I was capable of achieving far more than I realized, and took it up as his personal mission to make a civilized and well-groomed doctor, out of the cave-man that I was, and to an extend... still am! Your tireless efforts in making a difference in the lives of your students, is irreplaceable. The knowledge, guidance and love that you gifted me, will never be forgotten. You are a gentle-man and the epitome of a professional. Thank you dear sir.

I feel truly humbled to be given a *"Foreword"* by the distinguished **Dr. P. V. Majeed,** who has achieved, and contributed so much, not only in India, but also across many other countries, throughout his 32 plus years of service. Besides being a skilled and expert physician, he is also a very successful entrepreneur, whose energetic and motivating leadership qualities, are an inspiration to one and all.
Thank you dear sir, for taking the time to read this book, giving me your wise and honest suggestions, and for your heartfelt support.

I would like to express my deepest gratitude to my PhD mentor, **Dr. Manjula Shantaram**, for her unwavering support and guidance through my doctoral journey. Her expertise, wisdom, and patience have been invaluable, and I am truly fortunate to have had the opportunity to work under her mentorship. Thank you dear ma'am.

I want to extend my heartfelt thanks to my elder brother, **Mr. Aslam Muhyidheen.** for taking the time to read and critique my book. Your thoughtful insights and constructive feedback, have been invaluable. I deeply appreciate the effort you put into understanding my work, and providing such detailed comments. Your perspective has not only helped me see my writing from a new angle, but has also motivated me to refine, and improve my manuscript from its initial 90 pages, to this 400+ paged pile of information.

I owe a great deal of thanks to my younger sister, **Ms. Fadiya Muhyidheen**, for her tireless support and for helping me re-evaluate my work. Her insightful feedback and valuable tips have been instrumental in improving my work as she is currently a student in the medical field. I truly appreciate her guidance and encouragement throughout this process.

I would like to thank all my teachers, professors and seniors, who have been important critics, mentors and a great inspiration to me, from my schooling and college years, and during my time of clinical practice, namely,
Mrs. Manju Singh, **Prof. Dr. B.T. Chidananda Murthy**, **Dr. Reeves. R**,
Dr. Dilip. V. R, **Dr. Pradeep Nair**, **Dr. Deepthi. K**, **Dr. Srinivas Gupta**,
Dr. G. Sharmila, **Dr. Renjish. M**, **Dr. Vijayaraghavan**, **Dr. Venkateswari. K**,
Dr. Manu Pradeesh, **Dr. Aannsmol. V** *chechi*, **Dr. Muthu Pandian** *anna*, and
Dr. A. Gopinath *anna* who have all shared invaluable knowledge, and instilled a sense of curiosity, and the confidence to pursue my dreams. I am truly grateful for all that you have given me, and for being my role models.

I am forever grateful to **Dr. Venkatramana Hegde**, whose timely presence, was a pivotal moment, that forced me to pursue clinical practice, than academics and teaching (where my heart still is). More than that, his dedication as a physician, is honestly, inspiring. I truly believe that his work over the past twenty plus years across Karnataka-India, has been a foundation for the easy acceptance of holistic health on a larger scale. I am deeply thankful to you sir for all that you have done for me, and your commitment, to creating a positive change.

I would like to extend my deepest gratitude to my esteemed colleagues and seniors, namely **Dr. Manoj Johnson, Dr. Marian George, Dr. Satheesh Babu, Dr. Aparna Satheesh,** and **Dr. Akhila Vinod,** with their unwavering devotion to communal well-being and tireless dedication to patient care.
It is a privilege to work alongside these experts, and I am grateful for their guidance, support, and example in serving the community selflessly and wholeheartedly.

My heartfelt appreciation and gratitude goes to **Chef Arvind Joshi**, an exemplary chef and a very dear friend of mine. His innovative recipes, have not only changed my approach to cooking, but have also opened my eyes to the incredible potential, of combining health conscious ingredients with elite flavours. I am endlessly grateful for your friendship and the incredible times we shared together.

With all my heart, I want to thank **Mr. Sankar Babu** *appa*, **Mrs. Rani Sankar Babu** *amma*, **Mr. Rajkumar** *maamji*, **Mrs. Anushya** *maami*, **Mr. Vikram** *anna*, **Mrs. Sushmitha** *anni*, **Mr. Venkatesh** *thambi*, **Ms. Vedha Varsha** *paapa*, and **Ms. Shriya Krishna** *paapa*, who've embraced me as part of the family, blessed me with their immense kindness and love, celebrating each of my achievements like their own. I stride forward well and confident, knowing that I will always be protected by your prayers, and blessing.

I have been immensely blessed to always have so many friends during the various stages of my life, and naming them all over here would not be possible. Friends are a huge influence in shaping a person's character, and I am thankful that my path in life, turned into a positive direction. I love you all, and thank you all, for filling my life with happiness, and in helping me to keep going in the right direction.

I can't thank enough, my friends and colleagues, who constantly help in my growth and who have spared their valuable time, to help review this book. Constant discussions with namely **Dr. Sudarshan. S**, **Dr. Ramya. S. Babu**, **Dr. Shaheed Ali**, **Dr. Jaseera. M. A**, **Dr. Logeshwaran**, **Dr. Naeela. R**, **Dr. Sasi Vignesh**, **Dr. Swetha. R**, **Dr. Naveen Kumar**, **Dr. Monica Sun**, **Dr. Karthik**, **Dr. Amirthavarshini**, **Dr. Naveen Prasad**, **Dr. Aashitha. P**, **Dr. Gayatri Devi**, **Dr. P. Manikandan**, **Dr. V. Madhumita**, **Dr. Ellakya. P**, **Dr. Amritha. C. K**, **Dr. Sudarshanan. R**, **Dr. J. Varshini**, **Dr. M. Kavya**, **Dr. Anju Paul**, **Dr. Gowsika. V**, **Dr. Sanam Yusuf**, **Dr. Camila Jaleel**, **Dr. Ajay Prakash**, **Dr. Keerthana. V**, **Dr. S. Sidharth**, **Dr. S. Vidhyashree**, **Dr. Pooja Dayalan**, and **Dr. Preethi. P**, who helped shape this book. Without their valuable input and constant feedback throughout my practice, I wouldn't be able to confidently move forward. My heartfelt gratitude and prayers to you all.

With immense gratitude, I want to thank the families of my cherished friends namely, **Mr. Hashim. K. L**, **Mrs. Safoora** and family, **Mr. Abdul Sathar**, **Mrs. Arifa** and family, **Mrs. Omanakutty** amma, **Mr. Kannankutty** and family, **Mr. & Mrs. Shanmugam. K. M** and family, **Mr. Ravikumar**, **Mrs. Priya Ravikumar** and family, **Mr. Sakeer**, **Mrs. Bushra** and family, **Mr. & Mrs. Ali** and family, **Mr. & Mrs. Umer** and family, **Mr. Anil Kumar**, **Mrs. Soni. A**, **Dr. Prabhu**, **Mrs. Deepa**, **Mr. & Mrs. Rasheed** and family, all who have welcomed me into their lives with, warmth, hospitality, and become a source of encouragement, and wisdom, enriching my life in ways I cannot fully express. You have overwhelmingly uplifted me, and I am deeply thankful for each one of you.

I would like to express my deepest gratitude to my dear friends as well as business associates, **Mr. Sadiq. M** and family, **Mr. Al Ameen. A**, his wife **Mrs. Mubeena** and family, and all the staff of *ZiwaGroup,* for their unwavering support, and without whom, I would not be able to efficiently take care of all my patients, and spread the ever needed awareness of healthy living.
This team, their commitment and tireless efforts, of more than 200 dedicated individuals, and still growing, are what completes "Dr. Hamid Muhyidheen" by being my multiple arms.
Thank you all, from the bottom of my heart.

I would also like to express and share my love and gratitude, to all my **Patients**, and regular **Audience**, who in a way, are the real inspiration for me to set out on this, adventurous path, of compiling information, that has resulted into this book. My motivation has always been, to simplify everything, so that my patients can easily understand the complexities of their health issues.
I firmly believe, that education must come before treatment, as it is the true path to free ourselves from disease.

I found much joy and knowledge in writing this book, and for that, I am deeply grateful to one and all who inspired, supported, and guided me throughout.
I am truly thankful for your unwavering belief in me, and your invaluable presence in my life.

Foreword

by

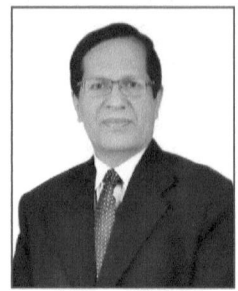

Dr. P. V. Majeed. BSc, MBBS, MBA.
Chairman, at **A. M. College of Pharmacy**
&
Executive Director, Paediatrician, Palliative Medicine consultant, Metabolic and Nutritional Medicine Consultant at
MIHRAS Multi-Speciality Hospital, Markaz Knowledge City- Calicut, Kerala- India
drpvmajeed@gmail.com

I am extremely delighted to write a foreword for the book written by Dr. Hamid Muhyidheen. In the acknowledgements of this book the author states that the name *"Hamid"* means *"One who is grateful."*
My name is *"Majeed"* which means *"Noble Glory."*
Incidentally, Hamid and Majeed are the commonly used words in the Muslim daily prayers. Hence, I have great pleasure to write a brief foreword for the book written by Dr. Hamid Muhyidheen.

This book is a worth reading compilation of science and facts, about food and energy. Each chapter covers the significance of food, focusing on nutrition, diet and calories. It also focuses on gut management, antioxidants and its healing properties, and many other exciting and relevant facts about nutrients and diet management.

The book can be read as a story, and one can finish the entire book in a single sitting. The central vision of this book is to spread the message of holistic living, promote scientific evidences of disease, and its prevention and control.

While going through the book, I am amazed to know that *"The Secret to Healthy, Long Life is - No Food"* which has no potential side effects on our health.
This book also has a sub-chapter about Autophagy, which is currently, of much relevance. The 2016 Nobel Prize in Physiology or Medicine, was awarded to Dr. Yoshinori Ohsumi, for his discoveries of the mechanisms for autophagy. Autophagy is a natural process in the body that deals with the destruction of cells in the body. It allows the body to recycle old cells, and regenerate new ones. This process plays a key role in maintaining cellular health, and it is found to have various benefits, including potentially slowing down aging, and preventing certain diseases. It's often associated with fasting and caloric restriction, as these conditions can stimulate autophagy.

Another chapter, that very much attracted me, is the one on mitochondria. Even though mitochondria are a small component of the cell, it is known as the power house of the cell. The strategic mission of the *Mitochondrial Biology Unit* (MBU), under Cambridge University, is to understand mitochondrial biology in health and disease, and to exploit this understanding, to develop new therapies and improve human health.
ATP is produced by mitochondria, and during ATP synthesis, the central rotor in mitochondria turns in one direction, and is shown to be about 150 times every second. In order to provide energy to sustain our lives, every day, each one of us produces a quantity of ATP, by this mechanism, that is approximately equal to our body weight.
German Scientist Dr. A. G. Fischer, invented an innovative equipment by utilizing QRS (*Quantum Resonance System*), which is used in my daily practices for pain management, and cellular correction based on, auto correction of mitochondria in cells. I had the opportunity to visit the institute of Dr. A. G. Fischer in Germany, and was able to understand more about mitochondria, and auto correction of ATP production in cells using QRS machine.

Obviously, this book is a good source of information to the common man, but it is also meant for the medical fraternity, researchers, and all who aims for a disease-free community. In short, this book is unique, and I'm sure that everyone will enjoy reading this book. Heartiest Congratulation Dr. Hamid Muhyidheen, for coming out with an informative compilation on food, nutrients, and causes of illness, which is the need of the hour.
I wish Dr. Hamid Muhyidheen all the success for his scientific endeavours.

With regards,

Dr. P. V. Majeed.

Preface

Ever since I can remember, I have always wanted to be a doctor. I'm pretty sure that it was solely by the influence of my mother, firstly, through her constant repetition that there was nothing better than being a doctor, which was imprinted on my mind (right now though, I do not agree with it, as I have witnessed, that all careers and jobs are of immense virtue). Secondly, she herself is a self-taught healer with many a trick up her sleeve. Her practical knowledge of medicinal plants is unmatched by anyone that I know, up to this day.

But my real quest for a more sustainable, and absolute health, started, when I felt devastated, humiliated, and defeated, when I was not able to successfully treat the Type-2 Diabetes, of one of my patients (**Mr. Mohammed Zaheeruddin**, an accomplished engineer, businessman, philanthropist and an esteemed gentleman), during my practice in Hyderabad. Even though financially, I was in a very comfortable stage at the time, despite being a fresher, that particular experience made me feel totally helpless, and restless. I felt like I couldn't stay there for a day longer, and so I resigned, packed my bags, and left immediately. I am extremely grateful to him, with whom I share a dear friendship even to this day, for being the reason, that set me out on this path of discovery.

Since then, I've been hungrier than ever, for knowledge, and to keep myself up to date with the latest advancements in medicine and health. Even though my main intention of writing this book, was for individuals from a non-medical background, to get a concise but clear picture of our body in relation to diseases, I am really satisfied with how this book has turned out to be, and can confidently say that even if you are a medical student, a practicing physician, a researcher, or anyone with a medical background, this book can help position you at a unique perspective, regarding health and diseases. Within these pages, you will find the collective efforts of countless individuals, scientists, physicians, researchers, and educators, who have dedicated their lives, to advancing the field of health and medicine. It is a combination of their expertise and research, through my personal experiences in the successful treatment of cases of metabolic syndrome, and auto-immune disorders, that has resulted into these pages, for the benefit of all who seek to expand their knowledge and skills, in the art of healthy living.

It is my sincere hope that this book will serve as a valuable resource and guide, on your journey through the vast and fascinating world of health. May it inspire you, challenge you, and empower you to make a positive impact in your lives, and in the lives of the ones you most love.

With warm regards,

Dr. Hamid Muhyidheen.

Introduction

In a world brimming with conflicting health information and ever-evolving wellness trends, where even harmful practices are promoted extensively, making informed decisions about your health can be overwhelming.
Even when it comes to healthy eating habits, there are still so many myths in this matter, that has become the biggest obstacle, for health seekers, from achieving a life of quality and health.

This book is designed to cut through the noise and provide clear, actionable guidance to help you make better health choices.
Through the complex working of the human body, the pursuit of a disease-free life, is an ever evolving journey, marked by a relentless pursuit of learning.
Drawing on the latest scientific research, expert insights, and practical strategies, my goal is to empower you with the knowledge and tools needed to take control of your well-being.
We explore key areas such as nutrition, exercise, mental health, and preventive care, offering evidence-based recommendations and real-life examples, to show you how these principles can be integrated into daily life. Whether you're seeking to improve your diet, adopt a more active lifestyle, or simply understand how various factors impact your health, this book serves as a comprehensive guide, to navigate the complexities of health and wellness.

Choosing a healthy diet is often frowned upon as it is considered a costly affair, but in truth, it is more cost-effective than facing the financial burden of surgeries due to extreme complications of various diseases, or the burden of ongoing medications.
For example, the average current rates for the medications or surgeries, for treating chronic lifestyle disorders and its complications, at a leading private hospital in Coimbatore-Tamil Nadu, India :-

- Insulin – ₹15,000 - ₹90,000 (Yearly).
- Dialysis – ₹1,50,000 - ₹3,50,000 (Yearly).
- Consultation charges for Special Surgeons – ₹3000 - ₹6000 per sitting.
- Diabetic retinopathy (injections, laser surgery etc.) – ₹30,000 - ₹1,00,000.

- CABG (coronary artery bypass grafting) – ₹1,00,000 - ₹5,00,000.
- Cancer treatments (including surgery) – ₹3,00,000 - ₹15,00,000.
- Kidney Transplant – ₹5,00,000 - ₹20,00,000.
- Liver Transplant – ₹18,00,000 - ₹25,00,000.
- Heart Transplant – ₹18,00,000 - ₹25,00,000.

For surgeries, these are the main charges, exclusive of medicine, anaesthesia, extra charges for transplant specialist surgeon, review and follow up charges, ambulatory, food, nursing and ward, ECG, ventilator support, pre-transplant investigations and evaluations charges, room charges (with increased charges for ICU), and much, much more.

Now the worst part of all this, is that these charges could skyrocket, to up to crores of rupees, depending on the availability, or rather 'unavailability' of these precious organs for transplant, especially the heart. When a donor becomes available, all the suitable candidates are informed, and the highest bidder gets to have a transplant.

It is worth noting that the average monthly income in India is just around ₹30,000 (₹3,60,000 per annum).

When it comes to healthcare, even struggling households with moderate incomes and little to no-savings, try to opt for the best hospitals and doctors (usually in expensive private sectors, in India), to try and give the best care for their dear loved ones, even when they are truly aware that they cannot afford it.
And so, the younger generations spend their lifetime trying to payback medical loans, that the elders would have racked up, and before long, they would find themselves in the same health situation…
loading their own children with even more financial burden, and sadly, the cycle continues, holding back young individuals from living a fulfilling life, away from heavy financial burdens, that was not their own to even begin with.

If you thought that was depressing, let me tell you that all of these organs are interdependent, and once you have a complication with one of these organs, like the kidney, it is highly likely that you have to get surgery for either the liver or heart in the near future.

It is estimated that up to **60%** patients suffer from multiple organ failures, if any one of these three important organs are severely affected. The emotional toll of dealing with chronic health issues and medical interventions can be profound, impacting not only the individual, but also that of their families.

Most patients suffering from these issues are not able to enjoy their life, or daily routine due to constant pain and discomfort, and even travelling short distances become a herculean task, that they feel, must be avoided.

Investing in whole, nutritious foods and preventive care, can significantly reduce long-term healthcare costs, and additionally, through prioritizing a balanced diet and an actively healthy lifestyle, not only do we safeguard our physical health, but also alleviate the stress and emotional strain associated with severe health complications, on ourselves, and our family and friends. Embracing preventive measures today, can lead to a healthier, happier, and more cost-efficient tomorrow.

If you are prepared with an open mind, and a thirst for knowledge, these chapters will be your guide, and each chapter will turn out to be a doorway, to new realizations.

Whether you're an expert or a newcomer, there is something here for everyone. I believe that the following information will be engaging, challenging, and inspirational to you, dear reader…

Contents

Chapter- 1 : Why Food Matters... 18

Chapter- 2 : A Story of The Biggest Lie Ever Told....................... 27

Chapter- 3 : The Lie Spread Like Wildfire To Kill **300 Million+**...... 33

Chapter- 4 : Low-Fat Diet Made Everyone **FAT**!......................... 36

Chapter- 5 : Heart Blocks and **FAT**!... 44

Chapter- 6 : The Real Culprit!... 49

Chapter- 7 : Designed To Process **FAT**!..................................... 54

Chapter- 8 : Choosing The Right Oil.. 65

Chapter- 9 : Counting **CALORIES** and When to Stop!.................. 78

Chapter- 10 : Stress & **CORTISOL**... 82

Chapter- 11 : Can You Really Avoid Bad Genetics?...................... 86

Chapter- 12 : Too Lazy To Exercise!... 88

Chapter- 13 : One Body, Shared by Two Friends......................... 94

Chapter- 14 : The Anti-biotic Dilemma..................................... 107

Chapter- 15 : One More Interesting Story................................. 113

Chapter- 16 : Pickle Body... 118

Chapter- 17 : Get to Know Our Major Food Groups................... 127

Chapter- 18 : The Secret to Healthy, Long Life is- **NO FOOD**...... 136

Chapter- 19 : Why Keto Diet is a Failure.................................. 144

Chapter- 20 : Protect Your **MITOCHONDRIA**....................... 153

Chapter- 21 : Is Organic Food Really a Scam?........................... 162

Chapter- 22 : Staple Food of the Future.................................. 182

Chapter- 23 : Treatment of the Future...................................... 188

Chapter- 24 : Diseases at Our Mercy....................................... 200

Chapter- 25 : Sample Diet Charts.. 374

Chapter- 26 : Sample Healthy Recipes..................................... 385

Chapter I – Why Food Matters.

The key to unlocking complete health in the modern era, is hidden in a few simple facts.

Humans had to majorly distance themselves from animals (as a food and nutrition source) twice in history, which was a vital catalyst, to bring about extensive positive and negative changes to our culture and health, as a society.

The first time was around **12,000** years ago,
and the second time… around **60** years ago.

The first time it occurred,

it was primarily circumstantial, due to mother nature's intervention, however, it had a more positive large scale impact, as it led to the vast expansion of the human population, paving the way for the emergence of more philosophically and technologically advanced civilizations.

But the second time though,

was due to our own doing, a decision, which led to a more negative impact, as it was the key factor in the emergence of the metabolic pandemic, that the world is engulfed in, and still suffers from, to this day.

Humans have been living on earth for more than **200,000** years!

And during this time, we have been farming, and consuming grains as our main food source, for only the last **12,000** years of it.

We humans depend on food for two major reasons, **Energy & Nutrition**.

Our energy is chemical energy (called ATP), which is like electricity. Our body must constantly create it, in order to function, and for us to stay alive.

Nutrition or Nutrients, are the building blocks in our body, which helps make hormones, immune cells, muscles, bones, carrier proteins, blood, skin, sperm, ovum, offsprings through reproduction… everything… even to make energy.

Let me state one other truly relevant fact, one to keep in mind…

*"All food that gives **Nutrients**, can give the body **Energy***

*But not all food that gives you **Energy**, can give you **Nutrition**."*

Try reading that again, before moving on to the next part.

Let us dig in a little deeper on why Nutrition must be given utmost importance.

The traditional classification of nutrients are as follows-

Macro-Nutrients (*Major*)	Micro-Nutrients (*Minor*)
1. Carbohydrates 2. Proteins 3. Fats	1. Vitamins 2. Minerals

The more accurate version for classification of nutrients, according to our body's needs should be as...

Macro-Nutrients (*Major*)	Micro-Nutrients (*Minor*)
1. Fats 2. Proteins 3. Water 4. Dietary Fibers	1. Vitamins 2. Minerals 3. Phyto-nutrients

You will have noticed that I removed the nutrient known as "most important" nutrient of all- **CARBOHYDRATES**.

Let me explain why.

A nutrient should be something that gives a unique gift to your body.
Something that none other can.
Without it, your body must suffer.
Only that particular nutrient should soothe the suffering.

We have all heard of deficiency diseases right?
If your body is lacking a single vitamin or mineral, there is a corresponding symptom or disease that follows.
For example-

Vitamins	Deficiency Disorders
Vitamin- A	Night blindness, dry, sticky eyes, increased risk of death in pregnancy and children.

Vitamin-B$_1$ (*Thiamine*)	Beriberi (cardiac and neurologic), Wernicke syndrome, and Korsakoff syndrome.
Vitamin-B$_2$ (*Riboflavin*)	Fatigue, blurred vision, dermatitis, brain dysfunction, impaired iron absorption, swollen throat, depression.
Vitamin-B$_3$ (*Niacin*)	Pellagra (causes dermatitis, diarrhoea, dementia, and even results in death).
Vitamin-B$_5$ (*Pantothenic acid*)	Fatigue, insomnia, depression, irritability, vomiting, stomach pains, burning feet, and upper respiratory infections.
Vitamin-B$_6$ (*Pyridoxine*)	Dermatitis, neurological disorders, convulsions, anaemia, elevated plasma homocysteine (high risk of atherosclerosis / heart block).
Vitamin-B$_7$ (*Biotin*)	Hair loss, skin rashes, brittle nails, fatigue, muscle pain, and neurological symptoms such as depression, lethargy, and tingling in the extremities.
Vitamin-B$_9$ (*Folate*)	Megaloblastic (few but abnormally large RBCs) anaemia, neural tube and other birth defects, heart disease, stroke, impaired cognitive function, depression.
Vitamin-B$_{12}$ (*Cobalamin*)	Megaloblastic anaemia (associated with helicobacter pylori induced gastric atrophy), gastric ulcers.
Choline (*formerly vitamin-B$_4$*)	Fatty liver disease, atherosclerosis (via lipoprotein secretion), neurological disorders, muscle aches, dysmenorrhoea, cognitive decline.
Vitamin-C	Scurvy (bleeding gums), fatigue, haemorrhages, low resistance / immunity to infection, biofilm formation by bacteria, leaky gut, anaemia.
Vitamin-D	Rickets, osteopenia, osteoporosis, abnormal colorectal growths, hair fall, endometriosis, frequent fevers and infection due to low immunity.
Vitamin-E	Low fertility, impaired in reflex, coordination, difficulty walking, and weak muscles.
Vitamin-K	Delayed clotting of blood causing significant bleeding, poor bone development, osteoporosis, and increased cardiovascular disease.

Minerals	Deficiency Disorders
Boron	Increased risk of osteoporosis due to low absorption of calcium and vitamin-D, hyperthyroidism, imbalance of testosterone and estrogen, neuropathy.
Calcium	Fractures, osteopenia, osteoporosis, rickets, dry scaly skin, brittle nails, pre-eclampsia, coarse hair, hypogalactia (low milk produced).
Copper	Leg muscle weakness, hair greying, saggy skin, loose faeces, anaemia (microcytic, normocytic, or macrocytic) and neutropenia. Thrombocytopenia (delay in wound clotting).
Iodine	Enlarged thyroid glands, reproductive failure, deficiency during pregnancy can cause cretinism, neonatal and infant mortality.
Iron	Dizziness, palpitations, breathlessness, fatigue, headaches, pale skin, Fanconi anaemia, aplastic anaemia, behavioural problems.
Magnesium	Infertility, poor growth, weak joints, muscle cramps, anxiety, insomnia, cardiac arrythmias, fatigue, constipation, depression, prolonged deficiency leads to diabetes, hypertension, coronary heart disease, dysmenorrhoea, osteoporosis.
Manganese	Epilepsy, infertility, lameness, poor growth, weakness, Mseleni disease, Down's syndrome, osteoporosis, and Perthest disease.
Phosphorus	Poor growth, rickets, soft bones, loss of appetite, anxiety, bone pain, fragile bones, stiff joints, fatigue, irregular breathing, irritability, numbness, weakness, and weight change. In children, decreased growth and poor bone and tooth development.
Potassium	Anorexia (eating disorder), arrhythmia (abnormal heart rhythm), incoordination, poor growth, hypertension, high risk of kidney stones, increased bone turnover.
Sodium Chloride	Nausea and vomiting, loss of energy / lethargy and confusion, loss of appetite. Serious cases can even cause seizures, coma and even death.
Selenium	Keshan disease (a type of cardiomyopathy, or disease of heart muscle). Kashin-Beck disease (a form of osteoarthritis). Nausea, vomiting, thyroiditis, headaches, muscle changes, hair-fall.
Zinc	Growth retardation, loss of taste and smell sensations, cheilitis (chapped & inflamed lips), thyroiditis, prostatitis, low sperm count, weak hair, dermatitis.

Nutrients	Important Functions
Dietary Fibers	We are talking about Soluble fibers / PREBIOTICS which essentially feeds and helps in growth of good microbiomes (bacteria, virus, fungi and a few worms as well) otherwise called as PROBIOTICS, which in turn produces essential nutrients, hormones and supports our body in various forms. A few examples- • Protects against colon cancer. • Prevents and helps alleviate gastrointestinal disorders (IBS, Crohn's, Ulcerative colitis, gastritis etc.) • Controls high bad cholesterol levels and manage blood pressure. • Reduces inflammation. • Protects against colonization of harmful microbiota, fungal overgrowth, parasites etc. • Helps in growth of micro-plastic digesting probiotics. • Treats piles, fissures, fistula and constipation. • Helps remove waste from the body. • Supports a strong immune system. • Helps control appetite and manage body weight, as well as actively aiding in weight loss. • Influences & benefit your mood & mental wellness.
Water	• The human body is 70% water. • It delivers oxygen & nutrients throughout the body. • Regulates body temperature. • Moistens tissues in the eyes, nose and mouth. • Protects body organs and tissues. • Major constituent of lubricating fluids of joints and cartilaginous discs in between the vertebral (back-bones). • Essential in waste excretion along with kidneys, liver, skin etc. • Crucial in digestion and absorption of nutrients to make them accessible to your body, and to be transported throughout. • Dehydration (low levels of water/fluids) causes dry mouth, sunken eyes, poor skin turgor, cold hands and feet, weak and rapid pulse, rapid and shallow breathing, confusion, exhaustion, and… • Loss of fluid constituting more than 10% of body weight will result in coma & eventually death.

Nutrient	Important Functions
Fats	<ul><li>Basic structure of each cell membrane (cell wall) to keep them fluid facilitate the exchange of nutrients, maintain cell integrity, fluidity, permeability and increases communication between cells.</li><li>Compose more than 70% of brain cells (the most crucial molecules that determine your brain's integrity and ability to perform).</li><li>LCFA are vital for brain and eye development during infancy.</li><li>Maintaining nerve impulse transmission - Myelin sheath.</li><li>Reduces inflammation and is also a potent anti-oxidant.</li><li>Produces messenger chemicals called cytokines, which are involved in the inflammatory response.</li><li>Crucial in absorption & transport of fat soluble vitamins A, D, E, K</li><li>Best fuel (Fat is the most concentrated source of energy with the least production of toxic by-products / free-radicals).</li><li>Provides insulation by maintaining body temperature in cold environments, by converting to energy, and the adipose tissue, where fat is stored, acts as an insulator by reducing heat loss from the body.</li><li>Fat pads around organs provide cushioning and protection, helping to prevent injury, and act as a buffer, absorbing shock & providing a layer of protection for vital organs like the kidneys and liver.</li><li>Essential for the normal growth and development and maintenance of the body as fats are the building blocks of steroid hormones (testosterone, oestrogen, progesterone, cortisol etc.)</li><li>Adipose tissue produces and stores hormones such as leptin, which regulates appetite, and adiponectin, which influences insulin sensitivity and metabolism.</li><li>Cholesterol is required to produce bile acids which in turn helps to digest other fats and fat soluble vitamins.</li><li>If our body cannot synthesize cholesterol, like in case of a disease called "Smith-Lemli-Opitz Syndrome"… it results in a number of issues to the body including autism, mental retardation, lack of muscle, and even death.</li><li>Plays a vital role in Human Immunity (explained in detail in Chapter- 7)</li><li>Body fat percentage lower than 3% for Men and 12% for Women can lead to multiple organ & system failure and eventually death.</li></ul>

Nutrient	Important Functions
Proteins	• Structure, growth & maintenance of the body. • Forms into enzymes that is crucial in various functions. • Hormones (Insulin, glucagon, growth hormone etc.) • Fluid and Acid-Base Balance. • Transport & storage of nutrients, hormones & fats. • Immunity & Protection (help form immunoglobulins or antibodies). • Wound Healing and Tissue Regeneration. • Energy Production. • Insufficiency of protein will lead to Kwashiorkor, Marasmus, impaired mental health, weakened immune system, oedema, leaky gut syndrome, wasting and shrinkage of muscle tissues, and organ failure, leading to extreme complications of the body.

So far, we have been able to list out some of the unique problems (diseases) that our body would have to face, when it is deficient in the corresponding Nutrients, be it Macro or Micro.

This is common knowledge to the medical fraternity, and to a lesser extent, to the general public as well.

If you would have noticed, I did not write about the deficiency disease that our body would have to face, if it was devoid of carbohydrates (or any other sugars from the diet).

Do you know why?

Because it doesn't have any... that's why!

If we were to make a table on the benefits of carbohydrates / sugars... all it would have to say for itself is "**Energy Producing Molecule**"...

Which is not something unique...
Fats & Proteins are a more efficient, and cleaner energy fuels than carbohydrates or sugars!

You see, the process of producing energy from carbohydrates / sugars, is just our body struggling to somehow, get rid of, or simply trying to throw away all that carbohydrates or sugars that we just ate…
out from our system!
We shall discuss about it in detail, in the chapter on Insulin Resistance.

Some may even point out that Hypo-glycemia (low blood sugar) is a deficiency disease of carbohydrates / sugars.
But it is **NOT**, and we shall discuss about this in detail too, while discussing Insulin Resistance.

Imagine that if our body was a house…
NUTRIENTS, are like the necessary materials needed to make a house, like the bricks, wood, stone, cement, metal, concrete etc.
ENERGY, is the "effort" done by workers or machines, in order to build the house.

Carbohydrates or sugars, only offer us energy (which can be obtained from other sources as well), and is not part of any fundamental or vital building material for the various physical or chemical aspects of our body (including organs, glands, hormones etc.)

But is it fair to villainize all sugars?
No, it really isn't fair.

I will tell you about a special, beneficial sugar, later on in the book.
But for now, keep reading, to understand why our current food habits, is not the right way for graceful ageing.

With that in mind, we have now established that –
Fats, Proteins, Dietary Fibers, Water, Vitamins, Minerals, Phyto-Nutrients (briefed in later chapters), and a unique form of sugar (not the ones we get directly from our food), are the only vital ingredients, required by our body for optimum health & functioning.

In the meantime, let me tell you a very interesting story…

Chapter II – A Story of The Biggest Lie Ever Told.

In 19th Century America, before road highways and railroads, the main system of transport for goods or cargo was by water-ways, through a system of rivers, canals, and lakes. Cincinnati, a city in Ohio state, was at that time, the heart and soul, of the **United States** of **America**.

The city of Cincinnati had a very fascinating nickname.
During that period, the most consumed meat in America was pork, and Cincinnati became the meat-packing hub, where livestock was butchered and sold locally or shipped to other states & countries. Cincinnati was the pork-processing center of the country, and so came to be called as "**Porkopolis.**"

Pig or pork was the popular meat source of the 19th century America and not Beef, as opposed to recent times, sheerly due to convenience of storage. You see, this was a time before refrigeration and the biggest struggle of 19th century butchers, was spoilage or rotting of meat.

Pigs are high in body-fat (around 25%), which makes them excellent for salt curing, which not only preserves the meat, but also helps in preserving its flavour.

Since pork meat was the main material for trade, the by-products of pork such as its skin, bones and fat were plentiful, which helped build an industry for *Tanneries*, *Boot Makers*, and *Upholsters* (soft, padded textile covering, fixed to furniture, like sofas), in Cincinnati. ***Animal Fats*** too, were valuable products, as they were made into soap and candles.

This is where I would like to introduce to you, two esteemed Gentlemen. They are first and foremost, Businessmen, before anything else.
Their names were **William Procter**, and **James Gamble.**

William Procter, a native of England, emigrated to America to start his candle-making business, after a fire destroyed his business in England. James Gamble, a native of Ireland, fled the country during the Great Potato Famine and became a soap manufacturer in the United States.

These two men happened to marry two sisters, Olivia & Elizabeth Norris, from Cincinnati.

Their father-in-law, Alexander Norris, is the one who first suggested, that the two of them, should go into business together.

And in 1837, a soap and candle manufacturing company, "**Procter & Gamble**" was born.

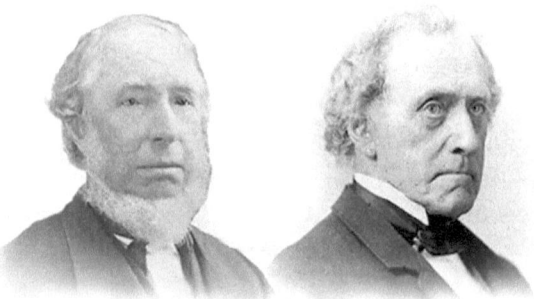

William Procter & *James Gamble*

In the 1870s, a major economic depression hit the United States and abroad which forced the two brothers, to somehow come up with a strategy, to survive this economic crisis.

And they did find a new strategy.

During that time, soap was manufactured as very large wheels, which were then sliced into smaller portions and sold at general stores.

Procter and Gamble's new strategy was, to mass-produce individually wrapped bars of soap, like we find in markets today.

But to make this happen, the brothers-in-law needed to reduce the price of their raw ingredients, and find a suitable replacement for the expensive animal fats (mainly pork fat).

They settled on a mix of palm and coconut oils, and created the first soap that floated in water.

This was seen as a very innovative invention at the time because, clothes and dishes alike, were washed in a basin filled with soapy lather (which was quite an inconvenience).

In a relatively short time, Americans all over the country came to know of this new and clean soap.

The **Procter & Gamble** company acquired a good reputation for purity, and started to be noticed nation-wide.

Procter & Gamble still kept pursuing the search for a lower-cost raw ingredient, which could further increase their profits.

> Let us stop here for now, and take a break on this lead.
> We will come back to this point soon.

During our short break,

I'd like to give you a very brief look on the **Cotton Industry** in the **USA**.

When Columbus discovered America in 1492, he found cotton growing in the Bahama Islands. A mere 8 years later, by the year 1500, cotton was known generally throughout the world.

The cotton market, which accounted for more than 50% of all American exports during the 19th century, supported America's ability to borrow money from abroad, and helped build enormous trade with the rest of the world.

But until the 1800s, cotton seed was considered as the waste of the cotton industry, as the oil extracted from cotton-seed, was not fit for consumption.

You see, cotton-seed oil is a very cloudy, red and bitter tasting oil, because it contains a chemical called **Gossypol**.

It is so dangerous, that even to this day, it is used in China as a method for male birth control, as it damages the male reproductive cells.

Gossypol is also toxic to most animals, and is shown to cause dangerous spikes in the body's potassium levels, cause organ damage, and even lead to paralysis of the whole body

And so, before the invention of the "**Cotton Gin**" (cotton engine- is a machine that quickly and easily separates cotton fibers from their seeds, giving much greater productivity), the cotton seeds were dumped into rivers, as an industrial waste.

Even after the invention of the Cotton Gin in 1793, most of these massive machines were set up on the banks of rivers, streams, or any other water source, so that the seeds could be easily dumped into the water source, and it would be washed away.

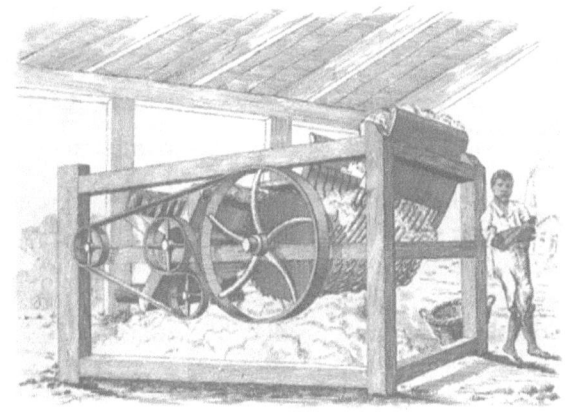

'Cotton Gin'

But since the toxic effects of cotton-seeds were well known by the 1790s, a penalty fine of **$200** was issued for dumping cotton-seed in any stream used for drinking or fishing, or if it was within an **800 metre radius** of a city or village.

So as you can see, this toxic waste of the cotton industry, was a menacing and looming issue at the time.

One of the good uses that they found for this oil, was to use it as an engine lubricant or fuel (like bow gasoline or petroleum is used).

Chemists of the time, tried to come up with various useful processes to use this waste oil, as fertilizers, soap, candles, cattle feed etc.

But even then, the toxicity in the seed still remained, which caused various health issues to those who used the products.

We can now continue with **Procter & Gamble**...

They, at last found their ultra-low-cost alternative oil, to mass produce their candles & soaps... which is the very same, toxic - Cottonseed oil, that we just discussed about.

And thanks to them, the United States economy, was boosted by the increase in production and sales of useful soaps and candles, from this ultra-low-cost raw ingredient (cotton-seed oil).

On the plus side, the toxic waste product of cotton farming, now got a new useful purpose.

A German chemist, Edwin Keyser, discovered a new chemical process, that could create a solid fat, from oils that are liquid.

Procter & Gamble immediately purchased the United States patent rights to this technology, and created a laboratory to experiment with the new process.

Soon the company's scientists produced a new creamy, white substance out of cottonseed oil, and it looked just like the most used cooking fat of that time... **Lard** (pork fat).

Procter & Gamble saw this as a game changing opportunity to grow their business venture, by entering the market for cooking oils.

Before long, they sold this new substance (known today as hydrogenated vegetable oil) to homes, as a replacement for animal fats.

This, my dear reader, was the foundation stone, responsible for the death of well over **300 million** people, up to date and still counting, due to metabolic related diseases.

Chapter III –
The Lie Spread Like Wildfire To Kill 300 Million+

An edition of the *"Popular Science"* Magazine from the 20th century, sums up the evolution of cotton-seed and its oil, precisely analysed as-

> *"What was **garbage** in 1860,*
> *was **fertilizer** in 1870,*
> ***cattle feed** in 1880,*
> *and **table food** and many things else in 1890."*

Garbage-- to engine oil-- to food-- happened over the span of 40 years.

Through the new food-processing invention of hydrogenation, the toxic cottonseed oil found its way into the kitchens of America's restaurants and homes.
Procter & Gamble came up with the name **'Crisco'** which was adapted as short for *crispness, freshness,* and *cleanliness*.

Convincing homemakers to replace butter and lard for a new fat created in a factory would be a difficult task, so the new form of food needed a new marketing strategy.
Never before in history, had any company, put so much money for advertising a product.

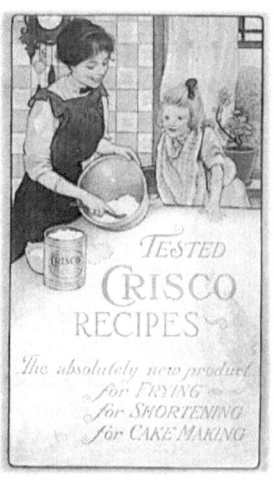

'Crisco Cook-book 1912'

They hired the **J. Walter Thompson Agency**, America's first full service advertising agency staffed by professional writers and artists. Various different marketing strategies were tested in different cities. Samples of "**Crisco**" were mailed to grocers, restaurants, nutritionists, and home economists. Doughnuts were fried in "**Crisco**" and handed out in the streets. Women who purchased the new industrial fat, got a free cook-book of "**Crisco**" recipes, where all recipes required three to four tablespoons of "**Crisco**."

Health claims on food packaging were unregulated at the time, and so, the copywriters claimed that cottonseed oil was healthier than animal fats, for digestion and health.
Heavy advertisements resulted in the sales of over **1.7 million** litres of "**Crisco**" in 1912, and over **27 million** litres, just four years later.

This new food was responsible for bringing in the age of, **Low-Fat** foods.

Procter & Gamble's Crisco was over 50% **trans-fat**. It wasn't until the 1990s that the health risks of trans-fats were understood. It is estimated that for every **2%** increase in consumption of trans-fat, the risk of heart disease increases by **23%**.

But the event that actually led up to give "*Scientific Support*" to this dangerous oil, responsible for the deaths of well over 300 million people and still continuing to this day, was the Heart Attack of then US president, Dwight Eisenhower in 1955, who later died from congestive heart failure in 1969.

Doctors and dignitaries from all over the country, came to visit the President after his first heart attack, and in attendance, was a founder member of the AHA (American Heart Association), Dr.Paul Dudley White. Also in attendance was **Ancel Benjamin Keys**, a physiologist with a PhD from Cambridge University.

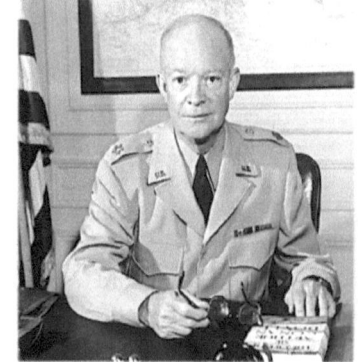

Dwight Eisenhower

During this event, **Ancel Keys** presented false research to Dr. Paul Dudley, which stated that '**saturated fats were bad because they increased blood cholesterol, which blocked coronary arteries and caused heart attacks.**'

As a result of this discussion, the AHA declared in 1961, that '**saturated fats were bad because they increased blood cholesterol, which blocked coronary arteries and caused heart attacks.**'

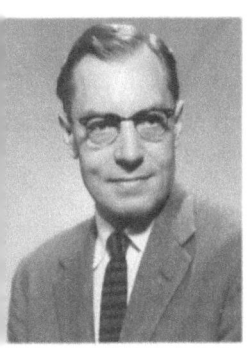
Ancel Keys

The AHA, was driven to this conclusion under pressure to uphold its reputation as a leading health authority, and was compelled to issue a decisive statement following President Eisenhower's heart attack.
Lacking a clear understanding of the actual cause, they relied on the only available (though flawed) research to appear credible.

With public trust and institutional credibility at stake, the AHA prioritized delivering **certainty** over **scientific accuracy**, ultimately shaping policy based on speculation rather than solid evidence.

An unbiased investigator would have realised the problems in Ancel Keys' hypothesis, as they have realized at present.
But the issue at the time was that,
- The AHA had not been presented with the complete data,
- And mainly because our friends, **Procter and Gamble**, had made a very small donation to the AHA, an amount worth around **USD- $20 *Million*** today.

The American College of Cardiology and even the World Health Organisation, followed AHA guidelines, and declared that fats in general, and saturated fats in particular, were to be strictly avoided to prevent a heart attack. Meat (red or white), cheese, butter, and egg yolk became prohibited foods.

The "Professional Advice" was to...
- Reduce fats to less than **30%** of the total calories per day.
- Reduce saturated fats below **10%** of the total fats consumed.

Even to this day, the global majority, including **Doctors**, follow these dietary commandments, because it was directed by the two most powerful, and respected cardiology associations...
not knowing that this advice was built on a lie.

This was the wind and fuel, that spread the lie like wildfire, causing a metabolic epidemic and the deaths of over 300 million people around the globe, up to date and still counting.

Chapter IV – Low-Fat Diet Made Everyone FAT!

So far, we have established that good natural sources of Fat, are essential for a healthy body, and anyone who still preaches that meat, fish, dairy and egg yolks will give you heart attacks, have been successfully misguided by Ancel Keys, William Procter, and James Gamble.

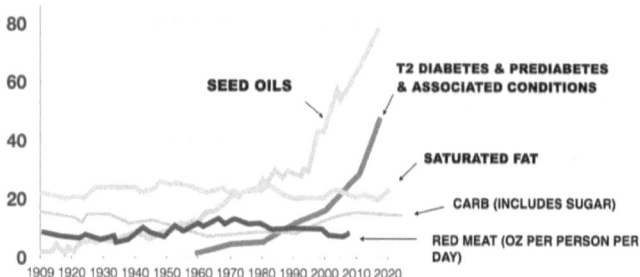

This is a graph representation, of how increased consumption of refined seed oils (cottonseed, sunflower seed, palm-olein, canola, corn, soybean, rice-bran, grapeseed etc.) since the 1960's, led to a direct impact on obesity rates, which have tripled, creating a public health crisis so widespread and damaging that, which started as an epidemic in the USA, is now a pandemic worldwide.

Why are we talking about obesity?
Does obesity have anything to do with heart attacks?

Yes it does, let me tell you how.

- **INSULIN RESISTANCE**

Insulin Resistance is the root cause for Obesity, Diabetes Mellitus Type-II, Fatty Liver, PCOD, Hypertension, Dyslipidaemia and many other Metabolic Disorders.

So *Insulin Resistance* is a bad guy right?
Well, in this age and time it affects us badly, but there was a time when we needed it dearly.

Yes its true... once upon a time, *Insulin Resistance* was the good guy, a vital tool for us, to survive a harsh time on earth, and which helped us get to where we are now.

We are alive now, because we are the descendants of people, who had in their body, superior process of *Insulin Resistance*.

12,000 years ago, before humans became settlers, and started farming grains for food, we were hunter gatherers.
During our hunting-gathering period, we had to rely solely on seasonal foods, as we were not advanced enough to store, or preserve food.

But by nature, our body had the technology to store and preserve food. This technology is what we call *Insulin Resistance*.

Our body would convert all the food that we ate in the summer season, into body fat, and store it. In the summer, we ate plenty of meat, fruits, and honey which would cause our body to secrete *Insulin*, which is the hormone that converts it all, into Fat storage.

And when the winter season arrived, and we had very little food to eat, our body would burn our fat stores for energy, and help us survive.

The *Summer* was a season of **Feasting**...
and *Winter* was the season of **Fasting**.

Since our ancestor's bodies were forced to use up all the extra stored fat in their body within 6 months, there was no time for the stored up fat, to cause damages to their body, in the form of metabolic diseases.

Two important things happen to sugars inside our body after we consume it. Insulin is released into our blood, where it either -

- Converts the sugar into Energy
(by triggering the appearance of a door called GLUT-4)

(OR)

- Stores it as glycogen stores, or as body fat.

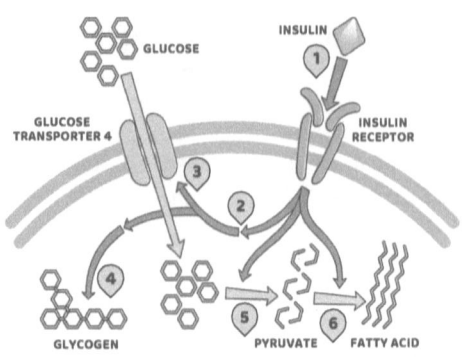

Mechanism of Insulin

Usually, the body stores the sugar as fat, into cells called as ADIPOCYTES, which are specially designed for storing fat. The main types of adipocytes that the body chooses for fat storage are *Subcutaneous Adipose Tissue* (**SAT**) and *Visceral Adipocyte Tissue* (**VAT**).

When we eat **adequate amounts** of sugar, the body stores the fat in the SAT type of adipocytes that are mostly located just beneath our layer of skin, especially in the thighs, arms, buttocks etc.

When we eat **more than adequate amounts** of sugar, our body starts to panic, and feels that there is not enough time to search for the SAT, to safely store this sugar as fat.

Now why does our body panic when so much sugar enters our body?

Because, as we all know, if high amount of sugar remains in the blood stream (as in the case of *Type-2 Diabetes Mellitus*) it will cause massive damage (called glycation or oxidation), around the body, starting from the most delicate of our organs, such as our kidneys, eyes and nerves, causing conditions like diabetic nephropathy, retinopathy or neuropathy.

So... when our body starts to panic, when we eat **more than adequate amounts** of sugars, our body feels that there is not enough time to search for SAT, and so it just hurriedly stores all this sugar, into the nearest adipocytes it finds, which are mostly **VAT** (*Visceral Adipocyte Tissues*). VAT are located deep within the abdominal cavity, surrounding internal organs like the liver, pancreas, and intestines.

Now the primary differentiating function that sets apart SAT from VAT, is that SAT undergoes '**hyper-PLASIA**' whereas VAT undergoes '**hyper-TROPHY.**'

Hyperplasia means that when there is excess of fat being stored, and SAT cannot take it anymore, SAT cells starts to multiply and increases the number of SAT cells, to help store more fat.
This helps reduce the stress on each cell.

Hypertrophy means that when there is excess of fat being stored, and VAT cannot take it anymore, VAT cells starts to grow larger to accommodate more fat storage.
But there is a limit to how much VAT can grow, so this can cause the increased amount of fat to squeeze the internal organelle of the cells, which causes extreme stress to the VAT.

And when *Insulin* starts forcing the sugars, as fat into the VAT cells, it becomes very uncomfortable and stressed.
Our body senses these stress signals, and sends out soldier cells to protect the VAT, but our body cannot exactly differentiate, if the stress is caused due to a harmful micro-organism or some other reason.

Our soldier cells then start shooting and firing out various signals, to start an inflammatory response from our body, in the form of something known as cytokines or interleukins, in the hope to kill whatever it is, that is causing the stress to the visceral cell.

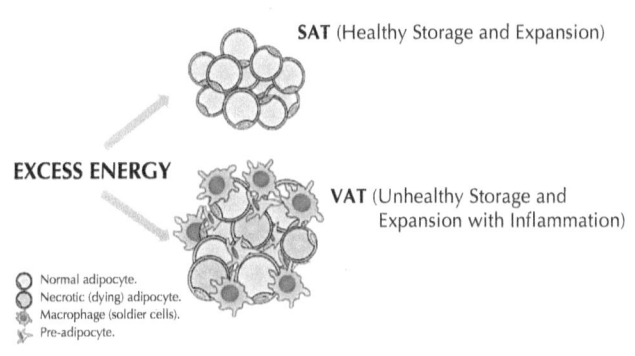

SAT (Healthy Storage and Expansion)

EXCESS ENERGY

VAT (Unhealthy Storage and Expansion with Inflammation)

○ Normal adipocyte.
○ Necrotic (dying) adipocyte.
 Macrophage (soldier cells).
 Pre-adipocyte.

Unfortunately, "**Fat**" cannot be "killed" like bacteria or viruses, so the soldier cells keep continuing to fire their inflammatory cytokines.

When this inflammation continues over a long period of time, it starts to damage a lock, that is present on all cells, called as INSULIN RECEPTORS, (the key to this lock is Insulin).

Once the *'insulin receptors'* are damaged, *'insulin'* will no longer be able to cause GLUT4 doors to open, which is responsible for taking sugars, and converting them into **Energy**.
This is called as INSULIN RESISTANCE.

When insulin resistance occurs, and the body cannot create energy from sugars, the body then has no other choice, but to re-direct all the sugar that enters the body, into storage, as Fat.
When fat keeps accumulating in different parts of the body, it leads to **OBESITY**.

When fat starts to accumulate in the liver, so much that the inflammation then affects the normal functioning of the liver, it leads to non-alcoholic **FATTY LIVER** disease.

When fat starts to accumulate in the ovaries, so much that the inflammation arising due to it, then starts to affect the normal functioning of the ovaries, and forms cysts, or causes hormonal imbalances, this is called as **PCOS** (*Polycystic Ovarian Syndrome*).

When all the locks (*insulin receptors*) are damaged, the body will not be able to make energy from sugars. As a consequence, we will start to feel dizzy and lose consciousness, which is known as - **HYPOGLYCAEMIA** or *'low blood sugar.'*

So this is, in fact an *'**energy**'* deficiency disorder…
and not a *'**sugar**'* deficiency disorder, as it is often misunderstood.
This only occurs, when we depend solely on sugar rich foods for energy.
It would not have happened, if we had given our body different options, to make energy from other foods as well.

When all our *Visceral cells*, are filled with sugars as fat, and cannot store anymore, and at the same time, when sugar cannot be converted into energy because all the doors (receptors) are damaged... then our body becomes helpless, and the sugar becomes stagnant in the blood, and this situation or condition, is called as **Type-II Diabetes Mellitus.**

The development of insulin resistance, causes a surge in insulin production called as hyper insulinemia, which in turn results in faster weight gain, and as the vicious cycle continues, it makes the insulin resistance situation even worse.
There are lots of symptoms of insulin resistance that are body shows us, but we are not too bothered about it to realise that it is in fact, the earlier signs of something deadly that is to befall upon our body.

Darkened skin in the armpit, back, sides of the neck, on cheeks, sides of the forehead etc. is something called *Acanthosis Nigricans*. It is one of the classic signs of insulin resistance. Skin tags or small skin growths are also commonly noticed along with fatigue and tiredness.

It is quite a common knowledge that the three primary symptoms of high blood sugar are increased thirst, increased hunger, and increased frequency of urination.

In the same way, one of the common symptoms of high blood sugar in children is ***bed-wetting,*** which is commonly blamed on lack of cognitive development or carelessness.
And when bedwetting persists after the age of 7 years, the kids are even taken to psychologists and swiftly labelled with borderline ADHD or a cognitive disorder of some sort. All this trouble could have been avoided if we had simply cut out their excess sugary drinks and sweets, saving both the children and the parents from the struggle and suffering.

But even though 12,000 years ago we started cultivating and consuming grains (rice, wheat, corn etc.), which are 80% carbohydrates / sugars, as our main food, and that too throughout the year, we still did not start suffering from metabolic disorders, until after the 1960s.

Why?

1. Only 40% of our total diet had carbohydrates / sugars. On top of that, the grains we consumed were whole-grains, mostly *'spelt'* grains with a 45% net carbohydrate content, (unlike the highly refined GMO grains available to us today with 70% net carbohydrate content), which helped in keeping the glycaemic index low.

    Moreover, it was a common practice to consume fermented carbs such as overnight porridge or sour bread, which again, drastically decreased its sugar content, and instead, created other highly beneficial nutrients (like soluble fibers).

2. Around 40% of our diet included good, beneficial Fats.
    Dairy products (milk, curd, butter, ghee, cheese etc.), nuts, fats from meat like lard and tallow, eggs, fatty fish were all consumed in plenty of amounts.

3. Around 20% of our diet included animal proteins (fish, mutton, beef, chicken, pork) which are complete and more bio-available (our body's ability to absorb and utilize it efficiently).

4. There was no constant snacking like we do nowadays, and even when they did snack, it was any seasonal fruit that was available, or sun-dried or preserved meat etc.
    There were mainly only one or two meals a day.
    Three or four meals a day was only possible for the privileged.

5. Almost everyone where farmers or in professions that required hard physical labour, which activates *'exercise-mediated glucose uptake'* pathways, that opens up GLUT4, and allows muscles to absorb glucose for energy without requiring insulin.

    This process reduces the risk of glucose being stored as fat, as *insulin* is typically responsible for promoting fat storage of sugars or carbohydrates. So there was no time for sugar to stay in the blood and cause its harmful deeds.

All of this came to an abrupt halt in 1961, when the AHA declared that saturated fats were bad, because they increased blood cholesterol, which blocked coronary arteries and caused heart attacks.
This caused a drastic shift in the diet of the general population-

1. Around 70% of our total diet shifted to carbohydrates / sugar rich, ultra refined, and genetically modified grains (which increased the glycaemic index, lowered the soluble fiber content, and modified the gluten content to become a more harsh version that triggers our immune system as well).

2. Consumption of dietary fats reduced to about 10% compared to the previously healthy amount of 40%.

3. The majority of good fats were replaced by the toxic waste, *Refined Oils*, which contained high levels of *Omega*-6 fatty acids and *Aldehydes* which are highly inflammatory and even cancerous, which was responsible for the sudden onset of **Insulin Resistance.**

4. We started to constantly snack on unhealthy ultra-processed options like deep fried chips or carbonated or sugary drinks. Three or four meals a day became possible for the lower income families as well.

5. Since technology had advanced by this time (grinders, washing machines, motor vehicles etc.), hard physical labour had reduced to a great extent, which meant less need for energy.

   Yet, we started consuming even larger amounts of food, as it started to become possible for the majority of the population, to be able to afford at least 3 meals a day.

> As we have just seen in the graph at the beginning of this chapter, the major shift in our diet occurred, after the AHA's declaration, resulting in the rise in usage of refined oils and refined grains, and avoidance of natural saturated fats, leading to a drastic increase of metabolic diseases, and the subsequent deaths of millions, from its complications.

Chapter V – Heart Blocks and FAT!

Why a special chapter for heart blocks?

Because the statement by the American Heart Association in 1961–

Saturated Fats Were Bad Because They Increased Blood Cholesterol, Which Blocked Coronary Arteries & Caused Heart Attacks-

… sent everyone into a frenzy and made them stop eating good fat, a vital and absolutely important nutrient!

So, what exactly is a heart block?

The majority of the population, to this day, believes that heart blocks or *Atherosclerosis* are actually hardened pieces of fat, from butter or ghee or coconut oils… that stops blood circulation, and damages the heart.

Actually, the yellow-coloured block shown in the picture below, is not fat, as many would assume. In fact, it is the buildup of **PUS**.

1- *Normal Blood Vessel*

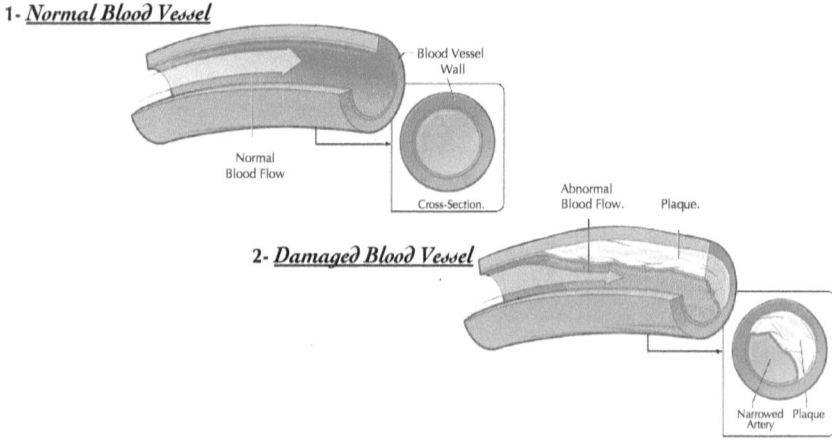

2- *Damaged Blood Vessel*

We have all, at least once in our life, had pus develop in our body either from pimples or wounds to the skin.

For pus to develop, we first and foremost need a site of wound or injury.

And then, if the injury is infected by harmful bacteria or virus, our immune system begins trying to fight it off, by sending soldier cells (white blood cells) to the area, to destroy the harmful bacteria.

Pus is the dead and decaying matter of a battlefield.
A battle between our soldiers (WBCs), and harmful bacteria.

In the same way, if pus has developed in our blood vessels, it means there must have been an injury first.

This injury on the blood vessel, is called as **Endothelial Dysfunction.**

Endothelial Dysfunction is mainly caused due to-

1. High blood sugar.
2. High blood pressure.
3. High blood uric acid levels.
4. High blood nicotine (due to smoking).
5. High blood leptin levels (Explained in Chapter- 6).
6. High blood triglycerides / VLDL (bad cholesterol).
7. High blood homocysteine (due to low Vitamin-B_{12}).
8. High blood oxidized-LDL levels (Explained in Chapter- 8).
9. High and uncontrolled function of mTOR (Explained in Chapter- 19).
10. High Inflammation from harmful metabolites (e.g. *trimethylamine*-N-*oxide*) due to gut infections, or diseases due to it, such as rheumatoid arthritis, SLE, IBS, IBD, eczema, psoriasis, etc.

Any of these ten major reasons, and other less common factors, can cause significant injury to the blood vessel, and result in the formation of heart blocks (Atherosclerosis).

Sixth on the list are triglycerides.
Even though they are fats, they are fats that have majorly been converted from sugars.

Yes... do you remember when I told you carbohydrates / sugars in the blood convert to fat?

Triglyceride is that fat, and they are just like blood sugars...
they are highly destructive.

Saturated fats on the other hand are highly helpful, because they are anti-inflammatory, and are also very potent **ANTI-OXIDANTS**.

> Speaking of anti-oxidants, let us side-track for a moment to know more about them.

- **Free Radicals & Anti-Oxidants** (Redox Health).

Free radicals are toxic waste in our body.
They are highly reactive molecules, with unpaired electrons, capable of damaging cellular structures, proteins, lipids, and DNA.

It mainly forms in our body as a by-product of the energy produced from our mitochondria. It also finds its way into our body from external sources like pollution, cigarette smoke, radiation, medication etc.

Free radicals do have a few useful roles in the body though, which is detailed in later chapters.

Let us imagine *Energy* as **Fire**...
and *Free-radicals* as **Smoke.**

Fire can be made through different fuels, like wood, petrol, diesel etc.
Some fuels burn clean, like petrol, with little, to no smoke produced.
Wood, however, burn with lots of smoke produced.
In the same way, for our body, clean fuels, are Good Fats (like petrol).
Bad fuel is Carbohydrate / Sugars (wood).

Using carbohydrate for fuel (energy) creates lots and lots of smoke (free-radicals), which is bad for the body.
These free radicals damage our body in so many different ways.

It can damage our skin and cause wrinkles, premature hair-greying, ageing, heart blocks, cataract, autoimmune disorders, neurodegenerative diseases and even become the causative factor for many types of cancers.

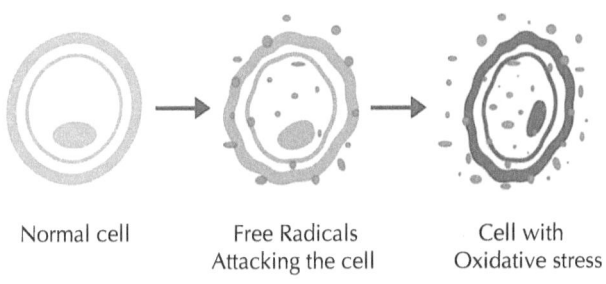

Normal cell   Free Radicals Attacking the cell   Cell with Oxidative stress

Oxidative Stress

You can compare the damage (oxidation) of free-radicals in our body, to that of rusting of iron or steel.
They are both the same process- **oxidation**.

> **Anti-oxidants**, are special molecules that protect our body from the damages (oxidative stress) by the free-radicals.

There are anti-oxidants created by the body (enzymatic), like, catalase, glutathione peroxidase, L-arginine, co-enzyme Q10, lipoid acid, metal chelating proteins, melatonin, uric acid, bilirubin, transferrin, etc.

And there are also anti-oxidants that we can take through external sources (non-enzymatic), such as vitamins and phytonutrients (mentioned in the first chapter as a vital, minor nutrient).

Phytonutrients are naturally occurring, potent anti-oxidants from plants and fruits. They are the compounds that contribute to their colour and flavour, and gives them their disease resistance property.

These bioactive compounds include flavonoids, carotenoids, and polyphenols, all of which help protect the body from oxidative stress and inflammation.

The functions of these compounds, while essential as antioxidants, are not limited to that role alone.

They are also involved in many other processes and pathways within the body, ensuring the smooth functioning and upkeep of our systems.

Natural fats are also very good anti-oxidants.

Did you know that it was common practice for centuries, before refrigeration, to pack raw meat with a generous amount of butter, or the fat of ducks, pork, mutton or beef?

This was an excellent way of preserving meat from spoilage because of the anti-oxidant properties of fat. It was also the reason why pork was the popular meat source of the 19th century America and not beef, as mentioned in the beginning of Chapter- 2.

The high body-fat (around 25%) of pigs, made them excellent for salt curing, which preserved the meat and its flavour.

In the same way, not only does good fats help in fighting against the damages from free-radicals in our body, but also creates only minimal levels of free-radicals when being converted into energy.

And even more, fats are an essential nutrient of utmost importance, which gives us numerous health benefits as listed in the first chapter.

Chapter VI – The Real Culprit!

If saturated fats are not to blame, then what is really the one responsible for creating so much damage in our body?

Ironically, our staple food, the one we consume the most (up to 80%), is the real culprit.
It is none other than, carbohydrates and sugars.
But they cannot commit their crimes by themselves.

They are only able to be highly efficient, in the presence of the highly inflammatory, *omega*-6 rich refined oils, their partner in crime.

Let us go through an interesting study called ***"The French Paradox"*** conducted in the 1980s-

	Indian Population	*French Population*
Carbohydrate	80%	40%
Dietary fat	15%	40%
Protein	5%	20%

If fat and cholesterol really was the cause for metabolic diseases, then Indians should have the lowest amount of diabetes, and heart attack deaths directly related to it...
because Indians only consume around **15%** of fat in their diet.

Other European countries enjoy an abundance of good fats, up to **40%** in their diet through dairy, meats and nuts.

Let the results speak for themselves!

	Indian Population	*French Population*
Average Blood Cholesterol Level	Below **200**	Above **250**
Diabetic Prevalence	**25%** of population	**4%** of population
Diabetic & Heart Attack Deaths	**400** in 100,000	**150** in 100,000

Diabetes related deaths in India, are among the highest in the world! With an alarming mortality rate of **400** *deaths in* **100,000** people annually, and a staggering **25%** prevalence of diabetes, India could even be described as the ***Diabetic Capital of the World***.

Compared to it, the fat eating, meat eating European populations, have only **150** *deaths in* **100,000** population, and a mere **4%** diabetic prevalence in total!

I have patients come up to me who are quite proud of themselves for keeping their total cholesterol below the level of $200_{mg/dl}$ and yet suffer from fatty liver disease, and do not even realize that keeping their cholesterol level below 200 means nothing, if you still suffer from metabolic disorders.
And even after realizing their mistakes, they still fear to eat the yolk of an egg or even to snack on cashews or peanuts, in fear of "Saturated Fats" and "Cholesterol".

This phobia... this fear etched in the subconscious mind, is the real villainous impact that *"The Biggest Lie"* had on the world.
Indians 50 years ago, even if from vegetarian families, used to enjoy plenty of fat and cholesterol from butter, ghee, milk, eggs, and fish, which kept them well and healthy.
For example-

- ***Havyaka Brahmins***, native to districts of North & coastal Karnataka, used to follow a Lacto-vegetarian diet.
  Butter, curd, and vegetables are the staples with Coconut used liberally in almost all dishes.

- ***Saraswat Brahmins*** from the Konkan region on the West coast of India, used to enjoy plenty of fish meat in their food.
  Konkani cuisine is usually Pesco-vegetarian, as according to the Konkani folklore, fish are regarded as sea vegetables.

- The ***Kashmiri Brahmins / Pandits*** native to the Kashmir Valley, have a tradition of consuming meat, including mutton and fish, along with all varieties of dairy.

The younger generations of these distinguished communities though, adopted the "**Low-FAT**" diet, as we all have, due to the relatively recent propagated information, and as a consequence, the majority suffers from diabetes and heart diseases.

The younger generations are so successfully manipulated, because of the infamous "*Food Pyramid Chart*" that we are all familiar with, starting from the second grade of our primary education system, which promoted that the bulk of our diet should be carbohydrate rich grains, and fats were supposed to be the least consumed food.

THE FOOD PYRAMID

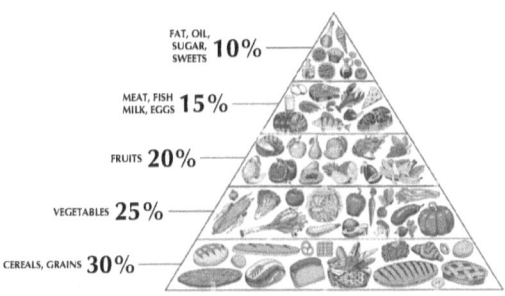

Fats are given least priority in almost all the textbooks of our Standard Education System, categorized along with sweets and refined sugars, leading to an untold fear of Fat (nutrient) to develop in the subconscious minds of the present generations as well. This is how the "Major Nutrients" are described in our textbooks...

- *<u>CARBOHYDRATES</u>*: Carbohydrates are also called energy giving food. They are the main source of energy.
  The main carbohydrates found in food are starch and sugars.

- *<u>PROTEIN</u>*: Protein helps in body growth and repairs the tissues so it is also called body building food.

- *<u>FAT</u>*: Our body stores the excess energy in the form of fat. This stored fat is used by the body for producing energy as and when required so fat is considered as energy bank in our body.

This description itself gives authority to Carbohydrates as the
"Major Energy Giving Food" and nothing could be more farther from
the truth, as we have discussed in detail until now.

Let us take a look, at a very interesting situation which can help us
understand better, that our body is truly designed to thrive on fats,
for health and longevity.

The Lake Nyasa region, located around Lake Nyasa (or Lake Malawi)
in East Africa, is home to several ethnic groups.
These tribes have historically relied on a diet rich in locally grown crops
such as maize, cassava, and millet, as well as fish from the lake.
The people also lead an active lifestyle, with physical labour being part of
their daily routine.

The Lugalawa Study was carried out within
the populations of two villages of the same
tribe around Lake Nyasa, who speak the
same dialect, have similar calorie intake
and lifestyles.

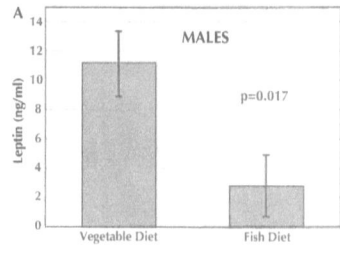

The only difference between these two
villages, was that, one was situated a little
further from the lake (*Madilu* village),
and so they consumed more grains and
vegetables, and the other village, named
Lupingu village, consumed more fish,
as they were more closer to the lake.

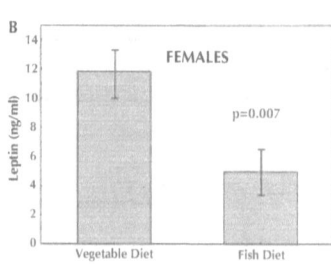

The important finding of this study, was
that the fish eating group, had very low
levels of **Leptin**, and the grain eating
group, had very high levels of leptin.

Leptin Variation

This extreme difference in levels of leptin,
was despite both of the groups having an almost identical BMI (body
mass index), similar calorie intake, and similarly active lifestyle.

What is **Leptin** and why is it important?

Leptin is a hormone, produced by adipocytes (fat cells), and it controls our hunger, by signalling the brain to stop eating, and promotes the body to start burning fat for energy.

But when a person develops *Leptin Resistance*, the brain doesn't respond to leptin signals, which leads to overeating, and poor regulation of fat stores, which then contributes to weight gain and metabolic disorders.

Higher leptin concentrations in the body, are themselves, an independent risk factor for stroke, coronary artery disease, and myocardial infarction (heart attack).

One other interesting statistics, provided by the FAO (Food and Agriculture Organization of the United Nations), according to which, the average annual consumption of meat of each individual in the year 2005 was-

5_{kg} in **India**, and

82_{kg} in **Europe!**

The average European eat 16 times more meat,
than an average Indian does!

The French Paradox study shows that the Europeans are yet,
vastly more healthier than Indians,
and it certainly looks like they

DID NOT

strictly follow
the "scientific advice"
of 1961 from the AHA.

Chapter VII – Designed to Process FAT!

Have you ever wondered which is the **FATTEST** *land mammal* on earth?

Is it an elephant? a hippopotamus? or perhaps a rhinoceros?

No… all of these animals have only less than **5%** of body fat.

The fattest animals are Brown bears, and Polar bears, with around **45%** body fat. But this is mainly to help them maintain their body temperature in their extremely cold environments, and also to give them energy, while they are in their long sleeps (Hibernation).

If not for those two reasons, it would be Humans that are the fattest land mammals… with healthy females having around **35%** body fat, and healthy males having around **25%** body fat.

Why do we need Fats in our body??

The first, and most important reason is, our BRAIN.
We are the most unique beings on this planet, compared to all other animals, for one very special reason, the human brain.

If you really think about it… we do not have wings like the birds.
But we humans fly so high and so far, even reaching outer-space.
We neither have large lungs, nor dense bones like the great whales, to support the high pressures of the deep sea.
Yet, we dive the deepest oceans, for hours on end.
We do not have the high speed of a cheetah.
But we outrace every animal on the planet.
We do not have the strength of an elephant or a lion, and yet…
We are the most powerful beings on earth.

All of this, and much more, because we were able to use this very unique gift of ours… **The Human BRAIN.**

Our brain is only around **2%** of our total body weight, and yet, it takes up around **40%** energy and nutrients from the total food we consume.

This brain of ours, is a fatty organ with almost **70%** of it, being composed of FAT. This extreme requirement, from our most valuable organ, which relies on fatty acids for its structure and proper functioning, is the first and foremost reason you need *Dietary Fats*.

Now when I tell you that we humans were designed to process fat, let us compare ourselves with the closest species to humans.
The Chimpanzee.

We are so much similar to them, that more than **99%** of our DNA match up to them!

You must understand that even very minute details, such as the colour and shape of our eyes, are all predetermined, and written down in the "Blueprint" of our body, our DNA... and only less than **1%** of DNA, differentiates us from the Chimpanzees.

Even though we are so similar... we are yet, so different in one, very important aspect.
The advanced ability of our body to process Dietary Fats.

And that is why, even though Chimpanzees have a so called "Healthy Lifestyle"- feeding only on fruits and leaves, while performing lots of physical activity, and with a muscular and toned body...
their average lifespan is only around **25 years**.

At the same time, we humans, were designed to enjoy and thrive on fatty foods and animal proteins, and live on average, for around **80 years**.

Humans are the only species known to produce **multiple** APOE isoforms (e2, e3 and e4), while there is only **one** APOE variant in our closest relative species, the Chimpanzee.

If you were wondering what an APOE means, let me explain...

APOE (Apo-lipo-proteins), are "Cargo Ships"
that carry the "Cargo" that are Fats,
through the "Sea" that is Blood...
for transportation to different parts of the body.

We all know that Fats cannot dissolve in water – *(Hydrophobic)*.
Blood is our transportation system, and since Fats cannot dissolve in blood… to transport this valuable nutrient that is Fat.
We humans went through an adaptation in our gene, where our body creates different forms of APOE (Apo-lipo-proteins), which acts as a bridge between fats and blood, to help transport the fats efficiently through our blood.

So basically HDL and LDL are the same thing… just cargo ships, travelling through the sea (blood), carrying a valuable cargo (Fats).

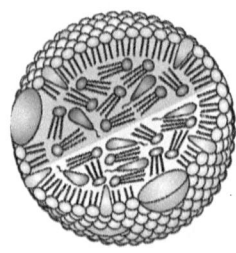

SURFACE COAT
- Unesterified Cholesterol.
- Phospholipids.
- Apolipoproteins.

LIPID CORE
- Cholesteryl Esters.
- Triglycerides.

This is the "Cargo Ship"… an ***Apo-lipo-protein (APOE).***

All APOE transports fat throughout the body.

Based on the amount, and type of Fat it is carrying which are *Cholesterols and Tri-glycerides*, the cargo ships are termed as high density, low density, intermediate density, very low density etc.

- ***HDL*** (high density lipo-protein)– Carries majority cholesterol than tri-glycerides.

- ***LDL*** (low density lipo-protein)– Carries slightly more tri-glyceride than cholesterol.

- ***VLDL*** (very low density lipo-protein)– Has vastly more tri-glyceride than cholesterol.

- ***Chylomicron*** – Transports the fats that are absorbed from the intestine, directly into the body's circulation.

- **Good Fat Bad Fat!**

'Good cholesterol' or 'Bad cholesterol' is just something that Doctors say, so that the people who find all this information very complicated, can understand it in a better way.

Even when I say this, I too have "over-simplified" the different APOE. For complete details, feel free to explore *'The Straight Dope On Cholesterol'* by Dr. Peter Attia.

All that being said... to put it in simple terms, let's just say that ***Cholesterol*** is good, and ***Tri-glycerides*** are bad.
But the truth is that there are good and bad ***Cholesterol***, as well as good and bad ***Tri-glycerides***.

The human body is designed to process *fat*... to stay alive.
Since *fats* are so vital for our body to function, if we do not eat enough saturated fats, or fats from natural sources like dairy, meat and nuts... our body creates its own fat, a duplicate or fake one, mainly from the sugars / carbs that we eat.
This duplicate fat can either be cholesterol or triglyceride.

But over **70%** of the fat created from sugars end up as triglyceride in the body's circulation. This is why I am referring to triglycerides as the bad fat, and cholesterol as a good fat (most of the cholesterol in the body is from natural sources, unless the person is a vegan, and doesn't consume animal meats, eggs or dairy).

ChREBP (*carbohydrate response element binding protein*), is what helps our body, to convert excess dietary carbohydrate into the type of fat called *Tri-glycerides*, for storage and usage. **ChREBP** is one of the major factor involved in the development of metabolic syndrome.

But the problem with this fat from sugars (duplicate fat), majorly *tri-glycerides*, is that they can never replace good, natural fat, because fat created from sugars, have the same nature as sugars.
They are highly inflammatory and oxidative, and are responsible for damaging our blood vessels which leads to heart blocks, and is one of the causes for *Insulin Resistance*.

Therefore, LDL or VLDL, our fat transporting molecules, with a higher ratio of *tri-glycerides* (for a person who consumes the typical modern diet, with excess refined carbs and seed oils), are of the same nature of sugar as well, highly inflammatory and oxidative.

If we take a look at the source of an infant's energy, from the mother's breast milk, the majority nutrition is *fat*.

	Baby Cereal	*Human Breast Milk*
Carbs / Sugars	88%	28%
Fats	5%	55%
Proteins	5%	7%
Soluble Fibers	2%	10%

The milk, rich in fats, helps not only in the perfect development of the brain and body, but also plays a vital role in our immunity during infancy, and also in our adult life.

It is a grave mistake on our part, to feed our babies *"Infant Formulas"* high in cereals, which are ultra-processed, and most importantly, high in carbs / sugar content. Instead, the best weening food for infants are fatty foods like bone marrow, cheese, egg yolks etc.

Dietary Fats help our immunity in several ways-

1. ***Energy Source for Immune Cells***- During an immune response, immune cells such as *Macrophages* and *Lymphocytes* require energy to carry out their functions effectively. Fat serves as the efficient energy source for these cells, supporting immune responses.

2. ***Cell Fluidity***- Fatty acids are crucial components of immune cells, playing a key role in maintaining the composition and fluidity of cell membranes. The fluidity of these membranes is vital for enabling them to recognize and respond effectively and allows for better communication and movement, and combat harmful invaders.

3. *Prostaglandin Signals*- Fats are essential for the production of signalling molecules called prostaglandins, which play a crucial role in regulating inflammation and immune function.
Specifically, *omega*-3 fatty acids, such as eicosapentaenoic acid (EPA) and docosahexaenoic acid (DHA), are known to give rise to anti-inflammatory prostaglandins. These prostaglandins help modulate the immune system's inflammatory responses, promoting a balanced immune reaction. *Omega*-3 fatty acids are primarily found in fatty fish and certain plant oils, and their intake has been associated with reduced inflammation and a lower risk of chronic inflammatory conditions, such as heart disease and arthritis.

4. *Immunity Vitamins*- Vitamins A, D, E, and K are immune supportive vitamins, which are also fat-soluble, meaning they require Fat to be absorbed, and transported in the body. These vitamins support the immune function, by enhancing the activity of immune cells and regulating inflammatory responses. Vitamin-D is also responsible for the direct production of immune cells, through its components called *Cathelecedin* & *Defensin*.

5. *Fat Tissue Regulation*- Adipose tissue, or our body's Fat Stores, serves as an endocrine organ that produces signalling molecules called *Adipokines*. Key adipokines, including adiponectin and leptin, play roles in regulating metabolism, immune function, and inflammation. Adiponectin typically has anti-inflammatory effects, while leptin, in moderate levels, is involved in energy balance and immune responses. Both contribute to the regulation of various physiological processes related to inflammation and immune modulation.

6. *Microbiome Support*- Fat intake can impact the composition and diversity of the gut microbiota, which in turn plays a vital role in regulating immune responses. Certain fatty acids, such as butyrate, are produced by gut bacteria through the fermentation of dietary fibers. Butyrate has been shown to support gut health by improving the integrity of the gut barrier, which prevents harmful pathogens from entering the bloodstream. Additionally, butyrate itself plays a role in modulating the immune system, in cases of infections.

Humans conquered the world, from the coldest regions of the arctic and mountains, to the harsh heat of the deserts, by surviving healthily on Dietary Fats.
And these Fats never resulted in heart blocks or metabolic diseases.

For example-

- The ***Caribou Inuits***, or most commonly called ***Eskimos***, natives of the 'Frozen North' (Siberia, Alaska, Canada, and Greenland), for more than 6000 years, lived by hunting animals, including birds, caribou (a type of deer), seals, walrus, polar bears, whales, and fish, which provided all the nutrition for the *Eskimos* for at least ten months of the year.
Only in the summer season, did they gather few plant foods such as berries, grasses, tubers, roots, stems, and seaweeds. The frozen, snow-covered lands are not fit for cultivation of plants.
Even with a diet rich in Saturated Fats, Eskimos lived free from heart problems, cancer, and other metabolic diseases.

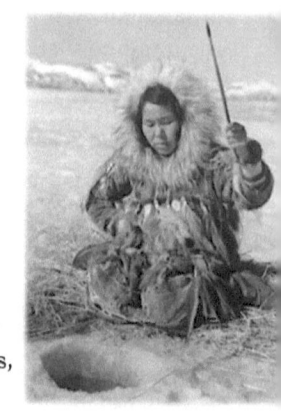

Eskimo

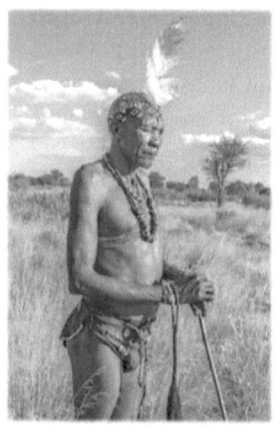

San-Bushman

- The ***San Bushmen*** tribals, indigenous to Southern Africa, are one of the oldest cultures, who are hunter-gatherers, and have survived their unique way of life to this day. Their staple food is the ***Mongongo nuts***, making up to **50%** of their diet. Their average daily consumption, about 300 nuts, provides an individual with **60%** Fat and **25%** Protein. The rest contains high amounts of Calcium, Magnesium, Zinc, Copper & Vitamin-E.
When the *San Bushmen* were asked why they hadn't taken up agriculture, they replied-
"Why should we plant, when there are so many *Mongongo nuts* in the world?"

- Two Polynesian Island populations, *Tokelauans* and *Pukapukans*, lives on a habitual diet high in saturated fat, and low in carbohydrates and sucrose. Coconut is the chief source of energy for both groups. Tokelauans obtain a much higher percentage of energy, up to **63%**, from coconut, compared to Pukapukans, who obtain around **34%**.
Vascular diseases are not common in both populations and there is no evidence of the high saturated fat intake having any harmful effect in these populations.

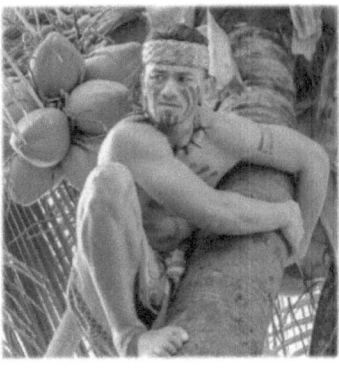
Aboriginal Polynesian

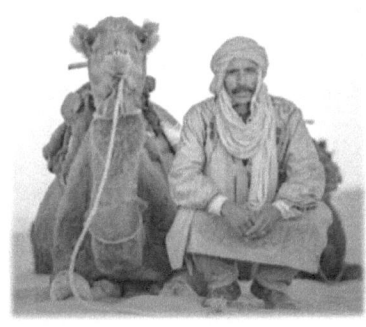
Desert Nomad

- The *Nomad Tribals of Deserts*, had no fixed home and wandered from place to place. Their indigenous diet was based on mainly meat, milk and other dairy by-products.
They dined on camel, rabbit, sheep and goat meat, and drank the milk of goats and camels.
Coastal tribes even had fish and bread in their diet as well.
But here too, the majority nutrients were fats and proteins.
There are still tribes who follow this way of life. Vascular diseases and metabolic syndrome are unheard of, in these desert nomadic tribal populations as well.

- Even where vegetations are plenty, as in the Amazon rainforest, tribals depended mainly on meat and fat for source of food.
The *Tsimane Tribe* of the Amazon, has lived almost completely free of heart disease, obesity, diabetes, and age-related cognitive decline. Based on decades of research, studying brain scans of 746 *Tsimane* from ages 40 to 94, they experience brain atrophying 70% slower than modern populations.

The *Tsimane* has a traditional lifestyle of hunting, gathering, fishing, and farming. They survive on a diet that includes tapir (a forest animal closely related to zebras), wild boar, other wild animals, vegetables, and fish caught from the river.

An 80 year old *Tsimane Tribal* has heart arteries better than that of a 40 year old American, scientists have discovered.

The *Tsimane* people have exceptionally low levels of visceral fat, contributing to their superior cardiovascular health, slower aging, and overall resilience compared to modern populations.

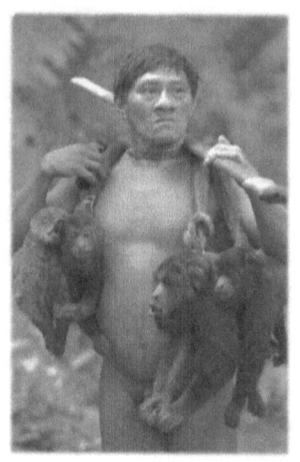

Tsimane Tribal

Did you know that there were much more than 60 species of elephants, including more than 10 species of Mammoths? Today there are only 3 species - *The African Forest* **Elephant**, *The African Savanna or Bush* **Elephant**, *and The Asian* **Elephant**.

Roughly around **13,000 years** ago, hundreds of thousands of the largest mammals on earth (*Mega-fauna*) went extinct, including species of very large deer, elephants and wild horses, to name a few, due to an event that caused ice sheets to rapidly melt, causing an increase in the ocean levels, leading to global floods, at a period in history named as- *"The Younger Dryas."*

Humans were forced to settle down to agriculture, from being **Hunter-Gatherers**, around 12,000 years ago, which switched our staple food from Meat and Fats, to Grains & Cereals.

Now we humans have started farming more sustainable animals like sheep, cattle, pork and chicken, but still hold on to eating more of Grains and Cereals, out of habit and *"Tradition."*

This *'tradition'* of depending on grains and potatoes for primary source of energy, was born out of extreme necessity such as famine or wars, if you look throughout human history.

Usually it takes around more than 2 or 3 generations to come out of the crisis, by which time, the existing generation, if not educated on the impact that food has on health, they would wrongly believe that meat and fats are bad for our health.

Human beings are indeed designed to process and thrive on Dietary Fats and Proteins. Following "traditions" is wonderful, but when we follow tradition without thought, we risk losing our health, as we can see it happening all around us, even in this *'modern'* era.

We can draw inspiration from South Korea's national efforts, particularly in their approach towards public health.

In the early part of the 20th century, South Korea faced significant poverty and hardship for several reasons, such as colonial rule by Japan, destruction due to the Korean war (which divided it into *South Korea* and *North Korea*), lack of natural resources, political instability and a rapidly growing population. But instead of exploiting the wealth and resources of their own land, the leaders and politicians, helped South Korea transition from an ***agrarian society*** into a major ***global economy*** by focusing on exports, industrial development, and education.
A movement that was later called "**Miracle on the Han River.**"

A century ago, the average height of South Korean women was just about **142 cm**. Since then, South Korean women grew an astounding average of 8 inches (20 cm), and presently stands at **162 cm** in height. The South Korean men grew 6 inches (15 cm) on average, while globally, the average increase of height in all other countries had only seen a rise of 3 inches (7 cm).

So what exactly happened?

One of the main issue targeted by the South Korean Government as soon as political stability was achieved, was to nourish the people with the best sources of food. Midday-school meals were revised by experts, and the children were given meals of bone broth or meat based soup, egg rice, kimchi (probiotic), protein dish (meat, fish, tofu), fruits, vegetable side dishes, and whole (full fat) milk.

Compared to it, the Indian midday meal consists of rice or flour (100_g), pulses or legumes for protein (20_g), vegetables (50_g) and 5_g of oil.
We will go through in more detail why this is not actually a balanced meal pattern, in Chapter- 17 and Chapter- 21.

But there are exceptions in India, in the states of Kerala, Haryana and Punjab, where their increased consumption of animal based proteins shows a significant difference in physical growth and health when compared to other states.
In Kerala, fish, beef and other meats, along with dairy, are consumed regularly, while in Haryana and Punjab, the rich intake of dairy produce like milk, paneer, ghee and curd ensures a steady supply of protein, healthy fats and micro nutrients, supporting bone growth and a taller physique. These regions consistently report taller individuals compared to other states, where vegetarian diets are more common, and animal protein is less prevalent.

Unlike many nations that prioritize solely on sophisticated medical technological solutions for health (not that it doesn't have its benefits), South Korea emphasized on the fundamentals, a healthy balanced diet and nutrition, while at the same time integrating them with advanced healthcare and infrastructures, which helped South Korea see an immense rise in the health of the population up until the late 2000s.

But as of late, the emergence of low-cost, more tastier and ultra processed fast foods, along with a more sedentary life-style due to advancements in technology, smart phone devices, and a culture of online presence rather than in the real world, has caused a rise in the cases of obesity, and metabolic diseases.
But thankfully their school meal system to this day, is still as nutritious as it was, helping in the healthy growth and development of South Korean children.

Our bodies are designed to thrive on fats and it is essential for our health and longevity. By embracing the wisdom of traditional diets that prioritize natural fats, we can reclaim our vitality, just as the resilient cultures of the past have done. The key, is to nourish our bodies, the way they were always meant to be nourished.

Chapter VIII – Choosing The Right Oil.

So far, we have been discussing a lot about Fats.
When it comes to cooking, traditionally, throughout all countries and cultures, the most commonly used oils or fats were *Butter*, and other animal fats like *Lard* or *Tallow*.

In India, since ancient times, our favourite cooking oil was *Ghee*.
It was understood that ghee contained properties that healed the body by relieving inflammations, assisting in digestion and by promoting a better immune system (just as we discussed in the last chapter).

It was said to enhance the *"Life Energy"* or *"Vitality"* and was used extensively in preparation of many medicines, by Healers of the ancient medical science- Ayurvedha.
It was so precious, that it held the nickname *"Liquid Gold."*

Cold pressed *Groundnut Oil* (also called *Peanut Oil)* was used widely in the northern parts of India along with cold pressed *Mustard Oil*, extracted from the seeds of the mustard plant... both of which have been used since hundreds of years.

When it came to coastal regions, cold pressed *Coconut Oil* was the most popular option, not only was it used for cooking, but even to be applied on the head and body, or be used as mouth washes and purgatives.
It was not limited to general wellness, but was also used as remedies for various specific diseases.
The Coconut was, and still is, an important segment of culture, religion and beauty in India.
Cold pressed *Sesame Oil* (also called *Gingelly Oil)*, from Sesame seeds are also very popular for cooking, in the southern parts of India.

Extra Virgin Olive Oil on the other hand, with its enumerous health benefits, even though used for cooking, is best used raw for garnishing or as salad dressings (the reason for it will be explained later in this chapter). Predominantly used in the *Mediterranean* region for almost all of their dishes, raw and cooked, now it has gained more popularity than ever, on a world wide scale.

If we really think about it, we have been consuming all these fats and oils since ancient times, and we have never had cases of strokes or heart attacks, or even obesity, like we do in the present time and present generation.

Why is it that **Refined Oils** are to blame?

What makes *Refined Oils* different from these *Cold pressed* **Natural Oils** or any other **Natural Fats**?

To understand why there is a difference, let me give you a very short and condensed form, of what Fats and Oils are actually made up of…

I know it can be a little too much *"Sciency"* and boring for some of you, but please read through and I'll try my best to make the "hard science" part, as simple as possible.

What makes these fats crucial for our basic physiology and health?

We have already gone through the many benefits of fats and why there can be no human life without it, in the first chapter.

Fats are actually made up of something called *Fatty Acids*.

More than 70 fatty acids have been identified in nature.

Based on their molecular structure, they are classified as –

- **SFA** (***Saturated*** *Fatty Acids*)
- **MUFA** (***Mono-unsaturated*** *Fatty Acids*)
- **PUFA** (***Poly-unsaturated*** *Fatty Acids*)
- *Trans-Fats*.

Fatty Acids and *Lipids* are related, but are distinct components of the human body, playing key roles in nutrition, energy production and storage, as well as cellular function, among many others.

Here are a few points that can help you differentiate between them-

Fatty Acids (FA)	Lipids
FA are organic molecules consisting of a hydrocarbon chain with a carboxylic acid group (-COOH) at the end.	Lipids are a diverse group of organic compounds that are not soluble in water (hydrophobic), and are made up of various molecules, including FA.
FA functions as one of the basic building blocks of lipids, essential for energy storage, forming cell membranes, and participating in various metabolic processes.	Lipids serve multiple functions, including energy storage, insulation, cushioning of organs, forming cell membranes (as phospholipids), and serving as essential components in various hormones.
FA can be categorized as *Saturated Fatty Acids*, *Mono-unsaturated Fatty Acids*, *Poly-unsaturated Fatty Acids* and *Trans-Fats*.	Lipids encompass a wide range of molecules like *Triglycerides* (composed of three fatty acids and a glycerol molecule), *Phospholipids* & *Steroids*.
FA are obtained through the consumption of dietary fats and oils, such as those found in animal fats, plant oils, nuts, seeds, and fatty fish.	Lipids are found in various foods, including animal fats, vegetable oils, dairy products, nuts, seeds, and fatty fish, dark chocolate etc.
Common examples of FA include *Palmitic Acid, Oleic Acid, Linoleic Acid*.	Common examples of Lipids include *Fats, Oils, Phospholipids*, and *Steroids*.

So even though all Oils look the same, inside them, there are many different types of fatty acids, that each serve a different purpose... just like *vitamins*. Even though there are many different types of *vitamins*, each gives our body unique benefits (refer Chapter- 1).

Our own body makes a few of these Fatty Acids, and so they are called *Non-Essential FA*. And then there are a few Fatty Acids that are very important for our body, but we cannot make them, and have to depend on different food sources for it.
These are called *Essential FA*.

Here are a few examples of *Fatty Acids*-

Name	Carbon Atoms	Type of Fatty Acid	Non-Essential Or Essential.	Common Source
Palmitic acid	16	Saturated FA	Non-Essential	Palm o
Stearic acid	18	Saturated FA	Non-Essential	Animal
Oleic acid	18	MUFA	Non-Essential	Olive o
Linoleic acid	18	PUFA	Essential	Eggs
Linolenic acid	18	PUFA	Essential	Flaxseed
Arachidonic acid	20	PUFA	Essential	Meat, d
Eicosapentaenoic acid	20	PUFA	Essential	Fish o
Docosahexaenoic acid	22	PUFA	Essential	Fish o

Now, based on the length of the molecular structures of *Fatty Acids*, they are classified as-

- **SCFA** (*Short Chain* Fatty Acids)
- **MCFA** (*Medium Chain* Fatty Acids)
- **LCFA** (*Long Chain* Fatty Acids)

I'm quite sure that you are all, well aware of the most famous essential fatty acid, a Long Chain FA, commonly called as **Omega-3 Fatty Acid**, which makes up about 30% of our brain and serve other greatly important cellular functions as well.

Extensive scientific studies have shown us the value of *Omega-3 fatty acids* as a therapeutic molecule, due to its immense anti-inflammatory properties. Proven to benefit patients with fatty liver, cystic fibrosis, heart blocks, dementia and much more.

Let us take a look at a few differences between **Short Chain** Fatty Acids, **Medium Chain** Fatty Acids and **Long Chain** Fatty Acids.

	SCFA *2 to 5 carbon atoms*	**MCFA** *6 to 12 carbon atoms*	**LCFA** *13 to 22+ carbon atoms*
Example	• Acetate (C_2) • Propionate (C_3) • Butyrate (C_4)	• Caprylic Acid (C_8) • Capric Acid (C_{10}) • Lauric Acid (C_{12})	• The *omega*-3s • Stearic Acid (C_{18}) • Oleic Acid (C_{18})
Natural sources	Produced by friendly bacteria, (Detailed in Chapter- 15).	Obtained from coconut oil, dairy produce etc.	Most common type of fats, can be found in all foods that have fat in them.
Uptake	Cellular uptake by ionic diffusion (40%). Non-ionic diffusion (60%).	Does not need enzymes, bile, nor chylomicrons, and is absorbed directly to the liver.	Requires bile, enzymes, and chylomicrons for digestion and absorption.
Storage	Rarely contributes to fat storage.	Rarely contributes to fat storage.	More likely to be stored as fat when in the presence of Insulin.
Health benefits	• Anti-inflammatory, anti-cancer, helps to maintain gut health, can be converted into energy sources.	• Converted into ketones, acts as an antioxidant, greatly improves metabolic health, supresses appetite.	• Essential for hormone production, cell health, and cell signalling. Each type has differing beneficial properties.

I have written down all this information, so that, even if you may not fully understand it, you will at least, still be aware of the complex structures, and functions that are actually taking place in your body, through something, we take so much for granted, ***Our Food.***

This is why, even the way and type of cooking, is as important as, choosing the right food. So that we do not change the beneficial chemical structures of these food, and lose its many health benefits…

or worse, change the chemical structure of the food so much... that it turns into a toxic compound, causing diseases as severe as hormonal imbalances, heart blocks and cancers!

So, when using animal fats for cooking, like butter, ghee, lard or tallow, make sure that it is natural, and not rancid. And when choosing the right cooking oil, the first thing to do, is to make sure that the oils are obtained, through the age old method of *Cold Pressing*.

Cold pressed oils are obtained by, slowly crushing oil seeds (groundnut, mustard, soybean, sunflower etc.) or by crushing the pulps, such as in cases of Olives and Coconuts, to extract oil from them naturally. Through this method, the chemical structure is preserved, and not only are the flavours retained, but also the nutritional contents.

Hot pressed oils are extracted by using high heat (more than *180°C*) and chemical solvents. Due to the extreme heat, the natural chemical structure of the oils are changed, which causes most of the nutrients and flavours to be lost, and more importantly, toxic carcinogens such as *Aldehydes*, are formed in the oils.

These cancer causing *Aldehydes*, are formed not only through the refining process, but also in our homes, when the oils are constantly heated to more than *180°C*.

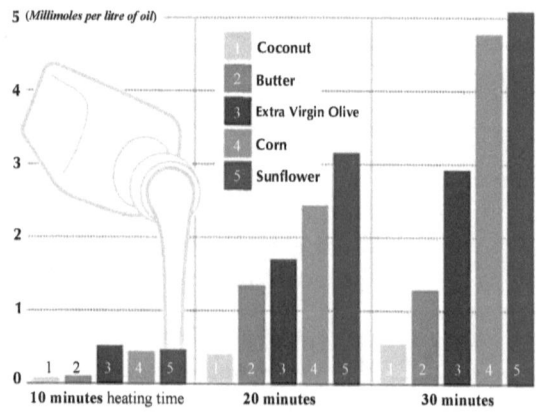

Concentrations of toxic aldehyde per litre of oil, when heated at 180° Celsius.

As you can see in the last graphical representation on a research, conducted to understand which oil can best maintain its chemical structure, even after long exposure to high heat, it shows that-

The *Undisputed King of Heat* is none other than **Coconut Oil**.
The next best cooking oil is **Butter**.

Even though **Extra Virgin Olive Oil** is a very healthy option, it cannot withstand high heat, so it is best used raw, for garnishing or as dressings, drizzled on top of salads.

This brings us back to the question, Why are *Refined Oils* to be blamed?

- Because the refining process itself uses high heat (more than *180°C*) to stabilize the oils, which leads to high levels of *Aldehydes*, a cancer causing agent. Studies have revealed that refined oils support the growth of tumours and cancers, including breast, colon, and prostate tumours in humans and animals.

- Refined oils and seed oils contain high amounts of the undesirable **Omega-6 Fatty Acids**. Excessive intake of *omega-6*, contribute to inflammations in the body, resulting in insulin resistance, allergies, atherosclerosis and even cancer. In the re-evaluation of the *"Sydney Diet Heart Study"* it was found, high intake of *omega-6* from vegetable oils resulted in a **62%** increased risk of death, from various diseases.

- Refining process uses harmful chemicals (such as hexane), for the complete extraction of oils from the source. Even though Hexane is volatile and will eventually evaporate, traces of it are known to cause nerve damage and paralysis of the arms and legs.

- Repeatedly heating oils to high temperatures can lead to the formation of oxidized fats, which, as we mentioned in Chapter- 5, is one of the leading causes for atherosclerosis or heart block formation. On top of that, *omega-6* is a very unstable molecule, and is more prone to oxidation. Refined oils, are mostly vegetable oils, high in *omega-6*... and since, by default they are made under high heat, they reach our homes, already as *Oxidized Oils*.

Last but not least, all refined oils are heavily adulterated with the extremely inexpensive **cottonseed oil**. As we have discussed in the second chapter, cottonseed is an industrial waste, and is unfit for consumption due to its toxicity, and the oil extracted from it, is the same.

The cost of one kilogram of sunflower seeds, it is around- ₹450.
It takes around 1.4 kilogram of sunflower seeds to be able to give one litre of sunflower seed oil.
If we were to include the costs of extraction effort, time and marketing, one litre of sunflower seed oil should come roughly around- ₹600.
By now you can guess where this is leading to...
One litre of sunflower seed oil in India, is available for around- ₹115.

This is the same case for all refined oils.
Heavily advertised, even to this day, as clean and disease free, refined oils are up to **70%** adulterated with this low-cost product of an industrial waste, that is cottonseed oil.
This is why it is important to check the method of extraction when purchasing oils, even if it reads on the label, Coconut oil, Extra virgin olive oil, Peanut oil, Bran oil, Palm oil etc.

- **Omega-6 Fatty Acids are Good and Bad!**

Without *Linoleic Acid* or most commonly called, the ***Omega-6***, our body would not be informed if there is an issue in our body.

For example, imagine that there are two switches, for controlling inflammation in our body.

Omega-6 Fatty Acids are the **ON** switch.
Omega-3 Fatty Acids are the **OFF** switch.

When a harmful bacteria enters our body, the *omega-6 fatty acids* help our body recognize this issue, by turning **ON** the inflammation switch.

And once this issue is resolved, our *omega-3* fatty acids help in letting our body know the same, by turning **OFF** the inflammation switch.

As you can see, the ratio between *Omega-6* and *Omega-3* in our body, must be ideally **1:1**

But the reality today, is that increased intake of refined oils, has changed this ratio to **50:1**

On average, the modern people are consuming far more *omega-6*, than at any other time in our history. Until the 1950s (as we have already discussed), most people didn't consume the 'seed oils' which are high in *linoleic acid* or *omega-6*, but still easily obtained the necessary amounts from nuts, meat, eggs, and dairy.

As stated in the *"American Journal of Clinical Nutrition"* they have found that consumption of Soybean Oil, increased to **1000 times** more, in just **90 years** (1909-1999), along with rise in other refined *omega-6* oils (that weren't widely used before the 1950s).

The following is a list of the most commonly used 'seed oils' today and the percentage of the 'inflammation causing' *Linoleic Acid* or *Omega-6* contained in it-

Vegetable Oils or Seed Oils	Linoleic Acid or Omega–6 Content
Safflower Oil	71%
Grapeseed Oil	71%
Sunflower Oil	66%
Corn Oil	60%
Soybean Oil	55%
Cottonseed Oil	53%
Peanut Oil	30%
Rice bran Oil	30%
Canola / Rapeseed Oil	21%

It is not just because of the increased refined oil usage, but also because we fear, and have altogether avoided saturated fats and animal fats, that are highly **ANTI**-inflammatory.

This is why, the obesity rates, and counts of death due to heart attacks, have sky rocketed in this modern era. The thought that *Linoleic Acid* or *omega-6* in 'seed oils' were *"Heart Friendly* and *Healthy"* originally came from experiments conducted in the 1950-1970s, just for the sake of plain and insensitive marketing for the *refined seed oil* business.

Luckily, both, *Omega-6* and *Omega-3* are *Essential Fatty Acids*.
So if we stop taking refined oils, slowly all of the extra *Omega-6* in our bodies will be used up, and at the same time if we consume lots of fatty fish such as *Sardines* or *Pink Perch*, we will be able to gain lots of *Omega-3 fatty acids*, and help reduce inflammations in our body.

Red meat such as beef, lamb, mutton and pork have better *omega*-3 to *omega*-6 ratios than white meat like poultry, and turkey.
'Grass-fed' animals have higher *omega*-3 ratio in their meat, and dairy produce, than ones that are 'grain-fed.'
Free range, pasture raised chicken, similarly, has higher *omega*-3 ratio in their meat, and eggs than mass produced, grain-fed broiler chicken.

Even if on a high grain diet, animals that are ruminants (with more than one stomach), such as cows, sheep and goats, have higher levels of *Omega-3* and lower levels of *Omega-6*, than monogastric animals (with one stomach), such as pork, poultry and turkey.

This is because the various chambers in a ruminants body, hold bacteria that metabolizes the *omega*-6 rich PUFA (poly-unsaturated fatty acids) from grains, into beneficial saturated fatty acids, and the other components of grains into various vitamins, amino acids (building blocks of proteins), and SCFA (short chain fatty acids).

This extensive microbial population in their gut, and the multiple stages of digestion, allow for better processing and helps detoxify harmful substances before absorption. This makes their meat significantly cleaner and healthier, even with a poor diet.

Whereas animals with monogastric system are '*homolipoid*' meaning that the fatty acid composition in their body, is a direct reflection of the diet that they consume.
Pork and chicken have been bred to accumulate *omega*-6 rich PUFA in their tissues because it makes them fatter faster, with fewer calories.

This means that they store *omega*-6 rich PUFA right in their fat tissue, sometimes in higher amounts than even seed oils.

Chicken meat is often considered a healthier option compared to pork due to its leaner profile, and lower fat content (where the *omega*-6 rich PUFA is highly accumulated).

Unlike pork, which tends to have noticeable 'marbling' fat interspersed within the muscle tissue, especially found in higher amounts in the fatty cuts of the pork, chicken meat is generally leaner, with less fat overall.

The fat that is present in chicken is more likely to be concentrated just under the skin, called white striping, and makes it easier to remove, for a low-fat protein meal.
These factors contribute to chicken's reputation as a better monogastric source of protein than pork.

In the case with *Omega-3 fatty acids*, there are three forms of it,
- ALA - Alpha-linolenic acid
- EPA - Eicosapentaenoic acid
- DHA - Docosahexaenoic acid

While ALA is technically an *Omega-3*... DHA and EPA are the biologically active forms of the *Omega-3* and, therefore, more important for our health in the long run.

Vegans usually opt for *Flaxseed* extracts, but it is mostly the ALA type of *Omega-3*, not EPA and DHA.
Even though ALA can be converted into EPA and DHA in our body, the conversion rate is quite limited, and so, it is better for vegans to opt *Seaweed*, that have higher, concentrated levels of EPA and DHA.

- **Yummy Deep-Fries are a Mistake.**

The flavourful and savoury, satisfying, crunchy bite of a samosa or a fried chicken is, to so many of us, the peak of food experience.
It certainly is a taste that one can get addicted to.
But this great taste brings even greater danger to our bodies.

Deep-frying involves submerging food in very hot oil, where the oil is soaked up by the food, and a crispy outer layer, or crust is formed. Now according to what we just discussed, if you are opting to deep-fry in refined oils, the resulting fried food is going to have various oxidized forms of proteins and fatty acids, which are most commonly -

- *Omega-6* and *oxidized omega-6* or *oxidized linoleic acids*.
- *Polycyclic Aromatic Hydrocarbons* (PAHs).
- *Hydroxy Linoleate* (HODE).
- *4-Hydroxynonenal* (4HNE).
- *Aldehydes*.

In 2019, studies found that levels of *Hydroxy Linoleate* were extremely higher in patients with *Glaucoma* (increased pressure within the eyeball, causing gradual loss of sight.)

Even if not ingested, the mere exposure to the cooking fumes from *omega-6* have found to be a high risk for cancer. When oils are heated during cooking, and especially overheated or heated to their smoke points, they not only produce harmful by products in foods, but also release dangerous fumes.
In a study of over 10,000 Chinese women who didn't smoke, researchers found double the risk of lung cancer, due to increased exposure to cooking oil fumes. The interesting part is, any overheated oil can create harmful fumes, regardless if the oil is rich in *omega-6* or not.

You could argue that, since *Coconut Oil* was found to be quite stable, why not deep-fry in it?

It would still contain toxic compounds.

How?

Because even though the oil is stable, the frying process changes the chemical structure of all our precious nutrients from the various foods that we are using to deep-fry, and increases the calories of the food up to 5 times higher, leading to premature ageing and metabolic diseases.

1. Usually the food used for frying are either meat, or batter, which is mostly made of grains or pulses. When in contact with very high heat, the chemical structure of the carbs / sugars changes into a cancer causing molecule called *Acrylamide.*

2. In the case of proteins, commonly found carcinogen, when the muscles of chickens, fish and other meat are exposed to high heat, are *Heterocyclic Amines (HCA)*.

3. And one more important toxic molecule you must be aware of, is AGE, the full form of which is, *Advanced Glycation End-products*. These are chemicals that are created in high heat, in combination with *Proteins-Sugars* or *Fats-Sugars*.
Fried chicken and Ice-creams are suitable examples.

The thing about "**AGE**" is that it speeds up *"Ageing"* and is also found be formed inside our body due to the excessive glycation effects of sugars on our body's protein and fat structures, and are found to cause many degenerative diseases, such as diabetes, atherosclerosis, chronic kidney disease, and Alzheimer's disease.

Even though our wrong food habits exposes us to various harmful compounds, our bodies are equipped with powerful counteractive mechanisms to neutralize these harmful substances, with the help of antioxidants, including those that are naturally produced by the body, and those that are derived from food.
But in the current era, the increased intake of excess carbs and sugars, junk and fried food, have tipped the scales to an extend where the body is not able to take control of the extreme amount of harmful substances that are entering the body, or being created in the body, majorly from our wrongful eating habits.

Thus, a balanced, nutrient-dense diet is key, to support the body's innate cleansing and healing abilities.

Chapter IX – Counting CALORIES and When to Stop!

*"If Calories Are More, The Food Is Bad.
If Calories Are Less, The Food Is Good."*

The majority of the population, look at food through this perspective. There is also an extreme version of this, where a group are adamant in their belief that-

"We can eat any kind of food as long as we stick to the daily caloric limit, and even if we by mistake, exceed the daily limit, we only need to exercise, and our body will turn out fine!"

No, our body will **NOT** turn out fine.
This is not the right way to categorize food, and solely counting calories and relating it to health is not scientific. Anyone with a basic knowledge of nutrients can easily understand that food in relation to health is more complicated than just calories.

As you have read in the first chapter, health is all about nutrition, and we have gone through the different *Macro-* and *Micro-*nutrients.
Calories on the other hand, is only a measurement of the amount of energy, that can be generated from the particular food.

To put it through a very simple example, the daily recommended caloric value is around 2200 calories for an adult.
One packet of instant noodles is around 350 calories. So according to the daily requirement, we would need to have around 6 packets of instant noodles to meet the daily quota.

Do you really believe that a person can live a healthy life, on nothing but 6 packets of instant noodles every single day?
They would start having all kinds of diseases and health issues in around 3 weeks itself.

So, we must only count calories as a secondary factor, in accordance with the primary factor, which is the nutritional profile of the food.

Traditionally, dieting solely based on counting calories have had its advantage and benefits, as it is a perfect stepping stone, to the path of healthy living, for someone who has no prior idea on the importance of food or nutrition.
Whether this kind of dieting is healthy or not, is another matter altogether, but it does definitely bring about visible results, through the loss of weight and reduction in extra bulk of the body.

The majority of the time, people who have started their diet based on just counting calories and gotten visible results, have had a boost in confidence, leading them to being more interested in dieting, and would continue on to inquire and improve their knowledge on proper healthy food habits, leading to a healthy inner as well as outer body.

In that sense, I feel that calorie counting has a done a lot of good for the general population.

But it is still my opinion, that if all other aspects of food and nutrition are known, then there is not much importance for calories in the picture. Calorie is one of the most over-rated, mis-understood, and mis-used detail in the health industry that is often used to deceive consumers.

Here are a few reasons why-

- *Calories Do Not Measure The Nutritional Value Of The Food-*

    The number of calories has nothing to do with the nutritional content of the food. For example, *zero-calorie soft drinks*, legally contain no calories, but contain artificial sweeteners which in fact do have calories. And sugars as we know, leads to all kinds of health problems as well.
    The actual information that we need to know are those such as, what minerals or vitamins are in the food?
    Or are there any toxic chemicals or preservatives in the food which could harm our bodies?
    The calorie count listed on the food label will not answer any of these questions. This type of labelling of calories on food packaging is designed to distract us from the only part of the package that actually matters- the **ingredients**.

- *Calories Cannot Accurately Measure The Energy That Food Can Provide To The Body-*

    If you were to eat a 1000 calorie pizza, theoretically it would mean you are full of energy that you can readily use. But in reality, how would most people feel after eating that very large pizza?
    Would they be ready to go straight to the gym or for a game of playing football?
    No they wouldn't.
    They would most likely be laying on the sofa and be experiencing low energy and would just want to go to a deep sleep.
    So something that has a lot of potential energy, shown as 1000 calories, doesn't actually have to give our body more energy.
    At the same time, less calories does not mean that the food has more health benefits, just as in the example of zero calorie soft drinks, given in the first point.

- *Eating Less Calories Does Not Always Mean To Lose Weight-*

    Calories do not give any information about the effects the food will have on our body. Calories are simply a measure of the potential energy, contained in the food.
    It all depends on the source of the calories.
    There is no optimum level of calories. There are foods which do good for our body, and there are foods that do bad. By choosing healthy foods that our body wants and needs, we will lose extra weight, regardless of how many calories we are consuming.

- *Counting Calories Takes Away the Joy and Pleasure Out of the Food Experience-*

    Food is more than just energy.
    It is nourishment, tradition, culture, pleasure, and joy, and it is mandatory that we celebrate the many roles that food plays in our lives. Counting calories, ignores this "Pleasure" element, and can make us feel like eating and cooking, as very stressful experiences. This usually put our body through negative effects instead of health.

Health doesn't need to be complicated.

A healthy, nutritious diet can be achieved through eating whole and natural foods, which not only help us lose extra weight, but also guarantee lots of energy, and most importantly signals our body that the food consumed is enough.

These whole foods helps in the production of hormones such as leptin and cholecystokinin, which makes sure that cravings are suppressed, and also keeps our body healthy and 'sensitive' enough to be able to receive the signals of these various beneficial hormones, in order to make sure that we do not eat more than our body needs.

So focus on learning and identifying food groups that contain vitamins and minerals that our body dearly needs.

It is definitely important to regulate the amount of how much we eat, but the best way to measure this, is by learning to understand the small signals, our body sends us in relation to hunger, as opposed to counting and measuring our caloric intake.

These basic changes can give you a healthy body, and you will start noticing a huge difference in your daily life instantaneously.

Chapter X – Stress & CORTISOL.

In both my practice and research, I have observed that while reducing insulin resistance and addressing inflammation can lead to significant improvements in health…
Uncontrolled emotional stress triggers the overactivation of the **HPA-axis** (*hypothalamic-pituitary-adrenal axis*), which causes an over production of **CORTISOL** (stress hormone).

This over production, occurring over a long period (chronic), results in something known as CORTISOL RESISTANCE… which is currently, one of the leading contributors to the global decline in health, affecting populations worldwide, regardless of age or gender.

A short *food for thought* –
[An interesting research revealed that refined oils can interfere with the production of *oxytocin*, the bonding hormone, which is essential for love, and emotional connection between partners.
This disruption could be a significant factor in the challenges that many couple face while trying to maintain loving, stable relationships today.
It can be a significant contributing factor to heightened emotional stress and an increase in cortisol levels, revealing a new perspective on the potential harms of refined oils beyond their physical ill-effects.]

Almost all tissues in our body have Gluco-corticoid receptors, because of which, high cortisol levels can affect nearly every organ system in the body, such as our –

- Nervous system.
- Immune system.
- Cardiovascular system.
- Respiratory system.
- Reproductive systems (both male & female).
- Musculo-skeletal system.
- Integumentary system (skin, hair, nails, glands and nerves).

In short, any and all diseases can be triggered merely, by excessive emotional or mental stress, and chronic (long-term) high Cortisol.

Headaches, heart disease, memory & concentration problems, digestive issues, repeated fevers and infections due to low immunity, sleeplessness, weight gain, thyroiditis, osteo arthritis, infertility, PCOD, allergies, skin diseases, auto-immune disorders, psoriasis and even cancers can start to develop, merely due to high Cortisol.

But cortisol is not a bad hormone.

In normal levels, it is necessary for our regular life, for maintaining a lot of bodily functions like, regulating metabolism in muscles, liver and bones, lowering inflammations throughout the body, regulating blood sugar and blood pressure etc.

Glucocorticoids are also the ones that control our *sleep-wake cycle* and *circadian rhythm*. This is why regular lack of sleep during night time can also be a triggering factor for high cortisol level and Cortisol Resistance. If a person have consistently high or low cortisol levels, it can have negative impacts on their overall health.

The three easiest steps to reduce high cortisol is to-

1. *Take Deep Breaths-*

   Deep-breathing exercises for at least 5 minutes, three to five times a day helps lower cortisol levels, ease anxiety and depression, and even improve memory. You can even try **Pranayama** techniques if interested in Yogic practices.

2. *Early Morning Walks-*

   30 to 50 minutes daily, especially in the early morning air, helps your body tune into your circadian rhythm and is one of the easiest ways to soothe your systems and reduce excessive levels of Cortisol.
   Quite similarly, an even easier tip that often helps to reduce cortisol is by merely gazing at the sky or sea.
   The natural vastness of the sky and the rhythmic movement of the sea helps the mind relax and reset.
   Just a few quiet minutes of gazing can make a noticeable difference.

3. *Just Have a Good Night's Sleep-*

    Easier said than done for some of us, but if your lack of sleep is due to pointless scrolling and addiction to cell-phones, gaming and social media, it's high time you start being responsible for your body, and give your body, sufficient time to heal. We need at least 7 to 8 hours of undisturbed sleep.

    I have personally had a great many patients, with a balanced and healthy eating habit, without any mental stress, but still suffers from metabolic disorders. And as you've guessed it, yes… the culprit is – *Not sleeping on time, or staying up late*.

    I cannot stress enough how much important this point is, because it puts a heavy stress on our system, and causes massive amounts of cortisol hormone secretions, to keep us up and functioning, during late nights, just because it is fundamentally against our body's circadian rhythm.

    When the body needs to make extra cortisol in emergency situations, it uses up the hormone progesterone to make cortisol, which then causes the body to react, and create more estrogen hormone, which results in estrogen dominance.
    This is especially more noticeable in women, as their bodies are more sensitive to the various hormonal changes that occur.
    Estrogen dominance, leads to uncontrolled weight gain, irregular periods, PCOD, fibroids, breast tumours, breast formation in males (gynaecomastia), and starts a vicious cycle of diseases.
    In short, just save yourself all the trouble and sleep on time.

While there are numerous medications available at present, to manage uncontrolled stress, they aren't always the best solution.
These drugs can help temporarily, but they often come with side effects and may lead to dependency. Relying solely on medicine can mask the root causes rather than addressing them.

But there are natural *'Adaptogen Herbs'*, which are plants that help the body reduce or manage the cortisol levels even if you are under uncontrolled emotional or mental stress. This can help prevent the subsequent ill-effects of high cortisol on our body as well.

The two most common Indian herbs used are,

- **Tulsi** (Ocimum sanctum) commonly known as *Holy Basil*.
- **Ashwagandha** (Withania somnifera) known as *Indian Ginseng*.

These are typically used today for regulating Cortisol levels, and not only have they been found to be very effective, but multiple clinical trials of these adaptogen herbs have not shown any major side effects from its prolonged use for treatment as well.

A great many scientific studies are still being conducted on these herbs' numerous benefits, and these herbs are widely available today in many user-friendly forms, making it easier for consumption, as in the form of capsules, teas, tinctures, and powders, making them easily accessible for those seeking natural solutions for stress management.

In conclusion, maintaining balanced cortisol levels is of utmost importance, when it comes to optimizing our health.

Keep in mind to revisit these proactive measures, throughout our discussion on various health conditions in later chapters, which are linked to cortisol dysregulation.

Chapter XI – Can You Really Avoid Bad Genetics?

Long story short...
Yes, you really can avoid bad genetics in the case of Metabolic Diseases.

How?

Epi-Genetics.

Epi-genetics is our own choices in life-style, and external environmental factors, that influences or even decides, how or whether your gene, expresses certain traits.

It does not change your DNA sequence, but epi-genetics can directly influence how your body reads a DNA sequence.

Factors that are considered in epi-genetics, can range from the type of diet that we follow or food we eat, physical activity, smoking, alcohol consumption, environmental pollutants like exposure to metals, toxic or polluted water, air pollution, radiation, organic pollutants, emotional stress, electro-magnetic pollutions, to even working during night time which deprives the body of sleep according to its circadian rhythm!

To understand this a little more easier...

Imagine that our genetics (*or* DNA) is a seed.

The plant inside the seed, is the disease (such as diabetes, PCOD etc.)

But, in order for the plant (disease) to sprout, and grow from inside the seed, it needs proper nourishment from external influence like sunlight, moisture, and the nutrients from a fertile land.
The various external factors, that caused the sprouting, and growth of the plant (disease) is ***Epi-genetics***.

It is a well-known fact, that has been proven through multiple researches that epi-genetics play a critical role in influencing the gene expression of *Metabolic Diseases*, such as diabetes, obesity, non-alcoholic fatty liver disease, osteoporosis, gout, hypothyroidism, PCOD and various others.

There are genetic diseases that are minimally, or in some cases, not in any way influenced by epi-genetics, such as Down Syndrome, Sickle Cell Anaemia, **Klinefelter Syndrome,** Turner Syndrome, Marfan Syndrome, **Duchenne Muscular Dystrophy,** etc.

But metabolic disorders are not as such, and are so highly influenced by our epi-genetics, that even the reversal of metabolic diseases are possible through the right lifestyle and diet choices.

The truth is that, the majority of us have actually given up.

Time and time again, we can find people who are fed up with the endless struggles due to their metabolic syndrome, who actually believe that there is no turning back, or that there isn't any remedy for these diseases. It is actually even taboo for the doctors to say that you can have a cure from diabetes, or any other metabolic diseases.

Now, the biggest challenge that patients face, when they decide to change their lifestyle is- **Exercise.**

They find it difficult to exercise either due to -

- Not physically being able to do exercises due to old age, diseases that cause joint or body pain, lack of time, etc.

OR

- Because they are just too plain lazy to do exercises.

This brings us to the next topic,

How important is physical exercise?

Chapter XII – Too Lazy To Exercise!

There's good news for those of you who are too lazy to exercise…

Even though exercise is essential for overall health, it only contributes to about **15%** of overall health and longevity. Healthy food and nutrition plays the leading role, contributing to around **85%** of your health.

This doesn't mean that we should give up on regular physical exercise… it is still very crucial in maintaining good health, improving muscle tone and bulk (essential for healthy ageing), preventing weak joints, and it helps relax your mind as well.

But regular exercise is a great responsibility on our part, to our body, because those who do it, are in more need of a healthy diet, than those who do not exercise.
This is because regular intense workout demands excess nutrition for our body. Nutrients such as potassium, vitamin-C, glutathione, etc. are a few of the many, that are drastically depleted during regular workouts.

One common mistake that people commit, is to try and imitate the diet pattern and workout routines of **'Professional Body Builders'** in the name of 'healthy living.'

What you must understand is that **'Professional Body Building'** is an extreme sport, which is strictly concerned with muscular size. Their only target, is to develop as much muscle mass as possible, with the least amount of body fat (which, as we discussed, can even lead to death.)

On top of that, this extreme way of exercise and high protein intake, activates the mTOR pathway (explained in more detail in Chapter- 19), which helps in the growth of cells and muscle.

But on prolonged and uncontrolled activation, especially when there are also underlying health issues, it can result in metabolic disorders, cardiovascular diseases, premature aging, and various types of cancers.

Organ health, athleticism, or fitness, is not considered by the majority of those following these routines, and neither can it co-exist with the kind of practices that body builders are going through, in their struggle to achieve massive bodies, in modern times.

The cases of heart attacks, strokes and deaths, among other numerous health issues keep rising in this extreme sport industry, and only a handful are aware of what they are actually doing to their body.

We can't solely blame these issues on the use of anabolic steroids (used for performance boosts) and their side effects. Even the seemingly 'harmless' bulking whey protein powders are often problematic, as only 15% contains actual protein, while up to 88% is merely sugar.
This is why buying and using bulking protein powders simply because you've started working out, might not be the right choice to be taking.

When you start using bulking proteins, you'll notice immediate muscle growth, which can be motivating. But remember, this growth is due to increased glycogen stores and enlarged muscle fibers. Once you stop the supplements and exercise, the size will shrink just as quickly.

This approach offers temporary satisfactions, like being able to admire your reflection in the mirror, or receiving compliments.
But this outward appearance is not necessarily a true indicator of health. The best option for good proteins are those from natural sources like eggs, dairy products and meat, which not only are pure sources of it, but are also more bio-available.

Physical Fitness, on the other hand, is what we really need to be achieving. Fitness prioritizes overall health and functionality.

You don't need muscles the size of large melons, nor six pack abs (not that a muscular body is not attractive) to prove that you are fit or healthy. If you do not have belly fat, and your body is flexible and strong enough, to be able to do your daily routines, without constant joint aches or pains, or any other diseases, then that itself is enough for a functional and healthy long life.

And to achieve this kind of *Functional Fitness*, regular physical exercise, along with a healthy diet is a must!

Now, in the case of individuals with a very active metabolism, or for those who have a very lean body structure, even though they stuff themselves with mountain loads of food, exercise is the right way to put on healthy weight.

Yes, the struggle to try and put on weight, is very real!
Just as real as the millions of people trying their hardest, to lose weight.

It is common in South India, for mothers and aunties, to force feed young teenage girls, a harmful amount of the so called "*Healthy*" weight gain formula of dates, jaggery and ghee.

This in fact, is trying to force the body to go into *Insulin Resistance*, which as we have just read about in Chapter- 4, can be the reason to drag in countless other unwelcome health issues and diseases, including PCOD or a dysfunctional thyroid in young girls.

This is clearly the wrong path to choose.

For those who are very lean, the right way possible, to gain healthy body weight, and that which does not give them diseases, is through-

- Eating a healthy and balanced, nutritious diet.
- Including regular ***Resistance Training*** (which is also called **Strength Training** or **Weight Training**) in your daily routine.

    This means, using of resistance bands or heavy weights like dumbbells, to create a resistance to the muscles, which will help to build strength, and increase the size of skeletal muscles.

    This in turn will help gain a healthy weight, and give the body a more fuller and healthy appearance.

So that is the take on exercise for very lean individuals, who cannot gain weight even after eating lots of food.

Now when it comes to losing weight... allow me to first highlight two common mistakes that we frequently encounter in our everyday lives.

- The Endless Walk of Vain.
- The Impulse "Attack" after a Quarter-Life Crisis.

1. *The Endless Walk of Vain* :–

This is the situation where we can see in every locality, uncles and aunties, who are overweight and most of the time with a belly (visceral fat), often during dawn, walking at a leisurely pace for around an hour, or around 5 kilometres in the firm belief that this "exercise" solely, will keep them healthy and rid them of their diabetes, obesity or fatty liver.

The more dedicated of them would walk a little more briskly, and would've changed their main dish from rice to wheat, and even go as far as to avoid their evening tea (a criminal offence in India), and also avoid all *'fatty food'* like dairy or fatty meat, in order to shed their extra weight.

If you have read this book up until this point, then I don't think I need to explain why these morning walks turn out to be as useless as changing the staple from rice to wheat.

Even if they were to join a gymnasium and perform heavy physical workouts for 2 hours a day, they still wouldn't be able to achieve proper health, without changing their diet along with their workouts.

2. *The Impulse "Attack" after a Quarter-Life Crisis* :–

Recently, we have seen a rise in the cases of untimely deaths due to heart attacks in young men, especially around the age of 35 years. Most of the time, these deaths occur, either in the gym, or during a heavy workout, or while doing some kind of physical activity, that we usually consider as healthy.

These are mostly cases where, the individuals, are those who have just settled down in life (financially or career wise), and have now, found enough time to focus on, and improve their physical health, which they have so severely neglected during their struggling years.

Usually after graduating college, up until they have gotten a decent income generating position, most of the middle class adult youths in India, struggle through this- "**Quarter-Life Crisis.**"

The physical impact that this neglect on their health, for roughly around 10 years, is not something that we can overlook. Little to no awareness about healthy food, is also a major reason for this failure to care for their body, and results in the regular consumption of highly refined or fried foods, carbonated drinks, flavoured juices etc.

I have personally known people who would do anything to save a few *Rupees*, even if it meant eating packeted potato chips or a packet of instant noodles for their daily meals.

But these kind of extreme deprivation of nutrients for the body, for years together can result in severe depletion of health, and even cause the formation of numerous, and quite severe atherosclerotic plaques, or as we most commonly call it - "Heart Blocks"

And as soon as these young men are able to afford time and money to start physical workout, they make the grave mistake of over-exerting themselves, on the initial days.
This intense strain after years of physical inactivity and neglect, causes cardiac arrests… which in truth, to those who observe closely, are neither so "sudden" nor "unexpected" as they seem.

As I have mentioned before, this doesn't mean that we should give up on regular physical exercise… but these are points to be noted,
to understand that even though the journey to good health is quite simple to follow, wrong knowledge could even cost a dear life.

It is also common to see people who are physically quite active, who regularly play sports, feel that they are in peak health just because they look athletic, and are physically flexible and strong. However, they will only truly be healthy, when they pair their physical activity with nutritious and healthy eating habits.

Frankly, people with poor eating habits who also engage in intense regular exercise, are far more at a health risk, than for those with unhealthy diets and sedentary lifestyles.

It is because the nutritional demand and requirement, is much more for those who perform intense regular physical exercise. And if they do not meet those demands with a nutritious and healthy diet, they are more likely to end up with extreme damage, and inflammations in their joints, along with unhealthy blood vessels, and an over-exerted body.

If you take a look at the life and diet of celebrity footballer *Cristiano Ronaldo*, the discipline in his diet, is as important (if not more important), as his physical training, which has allowed him to perform at the highest level, even at the age of 40 plus years, where normally, footballers retire around the age of 30 years, due to their body starting to show signs of decline and ageing.

Lionel Messi, the footballing **GOAT** (greatest of all time),
(as a Lionel Messi fan, I can't resist mentioning him), started seeing positive changes in his body, and performance after he changed his diet as well. It is famously reported that up until 20 years of age, Lionel Messi's major diet habit was mostly junk food, with pizzas and deep fried chicken with lots of soft drinks.
He would end up regurgitating and vomiting severely after each professional match, and was reported that he felt like he wouldn't be able to continue this career anymore.

So for those of you who are confused, or do not know where to begin, on taking the initial steps for a healthy life… you can first start by making changes in your diet (which we will discuss in detail in the following chapters), and after the inflammations have reduced, and there have been drastic improvement in your health and you feel energetic, only then comes the time to begin including daily physical exercise in your regular routine.

> This chapter should serve as an inspiration, to all those
> who have given up trying to change their lifestyle,
> who are too weak physically, either due to age,
> or a degenerative or inflammatory diseases of their joints,
> or any other similar diseases.

Chapter XIII – One Body, Shared by Two Friends.

If you ever thought that your body was your own, and is controlled solely by yourself through the help of your brain...
then you might find this chapter surprising.

You see, your body is only half you, in fact, less than half of you.
The majority of your body is occupied and controlled by trillions of friendly micro-organisms, also known as "**PRO-BIOTICS**"

Bacterial diversity analysis has shown that more than 1000 different species of bacteria, are present in our body.
A few of them are even friendly virus and fungus species.

Our body's total cell count is around- *70 trillion* (70,000,000,000,000 cells!)
Among those, human cells constitute around- *30 trillion*
Our friendly co-habitants make up the majority, around- *40 trillion*

These friendly bacteria are mostly found in our small and large intestines, which gives them the name *Gut Microbiome*.

Research has shown that a person is first exposed to friendly micro-organisms as an infant, during delivery through the birth canal, from the mother's vaginal fluids and then, through the mother's breast milk.

This shows another aspect of how important a mother's health is for the child. This is why there is a higher risk in children who were born through a caesarean-section, to have low immunity, and a subsequent higher risk to end up with diseases like eczema, allergies etc.

These friends of ours, Pro-biotics, control our body functions in so many important ways, that our digestive system, the GIT (gastro-intestinal system), also called as '**Gut**' is considered as our *Second Brain*.

The interesting fact is that, both of our brains are in constant interaction with each other via the *enteric nervous system*, which is a complex structure of nerves that transmit messages in the form of neurons.

The Human Brain	GUT (Second Brain)
85 billion neurons	500 million neurons
100 neurotransmitters identified so far	40 neurotransmitters identified so far
Produces 50% of all dopamine	Produces 50% of all dopamine
Produces 5% of all serotonin	Produces 95% of all serotonin

It is also a fascinating reality that scientists have found over *5 million* unique genes, which is part of the collective gut microbiota!

Comparing that to our own genome, humans have just around *25,000* unique genes as part of our biological body.

When you understand that even minuscule details, such as the colour and shape of our eyes, or the amount of hair follicles on our eyebrows, are all predetermined, and written down in the *"Blueprint"* of our body, in our 25,000 genes…
imagine the amount of information stored in those 5 million genes… which are **200 times** more genes than our own genome, and the countless functions and benefits that they provide for our body!

Some of the benefits of good bacteria (pro-biotics) include helping our body to digest food and absorb nutrients, and even to produce several nutrients that are completely unique (only made by them) in the intestinal tract.
They also help produce nutrients that are found in food as well, including folic acid, niacin, vitamin-B_6 and vitamin-B_{12}.

Beneficial friendly bacteria help protect the cells in our intestines from invading pathogens, and also promote repair of damaged tissue, binds and removes heavy metals (lead, chromium etc.), and having healthy bacteria in our body itself prevents the growth of harmful bacteria.

Here are a few examples of healthy bacteria (Pro-biotics) and a few of their known uses and benefits for the human body-

Bacteria	Important Functions
Lactobacillus Acidophilus & Lactobacillus Reuteri	• Used (in suppository form) to treat bacterial infections of the vagina. • In pill form, it can be taken to prevent and treat diarrhea, including traveler's diarrhea in adults and diarrhea caused by Rotavirus, Clostridium difficile bacteria or by over use of antibiotics in children. • Known to eliminate as well as degrade, hormone disrupting BPA and microplastics from the body, with more than 80% efficiency. • Used for preventing and treating diarrhoea in adults who are admitted in the hospital or receiving chemotherapy treatment for cancer.
Lactobacillus Rhamnoses	• Found to help prevent & treat eczema in infants. • Prevents colic (inconsolable crying) in babies.
Lactobacillus Salivarius	• Prevents the over-growth of H. pylori (Helicobacter pylorus), the bacteria that cause peptic ulcers, various types of gastric issues & migraine. • Helpful in prevention and treatment of intestinal diseases such as IBS (irritable bowel syndrome) and ulcerative colitis.
Lactobacillus Plantarum	• Improves the immune system against pathogens. • Helpful in Preventing and treating lung infections in young children.
Saccharomyces Boulardii	• It is actually a type of yeast, but it acts as a probiotic. Studies have found it helpful for preventing and treating traveller's diarrhoea, as well as diarrhoea caused by antibiotics. • Also useful for treating acne, and reducing the side effects of antibiotic treatment for H. Pylori bacteria.

Bacteria	Important Functions
Bifidobacteria Bifidum & Bifidobacteria Infantis	• When combined with Lactobacillus acidophilus, it helps prevent eczema in new-borns. • Increases our immunity against unhealthy bacteria and helps relieve IBS (irritable bowel syndrome) symptoms, such as abdominal cramps, pain, gas, and bloating.
Bifidobacteria Lactis	• Improve cholesterol levels in women and in people affected by type-2 diabetes mellitus.
Streptococcus Thermophilus	• These bacteria produce the enzyme lactase, which the body needs to digest the sugar in milk and other dairy products. Studies show that streptococcus thermophilus can help prevent lactose intolerance.
Akkermansia Muciniphila	• Helpful against development of auto-immune issues, diabetes, obesity, atherosclerotic plaques, IBS, IBD and aids in the treatment of cancer.

A very interesting organ in our body, the *Appendix*, was once considered a vestigial (useless) organ in the human body.

But in recent years, this view have been revised, and the appendix has gained its deserved recognition, as new research sheds light on its functions for the gut microbiome, and role in maintaining the gut health.

The delicate balance of microbes can be disrupted in certain situations, such as after a gastrointestinal illness, the use of antibiotics, or even stressful events, which can alter the gut environment and causes all sorts of physical and mental health issues.

The appendix play a key role in the recovery and maintenance of a healthy microbiome after such disruptions, through being a – *'Reservoir of Beneficial Microbes.'*

The appendix is home to a concentrated, diverse population of beneficial bacteria, kind of like a microbial vault, or a backup system.
When the gut microbiome is compromised, due to any issues, the store of beneficial bacteria, are reintroduced into the gut, which help re-establish, and re-populate the microbial balance in the gut.

The appendix also plays a role in immune function, as it contains lymphatic tissue, which is involved in the production of immune cells. These cells help recognize, and respond to harmful pathogens, in the event of an infection, which provide protection to the gut.

From an evolutionary standpoint, the appendix may have had a more prominent role in earlier human ancestors.
In those times, when diets and living conditions drastically kept changing, the appendix may have been critical for digesting various plant matter to extract its nutrients, and to maintain microbial health in the digestive system.
Even though this direct digestive function of the appendix may have diminished over time, its role as a *'safe house'* for gut flora remains of utmost relevance to this day and age.

Appendicitis or inflammation of the appendix, is a medical emergency that requires prompt treatment. But it is also important to recognize and evaluate, if the situation, calls for a necessary surgical removal of the organ (appendectomy).
And even though an appendectomy is generally lifesaving in cases of acute appendicitis, it could result in the slow and steady development of gastro-intestinal or auto-immune diseases.

On the note of auto-immune diseases, there's a high chance that you would have heard of any one of various auto-immune conditions, such as multiple sclerosis, S.L.E, vitiligo, ulcerative colitis, Crohn's disease etc., or even behavioural disorders like Autism and ADHD.

Up until recently, these diseases were believed to have no cure…
that it could only be managed through life-long medications (many of which, have heavy side-effects).

But since recent research started to focus on our gut bacteria and its various effects in our body, all the scientific findings implicated that these auto-immune diseases are not conditions due to a genetic default, but are in fact, initiated as a result of gut-bacterial dysbiosis and an issue in our intestine called as '*Leaky Gut*' (which is explained in detail at the end of this chapter).

It was discovered, that in the stool samples collected from patients suffering from auto-immune disorders, there were disproportionate amounts of bacteria. Which meant that, not only do harmful bacteria cause such diseases, but also, friendly bacteria.

When the friendly bacteria exceed their normal levels, or appear in places that they should not be in, it can result in conditions like-

- **SIMO** (small intestinal methanogen overgrowth)
- **SIBO** (small intestinal bacterial overgrowth)
- **SIPO** (small intestinal parasitic overgrowth)
- **SIFO** (small intestinal fungal overgrowth)
- **IMO** (intestinal methanogen overgrowth)

The excess neurotoxins from these over-growths dominate, and become the triggering factor for harmful diseases including metabolic, cardio-vascular and auto-immune disorders as well.

Even in the case of fungus, a healthy portion of 4% of our total gut flora must contain fungi. When left unchecked, and this percentage increases, and can result in SIFO (small intestinal fungal overgrowth) or Candidiasis (fungal infection) of our gut.

This infection can show symptoms such as leucorrhoea (foul odour vaginal discharge in women), dandruff, white coated tongue, oral thrush, and halitosis (foul mouth odour).

It has also been commonly found to cause cases of *Alopecia Areata* (round, smooth, bald patches of hair loss, that affects scalp, eyebrows, beard etc.) where regrowth of hair have been noticed, once the infection is controlled. The fungal infection is also one of the leading causes for **PID (pelvic inflammatory disease)**, which is often overlooked and instead, mistakenly treated for disc prolapse or muscle stiffness without any success, as it the infection, that needs to be addressed.

Here are some of the common auto-immune diseases and the most identified bacteria or virus found excessively in stool samples, in the patients suffering from it -

Disease	Dominant Bacteria
Rheumatoid Arthritis	Prevotella copri & Subdoligranulum didolesgii.
Ankylosing Spondylitis	Klebsiella pneumoniae.
S.L.E (*Systemic Lupus Erythematous*)	Ruminococcus gnavus & EBV (*Epstein-Barr virus*).
Multiple Sclerosis	Desulfo-vibrionaceae & Clostridium perfringens.
Autism	Several Clostridium species.
Hashimoto's Thyroiditis	Klebsiella pneumoniae.

Probiotic supplements (capsules with live beneficial bacteria) have become a widespread craze, with a product available for nearly every condition, from digestive issues to skin health.

However, a more innovative approach, FMT (*faecal microbiota transplantation*), goes beyond just supplementing with bacteria, and involves transfer of healthy donor stool into a patient's gut to restore a balanced microbiome.

This has shown significant promise in treating inflammatory bowel diseases like ulcerative colitis, *Crohn's* disease, and other forms of colitis.

By replenishing beneficial gut bacteria, FMT helps reduce inflammation, strengthen the gut barrier, and restore immune balance.

Recently, scientists have gone one step further, and made something called **Post-Biotics** available to us, which is the metabolic byproducts produced by the beneficial microbes.

These by-products include those, such as SCFA (short chain fatty acids), exopolysaccharides (complex sugars), peptides (short chains of amino acids), urolithins, bacterial cell wall fragments, and other lipids, which are all secreted by beneficial bacteria.

These by-products help with muscle building, gut barrier integrity and immune modulation. It also possess anti-inflammatory properties, and is an avid promoter of our metabolic and mental health.

Unlike probiotics, which require live bacteria to exert their effects, post-biotics can have similar health benefits without needing to introduce live microorganisms into the body.

This can be advantageous in cases where immediate result might be required, without having to wait for the healthy bacteria to colonise, and then start with its functions on a large scale.

This is where I would like to introduce the ***Beneficial Sugars***, that our body requires… that I did not mention in the first chapter.

It was not mentioned separately because it would come under the category of **'*Dietary Fiber*'** classification, which is food for the friendly bacteria, that is then metabolized as special type of fat (SCFA), small proteins (peptides), and **special complex sugars** or **exopolysaccharides**.

Exopolysaccharides (EPSs) are high-molecular-weight carbohydrate polymers that are secreted by the micro-organisms, and have many biological functions, including the protection of our friendly gut microbiome from harsh environmental conditions, such as dehydration, toxic compounds, and changes in pH and osmolarity, by helping to form protective biofilm complexes.

EPSs also helps our friendly microorganisms to attach to surfaces, concentrate nutrients for growth, and even helps them evade our body's immune response.

EPSs have become valuable in the food, pharmaceutical, and nutraceutical industries, as they are being used in drug delivery systems because of their biocompatibility, biodegradability, and lack of irritation.

Moreover, EPSs itself becomes a source of prebiotics, which help beneficial bacteria in the colon to grow and survive, and also play a role in increasing our body's immune system response, regulate blood pressure, and induce apoptosis and autophagy in cancer cell lines (explained in later chapters).

Some examples of EPSs include pullulan, botryosphaeran, scleroglucan, and fungal β-glucans (found to be beneficial in the treatment of sinusitis or fungal infections).

Similarly, *urolithins* are bioactive compounds produced by the gut bacteria, as a result of metabolizing foods that contain 'ellagitannins.' Urolithins are powerful antioxidants, which have anti-inflammatory effects, and promote autophagy.

It also play an important role in muscle building, and increasing the mitochondrial efficiency (explained in later chapters).

However, the ability to benefit from these various compounds depends on an individual's gut microbial flora, making the consumption of foods like pomegranate, berries, and walnuts extremely beneficial, even beyond their typical nutritional contents, only for those, with a good bacterial flora, that can metabolize it.

The relationship between humans and the gut microbiota is nothing short of symbiotic.

Friendly bacteria help us, and in turn, our bodies provide a stable environment and nutrition for these microbes, creating a mutually beneficial partnership.

As scientists continue to discover new nutrients, metabolites, and microbial interactions that contribute to human health, it is clear that our understanding of nutrition and health cannot be complete without the gut microbiome. Without our life partners, the gut microbiome, human life as we know it would not exist.

- **The Myth of The Leaky Gut.**

Now the issue with *"Leaky Gut Syndrome"* is that, it is still not officially recognized, and is still considered a hypothetical condition, because there is yet no 'exact' diagnostic method invented, to confirm this condition in patients suffering from its symptoms.

Everyone's gut is semi-permeable, meaning that the walls of our intestines are designed to absorb nutrients and water from our intestine, to our bloodstream.
Our intestinal lining also has the function of, acting as a barrier which prevents harmful bacteria and other infectious agents, and the toxic substances created by them, from entering our bloodstream.
This barrier is an important part of our immune system.

The conditions that weakens the intestinal walls, causing toxins to enter our bloodstream are, inflammatory diseases of our *Gastro Intestinal Tract* (GIT) such as, *Inflammatory Bowel Disease* (IBD) and various infections like bacterial, viral, fungal and even the infections of parasitic worms.

There have been cases where scientists found intestinal permeability in people before they were diagnosed with these diseases, which means that intestinal permeability can develop independently, due to a poor diet, alcohol abuse, long term drug use and even chronic stress.

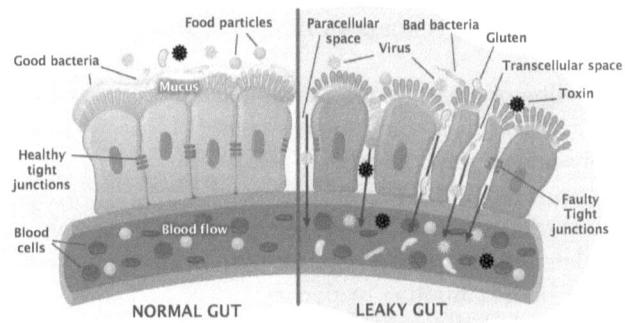

Leaky Gut Syndrome

One interesting factor that can be considered as a diagnostic factor, is **Zonulin**, which is a protein that regulates the permeability of the small intestine, by modulating the tight junctions between epithelial cells in the digestive tract (effectively modulates the permeability), and is involved in balancing the tolerance and mucosal immune response of the body.

Zonulin is produced in the small intestine, liver, kidney, heart, brain, and immune cells, and is also found in many foods, including wheat, dairy, legumes, nuts, and seeds.

This is why individuals with auto-immune tendencies and a delicate gut, have flare ups of these issues, when consuming wheat and other high-gluten grains, which contain gliadin, that stimulates the release of luminal zonulin, and leads to the increase of the intestinal permeability.

Increased serum zonulin levels are noted in majority of individuals with auto-immune diseases, and can be considered a diagnostic factor for the gut related auto-immune issues.

Levels of lipopolysaccharide-binding protein, soluble CD_{14}, bactericidal or permeability-increasing protein, and peptidoglycans are also currently being relied upon as markers to identify a leaky gut issue in patients.

Many other diseases that cause long term, low-grade inflammation have also been found to cause leaky gut syndrome, like Diabetes, Arthritis, Chronic fatigue, AIDS, Asthma etc.

A burning feeling of ulceration in the stomach, indigestion, loose stools, stomach pains, diarrhoea with mucus or blood, bloating, low energy are all commonly seen in cases of a *Leaky Gut*.

Our intestinal mucosal membranes, serve as barriers which are a critical first line of defence that protect against pathogens, and also helps in regulating the body's immune responses.
When there is an imbalance in the mucus membrane, it can contribute significantly to the development of leaky gut.

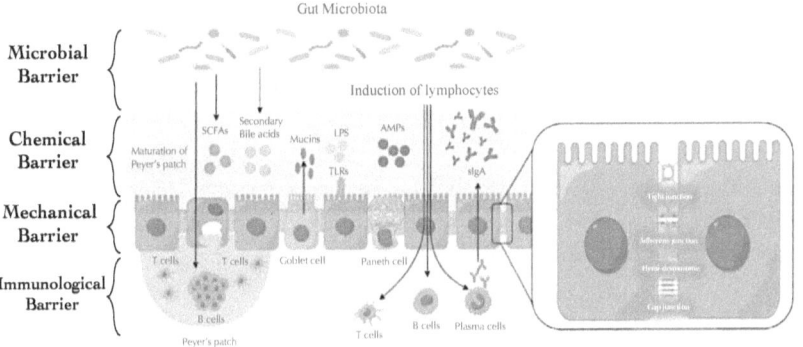

Main Layers of Intestinal Barrier

One key factor in maintaining the balance of the mucosal layer (shown as *chemical barrier* in the above image), is a gut bacteria named **Akkermansia muciniphila**.

This bacteria plays an essential role in maintaining the integrity of the gut's mucus layer, by feeding on mucus, specifically the mucin proteins that make up the mucus barrier. By breaking down mucin, this bacteria stimulates the gut to produce more mucin in response, thus ensuring that the mucus layer remains thick and protective.

When the balance of beneficial bacteria is disrupted, mucin production can decline, which leads makes it easier for pathogens to breach the intestinal lining and enter the bloodstream.

As mentioned before, the best way to preserve the mucus layer and repair a *Leaky Gut* is by bringing back the balance of the microbial flora in our intestines, and also, eating a healthy and balanced diet.

It is also quite fascinating how something as simple as proper chewing and safe swallowing can have a profound impact on gut wall integrity. EGF (*epidermal growth factor*), a polypeptide, plays a crucial role in this process by stimulating cell division and differentiation, particularly in the gastric mucosa (which is the lining of the stomach).

EGF helps protect this delicate lining from damage and is vital for maintaining the gut barrier function and preventing harmful substances from leaking into the bloodstream. EGF also helps in the transport of various substances through the various layers of the intestine, and plays a vital role in glucose metabolism.

Science has advanced significantly in identifying various irregularities in the gut microbiome and an innovative diagnosing method, known as the Metagenomics, are available to the public.

Metagenomics is the study of the structure and function of DNA, extracted from microbes like bacteria, archaea, fungi, worms, virus, etc. from the human gut, which helps to predict or even diagnose certain diseases that are associated with or caused by the specific bacteria or microbes, which in turn provide the potential to provide specified treatment options for human health, and treatment.

Clinical studies from organisations that recommend lifestyle changes based on results from metagenomics have shown-

- **19.5%** reduction in HbA1c in Type-2 Diabetic patients.
- **14%** reduction in systolic pressure in hypertension patients.
- **20%** reduction in general and specific inflammations.

BugSpeaks® is a brilliant organisation that helps in such assessment and diagnosis, and are a leading organization in their field, gathering various national and international awards, and recognition for their innovations, research and contributions in this sphere.

I am not sponsored by them, nor do I gain a profit from mentioning them here. But they are a genuine find for me, and I appreciate the good work that they do. You can visit their website, and get your *Metagenomic Test* done from the comfort of your home, at a time of your convenience.

Chapter XIV – The Anti-biotic Dilemma.

When we think about harmful bacteria in our body, or any kind of infection, our first option is almost always anti-biotics.
Synthetic and semi-synthetic anti-biotics are one of the greatest advances in modern medicine.

But over-prescribing, and usage without prescription (antibiotic abuse) is a very serious issue faced all over the world, and particularly in India, where it has been calculated that over **85%** of anti-biotics bought from pharmacies, are without a prescription from a licenced physician.

Even though it is highly effective in controlling infections, given below are a few reasons why its over-use and abuse, leads to further health complications, and worsens the disease it was supposed to treat -

1. *Anti-biotic Resistance*- Bacteria have the ability to adapt and develop resistance to anti-biotics over time. Overuse of antibiotics can speed up this evolution, leading to survival and thriving of mutated strains of bacteria with higher immunity, that can overcome the effects of the anti-biotics, and become more harmful.

2. *Destroys Even Friendly Bacteria*- Anti-biotics not only target harmful bacteria but can also disrupt the balance of beneficial bacteria in the body's microbiota. This disruption can lead to conditions such as antibiotic-associated diarrhoea or yeast infections, because friendly bacteria keeps the yeast or fungal population under control, the health amount of which is around 4% of our total gut flora.

3. *Secondary Infections*- Destruction of beneficial bacteria by the effects of anti-biotics, can create an empty environment where other opportunistic pathogens can flourish. This can lead to secondary infections that may become, more difficult to treat, or be more severe than the original infection.

4. *Side Effects*- Gastro-intestinal upsets, nausea, vomiting, headaches, allergic reactions ranging from mild rashes to severe hypersensitivity reactions, which can worsen the patient's condition and may require immediate medical attention.

5. ***Low Immunity*-** Prolonged or repeated courses of anti-biotics can disrupt the body's immune system and its ability to fight infections naturally. This can increase the risk of frequently being the victim of various infections and diseases.

6. ***Anti-biotic Toxicity*-** Anti-biotics abuse can cause very harmful (at times irreversible) effects on all our organs, and especially on the kidneys, liver, or nerves.

In short, even though synthetic anti-biotics are a valuable asset for us, we must use them sensibly, only when necessary, and under the guidance of a licensed doctor, to minimize the risk of complications, and to ensure an effective treatment.

So what do we do in cases where the anti-biotics are out-dated?

For example, the success rate of anti-biotics against H. Pylori (bacteria that causes gastritis, ulcers & migraines), used to be above **90%** around the year 2003, when it was first introduced.
20 years from then on, in 2023, statistics have shown that the success rate of these synthetic anti-biotics have come down to less than **15%**.

A study published in The Lancet, found that more than **1 million** people died **each year**, as a direct result of anti-microbial resistance (**AMR**) between the years 1990 to 2021.
This death toll is projected to **increase** by **70%** or, to almost **2 million** deaths **per year**, which, by the year 2050, could tally the death tolls to more than **40 million** deaths, from now, until 2050.

Why are the anti-biotics not updated?

The time taken for developing and bringing a new medicine to the market, can vary significantly depending on several factors.
On average, it can take around 10 to 15 years for a medicine to be created and brought to the market.

So what should we be doing instead?

Recent scientific research suggests that combining natural antibiotics with probiotics (friendly bacteria) may offer a healthier and more effective approach to achieving complete remission from infections, with fewer side effects, a method I personally stand by, due to its immense success in my own practice.

Why are natural anti-biotics better?

For minor infections and allergies, it is better to use doses of vitamin-D and vitamin-C, with readily available herbs and natural medicines like garlic, ginger, honey, turmeric, cinnamon, black pepper, tea tree oil, oregano, thyme, neem, cloves, black cumin and even coconut oil among countless others, mainly because of their targeted effectiveness and specificity.

Natural anti-biotics target the majority of harmful bacteria and are able to avoid damaging the friendly microbes population. Secondly, all of these herbs and their medicinal compounds are adaptive by nature.

How?

Natural antibiotics are bioactive substances found in various plants that possess antimicrobial properties, meaning they can kill bacteria or stop its spreading. For example, one of the most important bioactive compound of turmeric, is *Curcumin*.

There are numerous scientific evidences on Curcumins powerful anti-bacterial, anti-fungal, and anti-viral benefits. It is so effective that curcumin is extracted, and now available in tablet form at pharmacies.

Unlike conventional antibiotics, which are synthesized in laboratories, natural antibiotics from plants are exposed to the evolutionary process. Plants produce these bioactive compounds as part of their self-defence mechanisms against harmful bacteria, virus and fungi.

Over time, bacteria and fungi develop resistance, and increased immunity to these natural antibiotics through genetic mutations.

As a result, the plants too, are forced to evolve according to the current strength of the pathogens, and only plants with the strongest bio-active compounds will survive, which we humans, can use for our own health.

Advancements in technology have allowed us to isolate and extract nutrients from their sources, and when administered in the right concentrated doses, they help combat diseases and maintain good health.

You might wonder, why not use the herbs as they are?
Why the need for extraction?

Extractions are necessary in modern times because heavy metals like lead, mercury, cadmium, and arsenic are naturally present in soil and water, especially in areas with high industrial activity.
These heavy metals can accumulate in plants, including medicinal herbs, and prolonged consumption of herbs with high levels of heavy metals lead to toxic effects, particularly on the liver and kidneys, when consumed in constant doses over a long period.

For example cilantro is known for its ability to chelate, or bind, heavy metals from the environment, a function which can also be used to cleanse the body from heavy metals.
But this also indicates that the heavy metals can accumulate in these herbs if grown in contaminated soil. When used medicinally, cilantro extracts should be sourced from controlled, contaminant-free environments, and any raw cilantro used for detox purposes should be carefully sourced, before other cleansing processes.

Certain herbs (such as turmeric, ashwagandha etc.) must be carefully processed with specific extraction methods and purification processes (like aqueous or ethanol extraction, solvent extraction, supercritical CO_2 extraction etc.) to separate active compounds and at the same time, to reduce metal impurities as well as minimize toxic elements, before they are used for medicinal purposes.

Therefore, to ensure safety, look for herbs that are tested for heavy metals, and which are sourced from reputable suppliers that undergo regular testing and certification to provide assurance, that the products meet safety standards for heavy metal content, which helps to achieve the intended health results in patients.

Similarly, nutritional supplements are often a better option than conventional medicines for many diseases, as they are highly effective with minimal side effects, and work in harmony with the body, encouraging the body's natural ability to combat diseases and maintain overall health.

However, it is crucial to ensure that nutritional supplements are sourced naturally, rather than being synthetic, as the latter can sometimes cause harm rather than provide healing (of course, there are exceptions). There have been instances of severe complications, and even fatalities, resulting from its improper use.

For instance, vitamin-C in its natural form is much more intricate and is actually a 'vitamin-C complex' which contains numerous compounds that interact with each other to provide its benefits without any side effects. However, over **90%** of vitamin-C supplements available on the market, focus solely on isolating ascorbic acid from this complex.

The synthetic version of ascorbic acid is typically derived from a combination of primarily corn starch, which even though molecular structure-wise, may resemble the natural form, it lacks the accompanying bioflavonoids and other compounds that aid its absorption and utilization in the body, and could even be unfavourable to our body.

Or as in the case of calcium supplements, the "OG" supplement used by Doctors, many companies use calcium derived from limestone, which are not effectively absorbed by the body, and when not properly formulated or balanced with other nutrients, it mostly end up forming into kidney stones, gall-bladder stones, and atherosclerotic plaques (heart blocks).

Personally I do not recommend or prescribe calcium supplements, instead, I concentrate on other vitamins and minerals that help the patients increase their normal absorption of calcium, and deliver it to the targeted area in the body, so that our food itself is enough for the required amounts of calcium.

The issue with calcium supplementation is that, if it is not consumed along with sufficient dosages of vitamin-D, vitamin-A, vitamin-K, vitamin-C and adequate amounts of magnesium, it will not be effectively transported into the bones, and instead contributes to the formation of atherosclerotic plaques, or renal caliculi, as mentioned before.

This issue isn't limited to calcium or vitamin-C alone. Every nutrient is co-dependent, and rely on each other, for absorption and transportation.

One of the main challenges in the medical field today, is that Doctors, due to their busy practices, often lack the time to stay fully updated on the latest research and medical advancements.

Much of their knowledge and updates are from 'medicine sales representatives' who themselves, are only aware of what they are taught by the large corporate pharmaceutical companies that employ them.

This is why it is more crucial than ever, to hold regular CME (*continued medical education*) sessions for health practitioners, whether in large hospitals, or smaller clinics.
These sessions must include the evaluation and discussions of unbiased researches, as well as studies that may not receive widespread attention because of limited funding (due to its lack of business potential), to help enhance medical practice, and the art of healing.

Last but not least, it is important to remember that, even though nutritional supplements are highly beneficial and advantageous, they are never going to be a complete substitute for a balanced diet and healthy lifestyle. So don't even think about eating junk food along with your multi-vitamins, hoping for the best to happen!

Chapter XV – One More Interesting Story.

Now it may seem unfair that we blame the modern pharmaceuticals for a lot of side-effects and complications.

In truth, modern medicine has offered us a lot of benefits, but it is our own lack of knowledge, on where to draw the line, when it comes to the usage of such powerful synthetic drugs, that is the main reason behind all these diseases and complications.

Billions of dollars, and even lives and reputations have been sacrificed to build up the formidable *Pharmaceutical Empire* that currently dominates the global economy of our planet.
And so, it is obvious that they expect monitory returns from it, and will do whatever it takes to somehow try, and maintain their dominance in the medical sector and beyond.

In the second chapter, we have discussed about the biggest lie that was ever told... similarly, here let us discuss the incidents, that entirely changed the field of medicine and treatment.

But this story is not as bad as, what refined cotton-seed oil did to our lives, because there were lots of benefits for us, from the emergence of synthetic medicines.

It is essential though, to be aware of these facts, in order to realize, that not everything that is done for us, is with the best of intentions, and that we must understand the importance of being mindful, and to be able to choose appropriate treatment, for each health issue.

This is a very short version of how **John D. Rockefeller** influenced *Modern Medicine*, and dominated the medical sector.

John D. Rockefeller, at the time of his death, was estimated to be worth around 400 billion dollars, making him the -

"Richest Man In Modern History."

He had control of over **90%** of oil refineries in the United States of America, and was a rigorous monopolist, meaning that he solely controlled that industry.
He gained this position by simply cutting out his competitors through illegal methods, and sometimes through legal, yet unethical tactics.

In 1911 though, the U.S. Supreme Court, in an effort to stop his monopoly, ruled that John Rockefeller's company *'Standard Oil Trust'* must be dissolved.

And so Rockefeller split his company *'Standard Oil Trust'* into **thirty four** different companies.

But Rockefeller being the ruthless businessman he is, knew that he had to venture into other fields of business to stay atop, and long before the 1911 ruling, he had already started pulling the strings, to bring the medical sector under his control.

This was quite easy for Rockefeller because around the same time period, the scientists of the time were just discovering the numerous potential advancements in technology, offered from the petrochemicals that were produced from the petroleum industry, such as the ones that Rockefeller owned.

It was also the time when numerous essential vitamins like vitamin-C, vitamin-A, vitamin-D, vitamin-B_1, vitamin-B_2, and its functions, were being discovered, along with the basics of human physiology, and there was a lot of research focused on recreating synthetic lab versions of these vitamins. This is where Rockefeller saw great potential to utilize his position as an oil tycoon, and a petroleum industry monopolist, to venture into the medical sector.

At the time, herbal and natural medicines were highly popular in the USA, which interfered with Rockefeller's plans for a monopoly.
But he had much elaborate, yet precise plans for it, and as his first step, he purchased a German pharmaceutical company.

Then, the *Rockefeller Foundation*, funded the *"Flexner Report of* 1910", authored by a man named **Abraham Flexner**, who was commissioned by the '*Council on Medical Education*' which was created by the *American Medical Association* (**AMA**).

The aim of this report was to help evaluate, and restructure medical education in the United States of America. The report concluded that all natural healing modalities were '*Unscientific*' and decided that there were too many medical schools, as well as too many doctors in America, and called for the ***Standardization*** (the process of establishing and applying rules or guidelines to ensure consistency and uniformity) of all medical education in America.

This was with the hidden intention to give the AMA, the power to be the sole entity that could approve medical school licenses in the U.S, and in effect, be controlled by the person who funds the AMA, none other than Mr. John. D. Rockefeller.

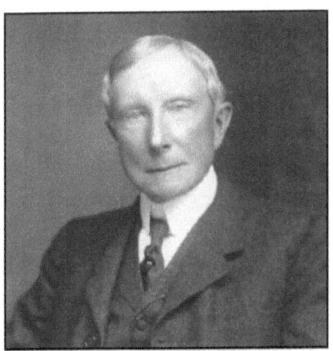

John D. Rockefeller

Based on **Flexner's** recommendations, the U.S government implemented changes, and helped modern allopathic medicine to become the standard medical system in USA.

Next, Rockefeller started to fund medical schools all across the USA, with the condition that, only *allopathic* or *modern medicine* be taught, and extra bonuses were offered in order to strictly adhere to these conditions.

This funding, systematically removed teachings on nutrition and diet, and any mention of plant-based natural treatments, from the medical education curriculum.

Rockefeller's influence on the media of the time, were also used to discredit, and demonize other systems of medicines, through targeted media campaigns.

Rockefeller then started funding the *American Cancer Society* (**ACS**), which later on influenced the government, to bring in the law, that made it illegal to use any treatment, other than chemotherapy, radiation, or surgery, for the treatment of cancer.

Now, Rockefeller was the happy and proud monopolist of so many businesses, that heavily relied on his petrochemicals industry.

Antibiotics, antibacterial products, analgesics, rectal suppositories, cough syrups, lubricants, topical ointments, creams, and gels, are all to a major extend, extensively dependent on the petrochemical industry.

Long term use of petrochemical-based products present major risks for our overall health, and well-being.
Allergies, birth defects, cancer, infertility, hormonal imbalances, and much more, are potent risk factors for frequent and heavy users.

The most harmful way that synthetic chemicals can cause issues in our body, is when it is absorbed into our bloodstream, when it enters through skin absorption, or inhalation.

Petrochemicals in skincare products, have been shown to contain neurotoxins, known to be toxic to the brain, respiratory system, and kidneys, and is known to contribute to many different types of cancers. The petrochemical ingredients that harm our body, which are commonly found in skin care products are parabens, benzene, PEG, DEA, TEA, MEA, toluene, butanol, silicone, synthetic emulsifiers, synthetic dyes or synthetic fragrances, and any other ingredient that ends in *-propyl*, or begins with *butyl-*... all of which, must be avoided.

It is an undeniable fact, that as a direct result of the petrochemical industry, we have been able to make major advances in medicine, healthcare technologies and surgery over the years.

Advancements in diagnostic machineries, surgical equipment, and even the lifesaving emergency medications, were all possible, only due to this system of medicine, and to a great extent, because of the petroleum industry.

However, it is unfortunate that our health as a society has also drastically decreased over the years, with conditions such as diabetes, cancer, heart disease, strokes, Alzheimer's, and respiratory diseases becoming the norm, even at relatively young ages.

Without a doubt, this situation can be blamed on, removal of subjects, that taught about the importance, and the influence of healthy diet and nutrition, on our body and overall health, from the medical schools, which have left the up-coming medical professionals almost clueless on what actually healthy food is.

It has also limited their view of treatment options, making them entirely dependent on synthetic medications and highly sophisticated machines, in their pursuit of treating diseases.

Fortunately, there is growing education and awareness, not just within the medical community, but also among the general public, and people are increasingly seeking to understand all the details of a disease, and all of their possible options, before deciding on treatments.

Chapter XVI – Pickle Body.

Recently, we have come across a trend called as the 'Alkaline Diet.'

The basis of the claim that we should alkalise our body, started from the idea that since our blood is of almost neutral pH (around 7), we should be consuming food that are either of the same pH, or that which stimulates it... thereby improving health and preventing diseases.

The alkaline diet was promoted by advocating the restriction on foods like meat and dairy, while claiming that *'alkaline foods'* such as fruits and raw vegetables are the key to good health.

As you can imagine, devoted followers of the *alkaline diet* began to experience severe nutritional deficiencies and related health issues, as mentioned in the first chapter.

Just as the **Procter & Gamble** business had done for their refined oils, the 'alkaline diet' was the commercial exploitation and lie created majorly by **Robert O. Young.**

But this lie created by **Robert O. Young**, is to this day, being extensively used, by other companies, to promote their sale of 'alkaline water' and other 'organic alkaline products' claiming to alkalize the body, and promote health. Not only are these products extremely expensive, but are also unsupported by any scientific evidence as they claim, and actually cause harm and disease instead.

Let us take a look at the stomach pH of different trophic groups...

Trophic Group	Stomach pH
Herbivores	4 - 6
Omnivores	3 - 4
Carnivores	2 - 3
Scavengers	1 - 2

Humans consume both plants and meat, and are generally referred to the *"omnivores"* category, and so naturally, we would assume that our stomach pH is in the 3 to 4 range.

But physiologically, our pH stands in the 1 to 2 range, which is the same range as that of scavengers (such as vultures, crows or hyenas).

We have evolved with such powerful acids in our stomach for the same reason as scavengers. As you may know, scavengers feed on dead and decaying meat, and so are highly vulnerable to infection from harmful pathogens (disease causing bacteria, virus etc.)
But their very strong stomach acids protect them from this issue.

In the same way, this powerful acid in the human stomach, most importantly evolved as a primary defence system for our body.

You see, no pathogen or harmful bacteria can thrive, or build large colonies, in an acidic environment.
They need a comfortable environment with a pH level above 5, to feel at home, and reproduce in vast numbers. But at the same time, our friendly microbes, are able to flourish and prosper in acidic environments.
Let me tell you how, with a simple example.

- **The Pickle Mechanism**

If we place a carrot in a jar of water and let it rest in room temperature for two weeks, we would surely find that the carrot and the water would be in a state, **NOT** fit for consumption. There would be visible signs of decay and rotting, along with moulds and fungi.

Now if we place a carrot in a jar of water, add few spoonful's of vinegar, and let it rest in room temperature for the same two weeks, we wound find that the carrot is still fit for consumption, and it would stay that way for a longer period as well.

The only difference here in both cases, was the pH.
The first jar contained only water, with a pH of around 7.
The second jar had vinegar in addition to the water.

It is a common fact that vinegar is acidic with a lower pH, and thus, by merely lowering the pH in the second jar, we were able to preserve the carrot from harmful pathogens, but at the same time, were able to harbour beneficial bacteria, particularly, strains of *Lactobacillus* species.

These friendly bacteria thrive by feeding on the sugars or carbohydrates present in the carrot, and as they metabolize these sugars, they produce lactic acid, which further lowers the pH.

This creates a self-sustaining loop that preserves the carrot and encourages the growth of more beneficial bacteria. This process is the foundation of fermentation, which not only helps preserve the food but also enhances its nutritional value.

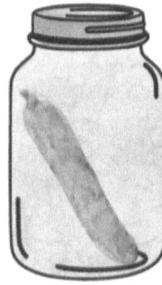 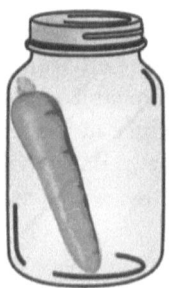

Water (neutral pH).   *Water + Vinegar (acidic pH).*

In the same way, our body naturally creates a barrier against harmful pathogens, while at the same time, maintaining a safe environment that support the growth of our friendly, beneficial bacteria by keeping our gastro-intestinal tract (GIT) acidic.

In Chapter- 13, where we had discussed about our friendly bacteria and their numerous benefits, there was the mention of one of the most impressive function done by them.

They produce something called as- **SCFA** or Short Chain Fatty Acids which play several crucial roles in maintaining our health.

SCFAs are produced when **Soluble Fibers**, are fermented by beneficial bacteria in the gut (particularly in the small and large intestines).

These fermentable fibers, mostly from vegetables and fruits, which include types like inulin, pectin, oligo-fructose, resistant starch etc. are broken down by the gut microbiota (such as those from the *Ruminococcaceae* and other such species), to produce SCFAs like butyrate, acetate, and propionate as byproducts.

In contrast, the current staple diet provides us predominantly with **Insoluble Fibers**, such as cellulose, chitin etc. (mostly from grains), which cannot be fermented by gut bacteria, and it passes through the digestive system largely unchanged.

Even though insoluble fibers help with our regular bowel movements, and supports in cases of constipation by adding bulk to the stool, they do not contribute to SCFA production, which benefits us beyond merely bulking of the stool.

Acetate is the most abundantly present SCFA (**60%**), and along with butyrate (**20%**) and propionate (**20%**), these three SCFAs are produced in the human intestine when anaerobic bacteria ferment non-digestible carbohydrates. A few benefits of these SCFA include-

1. *Energy Source*- Acetate, propionate, and butyrate, are types of SCFAs that serve as an energy source for the cells lining our large intestine, helping to maintain gut health and its various functions.

2. *Anti-inflammatory Effects*- Butyrate, in particular, is a potent anti-inflammatory SCFA, and helps to reduce inflammation not only within the gut, but also across all systems and organs of our body, including joints, which contribute greatly to our overall health.

3. *Protection Against Pathogens*- Short chain fatty acids are, as the name suggests, acidic, and helps to create an environment in the gut that is of a lowered pH, which is inhospitable to pathogenic bacteria, yet is a haven of abundance for beneficial bacteria.

4. ***Regulation of Immune Responses-*** SCFAs can balance the immune system, by regulating the differentiation and functions of our T-cell (which is where our body's soldiers come from).
Targeting GPCRs (G protein-coupled receptors) regulators by SCFAs is vital in maintaining immune tolerance, and prevents mistakes in immune responses, which protects us from autoimmune reactions, and diseases like Rheumatoid arthritis or S.L.E.

5. ***Maintenance of Gut Barrier Function-*** SCFAs are responsible for the integrity of the intestinal barrier, by increasing tight junction proteins (zonulin, occludin etc.), which prevents the leaking of harmful substances from the intestines into the bloodstream.
This barrier function is essential for preventing *'leaky gut'* which protects us from autoimmune reactions and diseases like ankylosing spondylosis or multiple sclerosis.

6. ***Absorption & Metabolic Effects-*** SCFAs increase the height of villi, allowing more space for nutrient absorption in the intestine, and SCFA also influence our metabolism in many ways, including regulating our hunger and appetite, through supporting leptin sensitivity. This helps for weight management, and issues related to insulin resistance and leptin resistance.

Gut bacteria (***Pro-****Biotic*),
produce SCFA (a type of ***Post****-Biotic*),
by feeding on soluble fibers (***Pre-****Biotic*).

Pre-biotics are found in many fiber-rich foods, including fruits, vegetables, and grains. But the amount of prebiotics in grains, such as 'resistant starch' are negligible in amount, for grains to be considered a gut healthy option.

This can surprisingly be changed though, by simply fermenting the grains. The common traditional practice of consuming overnight porridge of staple grains, was one of the main reasons why our older generations were not affected by the carbohydrate content in the grains, nor were they suffering from obesity or other metabolic issues.

Not only does the total carbohydrate content decrease to around 25%, but the increase in resistant starch, as well as beneficial bacteria in the food, when fermented, helped our older generations sustain themselves with optimum health.

The traditional method of fermenting the flour before baking, helped create 'sour breads' which was similar in health benefits.
Even though the baking heat would not allow pro-biotics to survive, the bread would still be a good pre-biotic, have much more nutrients (from the by-products of the pro-biotic metabolization).
They also contained decreased levels of carbohydrates and gluten (which is an indigestible protein that often triggers allergic and auto-immune tendencies in the body).

Traditional Italian pizzas are a wholesome food and a perfect example for a balanced diet, as it is made with a sour-bread base, with home-made tomato paste, large amounts of different variety of cheese, lots of different vegetables and pickle toppings, added with meat for proteins in the form of pepperoni, sausage, bacon, and even meat balls.

Finally garnishing the pizza with generous amounts of olive oil, and herbs such as cilantro, rosemary and thyme, created a food, that not only has all the nutritional elements required for the body, but also one that makes our taste buds dance around with joy.
Likewise, traditionally made burgers, were also a healthy staple.

But these once healthy foods, are now ultra-processed, refined, and commercialised, and are made with the most unhealthy ingredients and cooking methods.
As a result, they have lost their status as a nutritional powerhouse, and instead, have become an image that symbolize the growing health crisis of our generation.

Fermented vegetables and fruits such as pickles and kimchi are also rich sources of pre-biotics as well as pro-biotics. Apples, bananas, artichokes, asparagus, onions, radishes, pomegranate seeds, are all rich in different and unique kinds of pre-biotics that help flourish the gut flora.

It is important to have diversity in our food and diet, in the form of vegetables and fruits, as each offer a pre-biotic that varies in its form and function. In our gut, the intestines alone are roughly 20 feet long, and **to harbour the entire length of this area with beneficial bacteria is one of the greatest investment, one can accomplish for their health.**

Each pre-biotic have different layers in itself, so digesting some pre-biotics are harder than others.
This allows those particular pre-biotics to be able to reach the end of the colon and become feed for the pro-biotics in that section, and help in the abundant growth of friendly gut microbiome throughout the length of the gut, and not be concentrated in any particular section alone.

Over a 1000 different kinds of pre-biotics were found in the stool samples of wild orangutans, which showed the incredible diversity in their natural food choices.

Just because something is derived from nature, it doesn't necessarily mean that it is beneficial.

This is the case with *carrageenan*, a highly inflammatory fiber, derived from red seaweed. While it is plant-based, *carrageenan* has been known to cause various health issues, particularly inflammation in the gut.
It is commonly used as a thickening and gelling agent in processed foods due to its ability to create a smooth texture.

Carrageenan can be found in a wide range of products, including substitutes of dairy like almond milk, ultra processed coconut milk, and soy milk. Processed meats, salad dressings, ice creams, yoghurts, and even toothpastes and medicinal products like syrups and liquid medicines contain carrageenan as well, merely for its texture enhancing property.

Despite its natural origin, studies have shown that carrageenan can cause gastrointestinal discomfort, bloating, and even promote inflammation in the gut, harming the balance of the microbial flora, and causing leaky gut syndrome.

Carrageenan is a potent catalyst for inflammation, causing conditions like Irritable Bowel Syndrome (IBS), allergies and skin disorders.
It is so effective at triggering inflammation that scientists use it as a benchmark to test new anti-inflammatory drugs.

Its presence in many everyday products, especially those marketed as healthy or plant-based, makes it difficult for consumers to avoid this hidden danger, even when trying to follow an anti-inflammatory diet.

In the 1970s, the yearly average consumption of carrageenan was less than 90_{mg} per day, whereas today, it exceeds 250_{mg} per day.

Despite its inflammatory effects, *carrageenan* is widely used by food companies, because it is an extremely low-cost and effective emulsifier.

A loophole in its classification by the USA based FDA (Food & Drug Administration), have allowed it to remain in widespread use to this day.

The FDA has categorized *carrageenan* as GRAS (Generally Recognized as Safe) since 1959, allowing it to be included in foods without much scrutiny, and is listed as a dietary fiber on nutrition labels of food packaging, though it does not provide the health benefits that other healthy fibers offer.

Alternatives such as guar gum, agar-agar, and gelatine provide the same thickening properties for sauces and other foods but do not pose the same risks as carrageenan, and so, are better solutions for consumers to look for, and include in their diet.

Adopting certain traditional dietary practices also promotes better gut health and digestion. One such example is the Japanese practice of drinking vinegar before meals.

The Japanese are well known for their remarkable life expectancy, with their food habits playing a significant role. They are known to drink vinegar up to half an hour before each meal.

This has been found to significantly aid in digestion by increasing acids and digestive enzymes, promote gut health, reduce blood sugar spikes, and boost metabolism.

Beyond its culinary appeal, vinegar is also rich in acetic acid, as well as vitamins and antioxidants, which not only improves the functions of the internal organs, but also preserves the body from sudden ageing.

> In essence, the short chain fatty acids and
> the acidic environment of our gut, are crucial
> for our immunity, and overall health.
>
> If anyone has been misled by the false claims
> surrounding the "alkaline diet," you can set them straight
> with the reality of our -

PICKLE BODY.

Chapter XVII – Get to Know Our Major Food Groups.

The biggest confusion on choosing which food is healthy to eat, arises from being clueless as to which category of the **Food Group**, the particular food belongs to.

It is very important to at least have a very general idea of the various food groups, and the different foods included in them, and also the average nutritional content of each food group.

For example,
The most common mistake made by diabetic patients, is to switch their regular staple from rice, to wheat, oats or other millets.

I appreciate the fact that it is by now, common knowledge that eating various dishes made out of carbohydrate rich rice, is the primary culprit for Type-2 Diabetes.

However, the switch from rice to wheat, or other millets, does not make much of a difference because they are all in a sense, related to one another, and fall under the same food group – "Cereals & Grains."

If you take a look at the table given below, the finding of a scientific research study on the nutritional content of various grains, shows us the different percentages of carbohydrates / sugars contained in them.

	Pearl millet	Maize	Sorghum	Finger millet	Rice	Wheat
Energy (kcal)	361	362	339	328	358	349
Water	12.4%	20-32%	8-16%	13%	-	-
CHO	67.1%	68%	68-74%	72%	79.9%	74.1%
Protein	11.6%	6-15%	8-15%	8%	6.2%	12.3%
Fat	5.3%	5%	2-5%	1.3%	0.6%	1.5%

(Hulse et al., 1980). Food and Nutrition Center Tanzania Food Composition Tables, 2007.

> On average, the total carbohydrate / sugar content of any given cereal, millet or grain revolve around 70 to 85 percent.

One could argue that the Glycaemic index of each cereal, grain or millet would make a whole lot of a difference…

No, in the long run it doesn't.
Let me explain…

- ## **Glycaemic INDEX** vs. **Glycaemic LOAD**

Glycaemic index (GI) refers to, how easily and quickly the sugar in a particular food, is absorbed by the body, and shows up in our blood.

It is measured from zero to one-hundred, taking into account the rise in the blood glucose levels, 2 hours after consuming a particular food. Pure glucose has a glycaemic value of 100, and all the other foods are measured in reference to this particular value.

Rice has a GI of around **70** to **80**.
Oats which is of the same family (Grains), has a GI of around **40** to **50**.

This is merely an indication that the sugars in the oats, are absorbed more slowly into the blood, which prevents rapid spikes in blood glucose, and delays the occurrence of insulin resistance.

However, even if the sugar is absorbed slowly, all of the sugars in the oats (around 70%), will still end up entering the body, and be converted to fat storage, which nevertheless, will eventually lead to insulin resistance, even though it may take a little more time to do so.

Now, if at all this person who ate the oats is a very active person, and physically exercises a lot, then some of this sugar will not be stored as fat, but be used up as energy.

But even then, why consume food that primarily provides energy, only to burn it off through intense physical exercise?

As we have seen in the first chapter, the main thing that our body requires for health, is nutrition.

Why waste our time and energy, to eat bland energy giving foods, when we have the choice to eat nutritious foods that can give energy, and at the same time also help to repair, replenish and build the body?

We have also discussed how carbs / sugars damage our body in various ways (as sugars, triglycerides, free radicals, VLDL etc.) which again begs the question...

Why damage your body, waste your time and energy, to eat bland energy giving food, when you can choose to eat nutritious food?

This is why glycaemic index does not make sense.
It only indicates if there is an immediate rise in blood sugar.

But what about **sugar** that gets converted as the highly inflammatory triglycerides, forming into LDLs and the free radicals created from it?

What about the inflammation created by these residues that leads to issues such as insulin resistance and leptin resistance?

Therefore, "Glycaemic Load" (GL) is a more accurate measurement, of the long-term effects of the sugars, contained in particular foods, to our body and health. It is measured as...

- Foods with GL value more than **20**, does more harm in the long run.
- Foods with GL value less than **10**, is safer for our health.

For example-

Food	*Glycaemic Index* (GI)	*Glycaemic Load* (GL)
Carrot	75	2
Corn (Maize)	55	62
Eggs	0	0

When we take a look at the GI of a *Carrot*, it may seem scary, but in fact, it is a healthy and nutritious vegetable, which provides long term benefits and contributes to the health of our body.

At the same time, *Corn* (maize) may seem like a very good substitute for rice or wheat... but as you can see, the GL of it is quite high, and can contribute significantly, in the formation of insulin resistance, and cause lots of other harm to our body.

Note that, only the total sugars in a particular food, and its long-term effect, actually matter. But let us first, have a look at the different major Food Groups, and various examples of what kind of food comes under each category-

Food Group	*Examples*
Cereals & Grains	Rice, Wheat, Maize (Corn), Barley, Oats, Rye, Millets, Sorghum, Buckwheat, Quinoa, Amaranth, Sago etc. Often consumed in the form of bread, pasta, noodles, porridge, pastries, and more.
Pulses & Legumes	Lentils, Chickpeas, Black beans, Kidney beans, Lima beans, Mung beans, Black-eyed peas, Broad beans, Soybeans, Split peas, Green peas, Urad dal (Black gram), Masoor dal (Red lentils), Toor dal (Pigeon peas), French lentils (Puy lentils), Horse gram, Lupini beans, Bamboo beans etc.
Nuts & Seeds	*Nuts*- Almonds, Walnuts, Cashews, Peanuts, Pecans, Hazelnuts, Macadamia nuts, Brazil nuts, Pistachios, Pine nuts, Chestnuts, Hickory nuts, Kola nuts, Coconut etc. *Seeds*- Sunflower seeds, Pumpkin seeds, Sesame seeds, Flaxseeds, Chia seeds, Hemp seeds, Poppy seeds, Watermelon seeds, Fennel seeds, Basil seeds, Safflower seeds etc.
Fruits	Apples, Bananas, Oranges, Grapes, Strawberries, Watermelons, Mangoes, Pineapples, Avocados, Papayas, Kiwi, Blueberries, Raspberries, Blackberries, Peaches, Pears, Cherries, Lemons, Limes, Grapefruits, Plums, Apricots, Cantaloupes (Musk Melons), Figs, Dates, Pomegranates, Cranberries, Lychees, Passion fruits, Dragon fruit etc.

Food Group	Examples
Vegetables	*Gourd varieties*- Bitter gourd, Bottle gourd, Sponge gourd, Ridge gourd, Snake gourd, Wax gourd, Zucchini etc. *Roots varieties*- Carrots, Potatoes, Sweet potatoes, Beetroot, Turnips, Radishes, Parsnips, Rutabagas, Yams, Cassava, Ginger, Onion, Turmeric etc. *Stem varieties*- Asparagus, Celery, Rhubarb, Bamboo shoots, Kohlrabi, Broccolini, Scallions (Green onions) etc. *Leaf varieties*- Spinach, Lettuce (Iceberg, Butterhead, Red leaf), Kale, Bok choy, Mustard leaves, Beetroot leaves, Turnip leaves, Cabbage, Purslane, Chicory etc. *Flower varieties*- Broccoli, Cauliflower, Artichokes etc. ***Fruits of vegetable plant varieties***- Tomatoes, Cucumbers, Pumpkins, Bell peppers (Capsicum), Eggplants (Brinjal), Squashes, Chayote, Acorn squash, Okra (Lady's fingers) etc.
Meat, Meat Organs, Fish, Seafood & Eggs	*Meat*- Beef, Pork, Lamb, Goat, Chicken, Turkey, Duck, Rabbit, Deer, Bison, Moose, Buffalo, Horse, Camel, Quail, Goose, Emu, Ostrich, Turtle, Guinea fowl, Pheasant etc. *Meat Organs*- Liver, Spleen, Heart, Kidneys, Tongue, Brain etc. *Fish*- Salmon, Tuna, Cod, Trout, Sardines, Mackerel, Tilapia etc. *Seafood*- Crab, Shrimp, Lobster, Squid, Oysters etc. *Eggs*- Chicken, Duck, Quail, Goose, Turkey, Emu, Ostrich, Guinea fowl, Pheasant, etc.
Dairy products	Milk (from Cow, Goat, Sheep, Buffalo, Donkey, Camel etc.), Butter, Cheese, Yogurt, Cream, Ghee (Clarified butter), Buttermilk, Sour cream, Kefir etc.

This table that you have just gone through,
is a summary of the major food groups,
which was a major eye opener for me
when I was first studying about it.

The important thing to know about food, is that you don't actually need to specifically know every little detail about each food, but rather, we just need to have a general idea of the average nutritional contents of these 7 major food groups.

Average Nutritional Percentages of the 7 Major Food Groups-

Food Group	Carbs. (Sugars)	Fats	Protein	Vitamins	Minerals	Phyto-Nutrients	Solu Fib
Cereals & Grains	70 - 85%	1 - 5%	8 – 15%	5 – 8%	5 – 8%	1 – 2%	2 –
Pulses & Legumes	50 – 65%	1 - 5%	20 – 30%	10 – 15%	10 – 15%	2 – 4%	10 –
Nuts & Seeds	30 – 50%	40 - 70%	10 – 25%	15 – 25%	15 – 25%	1 – 3%	5 – 1
Fruits	15 – 40%	Lower than 1%	1 – 2%	20 – 25%	10 – 20%	2 – 5%	15 –
Vegetables	5 – 15%	Lower than 1%	2 – 3%	20 – 35%	20 – 35%	2 – 5%	15 –
Dairy Products	4 – 5%	5 – 40% Butter & Ghee 80 – 100 %	20 – 30%	20 – 35%	20 – 35%	Lower than 1%	Lowe 1
Meat, Meat organs, Fish, Seafood & Eggs	Lower than 1%	30 – 60%	20 – 35%	10 – 20%	10 – 20%	Lower than 1%	Lowe 1

This information is very essential for us to be able to mindfully choose healthy dishes for our day-to-day life.

Once you start eating healthy, you will feel addicted to how good your body feels… the ease at which you are able go about your daily routines, without any pain, fatigue or tiredness.

You will even feel less hunger.
One of the biggest fears that my patients have before starting a healthy diet, is about whether they will be able to control, or supress their excessive hunger.

Most of my patients try to convince me that they are merely victims of an insatiable hunger, which no matter how hard they try, never stops, and that this villain (hunger) is the reason that they over-eat.

GHRELIN- this is the hormone that makes you feel hungry. Normally, it is only produced when our body's energy is low. A less known fact is, that eating lots of sugars or fried food, causes our body to malfunction, and produce even more of this hormone, *Ghrelin*.

This is why, we can observe at Indian weddings, even after stuffing oneself to the point of explosion with yummy biriyani, there is still more appetite and hunger for lots of sweets like *Laddoos, Jilebi, Mysore-Pak and Gulab-jamun* after the heavy lunch.

Healthy and nutritious food, in contrast, produces **Cholecystokinin**, a hormone which tells the body, that it is happy, and content with the amount of food consumed, and that there is no more need for any sort of food, for the time-being.

As seen in Chapter- 6, the hormone LEPTIN, contributes to the feeling of satiety (fulfilment) as well, and it has been proven, that a grain-based diet, causes *Lectin Resistance*, a condition described as where –
'The Brain is Starving, But the Body is Obese.'

The resulting stagnation of high levels of leptin in the body, leads to overeating, and poor regulation of fat stores, which then contributes to weight gain, metabolic disorders, and high leptin concentrations in the body, which itself, is an independent risk factor for heart attacks.

But there are particular areas in our body which specifically uses **glucose** for energy, like certain tissues and organs that have a high demand for quick, accessible energy.

The following are commonly the ones in need -

- *Red Blood Cells*- The RBCs (red blood cells) lack mitochondria, so they cannot use fatty acids or ketones for energy. They rely exclusively on glucose for their energy needs and to maintain their crucial function of transporting oxygen and carbon-di-oxide.

- ***Kidneys** (specifically the renal medulla)* - While the kidneys can use fatty acids, the inner part of the kidneys (renal medulla) primarily relies on glucose for energy, especially when glucose is abundant.

- ***Muscle Tissue** (during intense activity)* - During high-intensity exercise or activities requiring short bursts of energy, muscle cells rely heavily on glucose (in the form of glycogen) because it can be rapidly converted to ATP or energy.

These tissues and cells listed above have the most significant and exclusive reliance on glucose for immediate energy. But to meet this very small requirement of glucose, we need not consume **80%** of carbs daily.

Around **35%** of carbohydrates that are offered by vegetables in our diet, are more than sufficient, for our sedentary and inactive lifestyle, that we currently lead in this technology dominated modern era.

If at all our body does require more glucose than that during any emergency, then our body converts the protein that we consume into glucose, and utilizes it for the necessary tissues.

As in the case with everything else in life, it is important to practice moderation when it comes to drinking water as well.
I've come to notice that the most abused health trend, is that which is concerned with drinking water.

There is one extreme group that claims, water need not be consumed necessarily if fruits are eaten... and then there is the other extreme group that drinks more than 5 to 6 litres of water, claiming water to be the *"healer"* of all known mental and physical ailments (diseases).

Too little water intake, can result in low energy, mental fog, an increased risk of stroke, moodiness, tendency to overeat, slowed metabolism, frequent headaches, dry and damaged skin, and weight gain among many other issues.
Too much water intake on the other hand, can cause **nausea, vomiting,** and **headaches due to altered pressure on the brain,** mental confusion or disorientation, drowsiness, extreme tiredness, muscle cramps and in extreme cases, can even lead to coma or death.

You see, our body feeling thirsty, or dehydrated with a dry and parched mouth, even after drinking adequate amounts of water, does not necessarily mean that it is asking for more water.

In this case, it is often, that our body is deficient in electrolytes.

So the best thing to do, is to have a glass of tender coconut water, or lime juice, or even a glass of store bought ORS (oral rehydration solution).

It is recommended to only have around **2 litres** of water a day (for those with a moderately active, or an inactive lifestyle), and the way to consume it is, slowly, with single mouthful sips, throughout the day.

Gulping down half a litre of water at a stretch, does not give our body enough time to absorb it. When we consume lots of water in a very short time, it mostly evacuates as urine, sweat or through our large intestine.

If we drink more than **4 litres** a day, it can cause a massive shift in our body's electrolyte balance. Electrolytes such as sodium, potassium, calcium, magnesium and other trace minerals, are essential for almost every function in our body.
Without it, our heart cannot pump blood, or maintain proper blood pressure, or transport nutrients to and from the cells, and many other similar, minute, yet extremely important functions.

Drinking large volumes of water, can cause these precious minerals to be excreted from our body. Hyponatremia is the common condition that occurs as a result, which means, that the body does not have enough sodium. This can cause the person to collapse, and even death may occur, as a consequence.

> Even though eating and drinking healthily is of utmost importance, it is even more important, to **NOT** eat...
>
> Let us discuss in detail, about giving our
> *Gastro Intestinal Tract* (**GIT**) a rest, and about
>
> **Intermittent Fasting**.

Chapter XVIII –
The Secret to Healthy, Long Life is- NO FOOD.

Fasting or specific periods of abstinence from food or water, is nothing new to humanity. It is a major part of almost all traditions, religions and beliefs, and has historical and cultural roots dating back to centuries.

Ancient civilizations had practiced fasting mainly for spirituality, and even to this day, the physical health benefits of fasting are only considered secondary, in various religions.

The so called "Modern Era" as a historical period, began in the 17th century. It is noted so because certain social changes occurred during this period, which also in turn changed the food habits of the people.

Before this time, the better part of the population were farmers, which only allowed time for meals either twice, or only once a day, which meant prolonged periods of empty stomach, with occasional drinking of water, or snacking on fruits, dried meat etc.

This was a time when the lifestyle was such, that even if conscious efforts were not put on intermittent fasting, the majority of the population, were still following it every day.

And before that, we were hunter-gatherers, living in a constant cycle of scarcity and abundance. Our ancestors would often go for extended periods without food, particularly between hunts.

Sometimes, they might fast for three days or more, depending on the success of the hunt. This natural fasting allowed them to survive periods when food was scarce, relying on their ability to go without eating until they could catch or gather their next meal.

During the winter season, fasting became even more inescapable for the hunter-gatherers, with fewer food sources available, in the colder climates, the lack of fresh fruits or meat, made regular meals impossible.

People would rely on stored food, like dried meat or preserved fruits, but even these food sources were limited. During this age, fasting was not a conscious decision but a survival strategy, as the body had to adapt to extended periods of food scarcity.

This way of living helped to tap into the survival and longevity mode of the human biology, and it was simply part of their rhythm of life, a natural way of being in tune with the environment.

But since we are living in an ultra-modern era, where all kinds of food are readily available (especially tasty, yet unhealthy ones), we must make a conscious effort to practice voluntary abstinence from food, to give a chance for our body, to rest and to heal.

- **AUTO-PHAGY**

The 2016 Nobel Prize in Physiology (Medicine) was awarded for the discovery of the process of autophagy…

Auto- means *"Self"*

Phagy- means *"To Eat"*

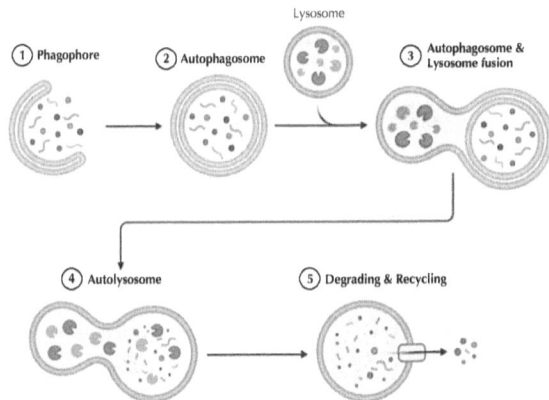

Mechanism of Autophagy

It is a process, where the cell destroys itself, and recycles it's damaged components. Removing old, faulty proteins and organelles, ultimately helps in forming fresh and renewed cells, and helps to maintain the efficiency and health of the whole body,

Intermittent fasting gained widespread popularity, particularly after the *Nobel* winning discovery in 2016, and the fact that it can switch on the incredible process of Autophagy in our body.

It is a relatively simple approach, compared to the other traditional calorie-restricted diets. The benefits of this seemingly simple, yet effective practice, and the subsequent onset of autophagy, is so much more than we could ever imagine.

Here are a few examples…

1. ***Increased Longevity*-** one of the best results of this practice is an extended lifespan. Studies prove that it is through promoting cellular repair mechanisms, reducing oxidative stress (damage from free radicals), improving our metabolism and effectively reducing the risk of age-related diseases. **Mitophagy** (explained in Chapter- 19), caused by fasting, is also an important reason for our longevity.

   Fasting causes a form of stress in the body, known as **'eustress'** or positive stress, which triggers several beneficial biological responses. The temporary scarcity of nutrients that our body faces while fasting, activates several survival mechanisms at the cellular level.

   The activation of DNA repair mechanisms, and enhancements in the production of certain proteins that protect the cells from damage, are key outcomes of this process.
   The secretion of an enzyme called **telomerase**, is one such crucial process. This enzyme works to repair, and lengthen **telomeres** (which are protective caps at the ends of our chromosomes).

   Telomeres naturally shorten with age, and their length is associated with cellular aging and lifespan. By promoting the lengthening of telomeres, intermittent fasting is essentially helping to slow down the aging process at the cellular level, which translates to, extending the natural lifespan of our biological body.

2. ***Improved Heart Health*-** By reducing high blood pressure and high leptin levels, regulating cholesterol levels (improves the HDL cholesterol, and lowers triglycerides and LDLs), it helps reduce the inflammations in atherosclerotic plaques, which results in reduction of heart blocks, improving cardiac health greatly, through fasting.

3. ***Stored Sugar (Fat) Loss*-** Fasting aides in weight loss and reduce our body fat by creating a need for energy, and increases leptin sensitivity. By reducing the total time we eat, we naturally consume less bulks of food, leading to lower calorie intake. Additionally, fasting forces the body to use up all of its stored fat, for energy.

4. ***Improved Insulin Sensitivity*-** By reducing inflammations, which gives the body enough time to repair *Insulin Receptors*, the *Insulin Resistance* is reduced… automatically improving the *Insulin Sensitivity*. This in turn is very useful for Type-2 Diabetic patients, where their blood sugar levels are reduced, and so are their triglyceride stores (which is the reason for the inflammations in the first place).

5. ***Healthy Neurons*-** Brain Derived Neurotrophic Factor (BDNF), a protein that support the growth and survival of neurons, was found to be high after periods of fasting.

    Enhanced focus and mental clarity was also observed during fasting, which was attributed to changes in neurotransmitter levels, protecting against neurodegenerative diseases like Alzheimer's.

    These changes are mainly caused due to compact and efficient energy derived from ketones (from fat stores). Significant improvements in sleep quality was also a noticeable point.
    Periods of fasting can help regulate circadian rhythms and promote deeper, more restorative sleep.

6. ***Healthy Gut*-** Fasting gives a time for our digestive system to rest, which then improve digestion and reduce gastrointestinal issues such as bloating and indigestion. It also starves harmful Gut bacteria, and gives a good winning chance for the survival and habitation of our friendly and beneficial Gut bacteria.

7. ***Enhanced Immunity-*** Studies prove that fasting boost our immune functions by increasing the production of immune cells, and reducing inflammation, giving our body a much required boost to help fight off infections and diseases caused by pathogenic micro-organisms.

Fasting is also found to have anti-cancer effects, reducing the growth of tumours and even supporting the effectiveness of chemotherapy treatments. Autophagy is found to occur in cancerous cells as well, which aids in the fight against cancer.

Fasting is easier to follow, than any other calorie-restricted diets, because it doesn't require any sort of strict calorie counting, meal planning, nor heavy physical exercises.

You can easily be flexible in your food choices, and can adapt fasting to fit a scheduled or busy lifestyle, or an inactive or lazy one as well.
It is also a sustainable practice in the long term, as it does not make us feel excessively deprived, or restricted.

One of the often-overlooked benefits of fasting is the spiritual experience it brings. Individuals often acquire a deeper sense of self-reflection, mindfulness, and heightened awareness of thoughts and emotions, which develops a stronger connection to others, particularly to those who are less fortunate than us physically, psychologically or even financially.

The experience of hunger and the absence of food, helps develop greater empathy and appreciation for the struggles that others face daily, which often deepens the sense of compassion and solidarity. These emotions are essential for building and balancing our overall health as well.

I prefer fasting each and every day.

Why?

Because it is basic cleanliness. I have seen gents and ladies who take utmost care of their skin, clothes and hair, using lots of moisturizers, skin and hair care products, keeping their rooms and surroundings extra neat and clean… except their gut and body.

Imagine what happens when you don't clean your house every day, the dirt and trash starts to pile up, and you will be faced with quite an unpleasant situation in the near future.

The same way, if you let your body have a bit of free time by fasting, our body will spend that much needed time by cleaning itself, and will bring about all of the various benefits we just mentioned, and more.

I prefer fasting each and every day.

How is it possible?

By eating your dinner early, and having your breakfast a bit later in the morning.

If you have your dinner by **7:00 p.m**, you can have your breakfast around **9:00 a.m**.

This gives you around **14 hours** of fasting time.

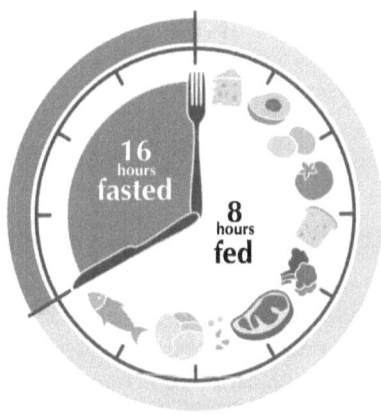

You can take it up to **16 hours** as well.

It is better **to not** fast less than **12 hours**.

This is to make sure that the autophagy completely sets in, and that it is able to give us its benefits to the maximum.

Total dry fasting (without even a sip of water), is the way to get best results, but beginners can slowly accustom their body into intermittent fasting, by eating small cut pieces of fruit, (only when extremely hungry, during the fasting hours), for the first 7 to 10 days.

For the next 5 to 7 days, they can switch from fruits to few sips of fruit juices. And during the next 5 days, drinking sips of water (only if extremely thirsty), will do the trick. One can begin total dry fasting, after following these initial days of tempering the body.

This begs the question…

"Isn't breakfast the most important meal of the day? How can you skip breakfast and just eat lunch!"

Firstly, if your lunch is your first meal of the day, it's not your lunch… it's your breakfast.

Because, just as the name 'BREAK-FAST' suggests…

breakfast is - '**Breaking** your **Fast**.'

And also YES, breakfast is the most important meal.

Why?

It is not about '**WHEN**' you have your breakfast,

It is all about '**WHAT**' you eat for your breakfast.

Those who do not break their *fast* the right way, have not gotten any benefits from their hours of starvation.

It doesn't matter if you have your breakfast at 6:00 a.m, 11:00 a.m, in the morning, or even at 3:00 p.m in the late afternoon.

If we do not give the body healthy, nutritious food during '**Break-fast**' we are only going to do more harm than benefit for ourselves.

It is best to have eggs or a combination of good fat with proteins, and cooked vegetables when breaking your intermittent fasting. A research conducted by the *Harvard Medical School*, published in 2012, looked at how three different types of breakfasts, with the same amount of calories, affected our biological system.

- In the *Refined Oats Group*, a staggering **81%** of participants, reported feeling hungry soon after breakfast and wanted more food. Additionally, their cortisol levels (stress hormone) were unusually elevated, indicating a metabolic imbalance.

- In the *Steel-Cut Oats Group*, 51% of participants asked for more food after breakfast. While not as high as the first group, they too experienced elevated cortisol levels.

- Participants of the *Omelette Group*, who had a protein and fat rich breakfast, were satisfied with what they ate and did not request more food. Interestingly, their cortisol levels remained balanced, indicating that the high fat and protein, with low carb meal, provided longer lasting satiety and stable blood sugar levels.

But I was taught during my medical college years, that eating saturated fats, led to heart attacks, and that meats, cheese, butter, coconut oil and egg yolks, were never to be even touched.

Repeated guidelines from the *American Heart Association* (AHA), the *American College of Cardiology* and the *World Health Organisation* (WHO), set a clear "*fact*" that fats in general, and saturated fats in particular, were to be strictly avoided to prevent heart attacks.

The advice since the 1960s, was to strictly reduce fat consumption to less than 30% of the total calories consumed in a day, with saturated fats to be kept well below 10% of the same.

> This is why most doctors who are not updated on current scientific research, blindly continue to follow this order, from the two most *powerful* and *respected* cardiology associations.

> But since we have already in detail, debunked this misinformation, let us take a deeper look at yet another one...

Chapter XIX – Why Keto-Diet is a Failure.

In 1911, the first modern use of starvation for the treatment of epilepsy was noted. Two physicians in Paris reported that seizures were less severe in period of starvation. This helped lay the foundation for the development of the ***Ketogenic Diet.***

But it wasn't until 1921 that any other physician tried this method, to generate ketosis. Dr. Rollin Woodyatt noted that under conditions of starvation, ketones appear in our body.

Around the same time, Dr. Russell Wilder found that ketones could be produced for therapeutic benefit, but with a low carb diet rather than starvation. He developed the term 'Ketogenic Diet.'

This diet then went on to become extremely popular in the treatment of childhood epilepsy, and as advanced epilepsy medications were developed and made available during the 20th century, the ketogenic diet slowly lost its place as an effective treatment for epilepsy.

So what actually is Ketosis?

Simply put... normally, our body mainly uses carbohydrates (sugars) for simple and easy production of energy.

When we eat less carbohydrates / sugars, our body first uses up glycogen (which is stored glucose or sugar) as fuel for energy.

But after three to four days, theses glycogen stores are depleted.

Our stores of body fat, is then the readily available fuel, and it is send to the liver to form *Ketones*, which are a much more efficient fuel than glucose, and also offers a wide range of health benefits for our body.

Most importantly, in normal ketosis, there is no change in our blood pH levels. But in a flawed ketosis (particularly in diabetic patients), when the blood ketone levels exceed so much that the pH of blood becomes acidic... it is called as ***Keto-Acidosis.***

Uncontrolled and untreated, *diabetic keto-acidosis*, can lead to extreme complications such as loss of consciousness and, eventually, death

This is the primary reason why the keto-diet often gets a bad reputation. Simply because the majority of people do not know the difference between **KETOSIS**, and **KETO - ACIDOSIS**.

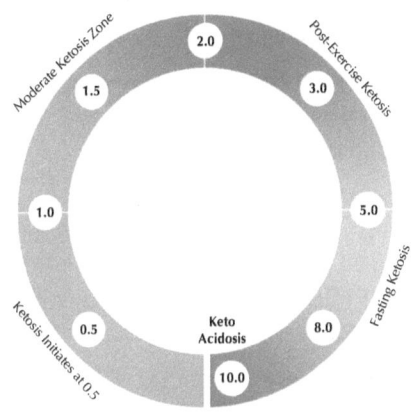

Ketosis Range Chart

The second most important reason why keto-diet has failed, is simply because, a number of incidences, were people without a complete understanding of the keto-diet... started dieting in a wrong way, and were left with severe cases of gastritis, ulcers, fatty liver disease, kidney stones, and extreme fatigue that eventually led to many reported deaths.

As it is often said, *"Half Knowledge is Worse Than Ignorance"*

This is especially true in the case of the ketogenic diet.

Even to this day, there are so many, who, on a daily basis, eat deep fried chicken from fast food chains, combined with sugar loaded soft drinks, claiming to have eaten "enough" vegetables (when all they would've had, were a few slices of cucumber & carrots, or a few shavings of cabbage), all in the name of following a "Healthy Keto-Diet."

Continuing this same routine for more than 3 months is what led to the above said issues, like severe cases of gastritis, ulcers, fatty liver disease, kidney stones, fatigue... and even death.

The third reason why keto-diet has failed in the minds of people, even though it is incredibly beneficial, is because of the fear created when, there is constant tiredness or fatigue, skin rashes, or a fruity odour or metallic taste in the mouth (keto breath), during the initial few days... when the body is in the ongoing process of shifting its energy source.

It is important to understand that these symptoms, are indicating various underlying issues that need to be solved.
Here are a few points that need to be known -

1. ***Blood Sugar Fluctuations*-** A spike in fasting blood sugar is noted, which is the fat stores being re-converted into sugars (*gluco-neo-genesis*), to be utilized as energy. Individuals who are uninformed, especially those with diabetes, may find this concerning or overwhelming.

2. ***Vitamins-B_1 & B_2 Deficiency*-** When there is a deficiency of 'B' vitamins, especially that of vitamin-B_1 and vitamin-B_2, which are involved in fat metabolism, it can be the cause for fatigue and most commonly, skin rashes. Since it is so vital for ketosis, it is depleted quite quickly, and require constant replenishing. Egg yolks and dairy, are good sources for both.

3. ***Sodium & Chloride*-** Our body loses water along with these essential minerals due to increased urination during ketosis. Make sure to include at least 1tsp. of salt daily.

4. ***Magnesium*-** *The Powerhouse Mineral* is vital to **ATP** (Energy) production. Include green leafy vegetables like spinach and lettuce, seafood, nuts (including almonds and cashews), seeds (like pumpkin seeds or sunflower seeds), coconut, dark chocolate etc.

5. ***Maintaining Electrolytes Balance*-** Sodium, potassium, magnesium, and calcium ensures successful entry into ketosis without discomfort. Avoid dehydration by maintaining proper fluid balance, and electrolyte intake through either ORS (available at all medical stores), or tender coconut or lemon honey water.

6. ***Vitamin Deficiencies*-** In addition to '**B**' vitamins, deficiencies of vitamins A, D, E and K (the fat soluble vitamins), can also cause keto-diet fatigue. Make sure to have enough consumption of foods rich in each of the vitamin mentioned.

7. ***Slow metabolism*-** Reasons include menopause, hypothyroidism, hormone imbalances, stress, genetic predisposition, and frequent inconsistent dieting, which can all lead to a slow metabolism.

   Intermittent Fasting, consuming ACV (*apple cider vinegar*) before meals, and even mild exercise can help by-pass this issue.

8. ***Alcohol Intake*-** Drinking alcoholic beverages, can cause fatigue, keto-breath and lead to quick weight gain. Because alcohol is a toxic compound, the liver prioritizes alcohol detoxification over other metabolic processes, including fat burning.

   Even small amounts of alcohol can stop ketosis, and it could take at least 2 to 3 days for the immediate harmful effects to settle, and the body to begin its normal functions.

9. ***Sluggish Fat Digestion*-** Our body requires plenty of bile to digest fatty foods, absorb fat soluble vitamins, and to eliminate waste. If the bile is not in its proper concentration, fatigue could set in.

   Skin rashes are also commonly seen when a sluggish bile is present. Make sure to include more MCT (*medium chain triglycerides*) like coconut oil and butter, because they are fats than the body can absorb and use even without the help of the bile.
   It also helps in restoring the necessary concentration of the bile.

   Bile salts are also essential for the proper concentration of the bile, and these are made, primarily from taurine and glycine (amino acids that can be best obtained from red meat and bone broths).

10. ***Imbalanced Gut Microflora*-** Although it may not seem obvious, your intestinal microflora can significantly impact your ketosis and cause skin rashes and fatigue. We can diversify intestinal microflora by consuming probiotic-rich foods such yoghurt and pickles, and consume multiple varieties of vegetables for diverse pre-biotics.

11. ***Lack of exercise-*** Regular physical exercise is important for increasing the metabolic rate, and to maintain ketosis. But for individuals incapable of exercise due to arthritis or similar painful health conditions, *intermittent fasting* is a healthy option.

12. ***Underlying Health Issues-*** Gastritis, fungal infections, thyroiditis and food allergies are some of the issues that can slow down ketosis and cause fatigue, skin rashes or keto-breath. But these issues can be solved through proper nutrient intake and medications.

13. ***Emotional Stress & Cortisol-*** As discussed in Chapter- 7, stress can disrupt the body in any possible way that you can think of, so it is crucial to take the required steps necessary, to keep it under control.

14. ***Electro-Magnetic Fields-*** Long-term exposure to electromagnetic fields (EMFs) from electronic devices such as smartphones, laptops, tablets, etc. lead to increased stress hormones within the body, resulting in fatigue and tiredness. This is a relatively overlooked cause, so make sure to spend some *'Device-Free'* time.

So these are some of the reasons why the ketogenic diet has a very bad reputation even among doctors, and why the keto-diet has failed to convince the majority of the population.

Our body will not always be in ketosis, but it will go through waves of it, during a 24-hour period, and that is how it is designed biologically.

There are so many factors around getting into healthy ketosis and continuing it in the right way, but there are chances that one can upset their metabolism if they practice ketosis the wrong way.

This is because even though we are biologically designed to rely on ketones for energy, our bodies have spent decades, relying on the easily accessible sugars for its major source of energy.

Transitioning to this healthy fuel source, would need a bit of fine tuning, before our body starts running on it efficiently.

But if you do choose to change your eating habits, and try to persuade your body into changing its source of fuel, you will find that-

- You start losing extra weight and unwanted fat around your belly.
- Feel more energized even while fasting.
- Start having better mental clarity, memory, focus, and attention.
- Decrease in inflammations and pain.
- Notice improvements in arthritis conditions.
- Feel satisfied after eating moderately, and do not have cravings, excessive hunger or the involuntary tendency to over-eat.
- Always in an uplifted mood, and do not suffer from depression (those that has no typical and specific reasons), anxiety or mood swings.
- Have normal blood sugar levels, regular periodic cycles, normal blood pressure and much more.

The list of diseases that is significantly reduced just by eating the right way, exceeds any other treatment method. We will be going through those diseases in the coming chapters.

Up until now, we have explored why **Fats** are the most essential nutrient for our body, offering maximum benefits with minimal harm.

We've also examined in detail why **Carbohydrates**, or sugars, are not the ideal fuel source for our body.

So let us next explore the last major nutrient **Protein**.

There are those who claim that proteins are the most important nutrient. However, let us discuss why this isn't entirely true, by highlighting a specific pathway in the body, that I believe, deserves your attention.

- **The mTOR Pathway.**

The mTOR (**mechanistic** target of rapamycin, previously known as **mammalian** target of rapamycin) pathway, regulates a wide variety of cellular processes, including growth, metabolism, protein synthesis, autophagy, and cell survival.

It is activated by, **mTORC1** (mTOR complex-1), and **mTORC2** (mTOR complex-2).

mTORC1 is mainly involved in cellular growth, and metabolism. It controls protein synthesis, lipid synthesis, and cell cycle progression.

mTORC2 is involved in regulating cell survival, metabolism, and the organization of the cyto-skeleton (a microscopic network of protein filaments inside many living cells, that allow cells to retain its shape).

This pathway is switched on, by reading signals from various processes in the body such as, nutrient availability, energy status of the body, growth factor presence, stress etc.

When mTORC1 is activated, after reading such signals, it starts to promote processes like protein production, cellular growth, and anabolic (constructive) metabolism, which are all processes that help in the building, and growth of the body.

Now this may seem harmless, but you must understand that uncontrolled multiplication and growth, especially that of damaged cells, is what *Cancer* basically is.

And an uncontrolled activation of mTOR can also lead to formation of acne, fibrosis, and a multitude of diseases.

You may ask why damaged cells are prompted to multiply and grow.

This is because, mTORC1 actively puts a brake on *autophagy* (which we just covered in the last chapter), the process that cleans off damaged, or unnecessary cells and components.

Several factors and conditions increases the mTORC1 activity, and the main factors are –

- High levels of amino acids (building units of proteins).
- High carbohydrate or sugar content, which not only causes the activation of mTOR, but also leads to the secretion of insulin, which is also a main factor for activating the mTOR pathway.
- Anabolic steroids can increase mTOR activity by mimicking the actions of growth factors in the body.

- Resistance exercise, and physical activity also activate mTOR, stimulating the muscle protein synthesis and promoting muscle growth. This is why, in the chapter on exercise, I mentioned that while exercise is essential for our body, vital nutrients and periods of autophagy are more important for overall health and longevity.

    Therefore, it is important to combine a healthy, balanced and nutritious meal plan, combined with intermittent fasting, when consuming more protein and engaging in regular exercise.

Factors that decrease the mTOR activity are -

- Restricting the total calorie intake.
- Consuming just adequate amount of proteins, only that which is necessary for the normal upkeep of the body.

There are also plenty of plant derived compounds which decreases the activity of the mTOR pathway, such as –

- *Resveratrol,* a polyphenolic flavonoid, found majorly in grape-skin.
- EGG (*epigallocatechin-3-gallate*), found majorly in green tea.

These compounds are significant in helping to reduce the size and formations of mTOR driven acne, papules, pustules etc. and furthermore, helps in stopping the growth of the harmful bacteria, and their biofilm formations, in these cases as well.

But if you are someone who would like to build muscle bulk, and gain strength through resistant exercise and consuming excess protein, it is crucial to approach it in a balanced way to ensure health.

To counterbalance the overstimulation of the mTOR pathway, which leads to unchecked cell growth (even harmful ones), it is vital to incorporate *intermittent fasting* into the routine, on a daily basis, which will give the body an opportunity to enter the state of *autophagy*, and allow adequate time for cellular maintenance and repair.

This combination helps strike the right balance, allowing you to build muscle bulk, while also promoting long-term health.

When mTOR is activated appropriately, it becomes an essential factor for the normal growth and development of the body in children especially during their early years.

It also supports essential biological functions, such as the growth and repair of tissues of the muscle and organs, particularly after intense exercise or some sort of injury or damage.
It also assists and supports the immune system by regulating the growth and function of immune cells, particularly during an immune response.

But when the mTOR pathway is operating in ranges that are more than required (particularly during insulin resistance or similar systemic defects in the body), it can lead to several health issues such as, cancer, metabolic disorders, cardiovascular diseases, premature ageing, and even neuro-degenerative diseases.

> Proteins play crucial roles in regulating
> many vital processes in the body.
>
> However, maintaining the right balance is
> key to achieving, and preserving optimal health.
>
> This is why relying solely on high-protein diets
> while neglecting fats is not the best approach.

Chapter XX – Protect Your MITOCHONDRIA.

The mitochondria, or more famously, the *'Powerhouse of the Cell'* generates 90% of our body's energy. Without these energy generators, our cells and our body, would stop functioning.

Our major fuel sources, fats and glucose, are converted into something called as an ATP, which contains energy... much similar to batteries. These ATP molecules are like supercharged batteries, ready to release their surplus energy, at any needful moment.

The ATP molecules travel to all the essential parts of the cell, and once they are at their destination, they break apart, creating a surge of energy for the body's components to use.

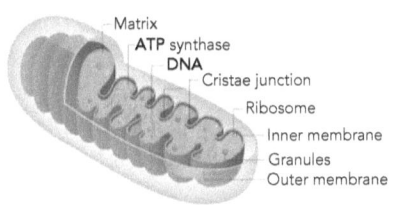

Each cell in our body can contain from around 5000, to about 100,000 (1 Lakh) Mitochondria!

Mitochondria plays vital roles in energy creation, cellular signalling, and maintaining the environment balance in a cell. When our body starts to lose large amounts of mitochondria, it leads to various issues that include neuro-degenerative and metabolic disorders, as well as diseases related to ageing. A few important roles performed by our mitochondria include,

- Cellular respiration or ATP generation based on the ever changing energy demands of our body. The mitochondria **regulates metabolism**, and adjusts the ATP production accordingly.

- Balances calcium in the cell, which controls functions like muscle contraction, controlled cell death, and cell signalling.

- Mitochondria can generate heat through a process called thermogenesis. Brown adipose tissue, are mainly used in this process, which keeps us warm even in the cold.

- Participates in synthesizing *'Haeme'* a component of Haemoglobin, and also other proteins involved in oxygen transport and metabolism.

- Plays a key role in initiating apoptosis, a process of scheduled cell death, which is vital for tissue development and removal of damaged cells. Mitochondria releases proteins like *Cytochrome-C*, which triggers apoptosis, leading to cell death.

- In steroid producing cells, like those in our adrenal glands and gonads, mitochondria are involved in synthesizing steroid hormones like cortisol, aldosterone, and testosterone.

As you can see, there are many vital functions in the cell, and our body, that require all of the effort and function from our mitochondria.

If those important functions were to be interrupted in some way, our cells, and our body as a whole, would be in deep trouble.

We can compare it to, the occurrence of a 'total electric power outage' or a 'blackout' in a metropolitan city!

This sudden loss of power and energy would obstruct the very vital operations in our cells. When our mitochondria cannot work in the way that it should, it is called as- *"Mitochondrial Dysfunction."*

And the side effect of the mitochondrial dysfunction that most intrigues me personally, is its direct impact on the *"Ageing"* of our body.

Ageing cannot be attributed to just one determining factor.

However, researches today have been focusing on the molecular level to figure out the ageing process more clearly, and it is the mitochondria, that scientists have figured out, which plays a vital role in ageing.

Here are a few points which you will find interesting -

1. Mitochondria have their own DNA known as *"MtDNA"*.
   According to the theory of evolution, it is theorized that the mitochondria used to exist entirely separate from cells, operating as single-celled organisms on their own, and sometime during our evolution, mitochondria and other cells decided to live symbiotically (a mutually beneficial relationship between different organisms.)

   Now whether this theory is true or not, it is a fact that without our mitochondria, we can never exist as this complex organisms that we currently are. Adding to their unique role in our body, mitochondrial DNA is inherited exclusively from the mother, making us genetically more similar to our mother than to our father in terms of mitochondrial genetic material.

2. MtDNA is now a popular subject of aging research in recent years, and studies strongly suggest that ageing is correlated to the damage caused by free radicals to our MtDNA as much as our other cells nuclear DNA. A review published in 'The Journal of Clinical Investigation' states that –

   "There is solid evidence that the amount of MtDNA mutations increases with age in humans. Deletions in MtDNA have been observed in the aged human central nervous system, skeletal muscle, and hepatocytes."

   To understand the importance of this statement a little better...
   You need to know, that our body is constantly recreating our DNA and MtDNA. Ideally, if there is a perfect copy created during every replication, then it means we will live forever.

   But of course this cannot happen.

   Telomeres (mentioned in the chapter for fasting), are protective caps at the ends of chromosomes that prevent DNA damage during cell division. Very minor errors will definitely occur in this replication process due to damage caused by ROS, micro plastics, chemicals, minor replication errors during normal MtDNA synthesis, or radiations etc.

   As it is commonly said, *"Little Drops Make The Mighty Ocean"* –

... the very small mutations can end up multiplying the errors in each consecutive replication process, causing the telomeres to shorten, which it eventually leads to 'cellular *senescence*' or death, when they become too short.

3. In the fifth chapter, we had discussed *Free radicals*. So even though these unstable molecules can find its way into our body from external sources like pollution, cigarette smoke, and radiations, the majority of it actually forms in our body as a by-product of the energy produced from the food we eat, which occurs in the mitochondria.

   Since free radicals are produced from inside the mitochondria, the mitochondria is also the major victim of the toxic effects of free radicals, due to its close proximity, which is the leading cause for *Mitochondrial Dysfunction*.

   A review published in "Cell" states that - *"In postmitotic tissue such as brain, the levels of ROS are significantly higher in mitochondria compared to nuclear DNA. Reasons for these differences are thought to include the proximity of mitochondrial DNA to the source of oxidants and the lack of any protective histone covering."*

   Even though our body has enough antioxidants to combat these free radicals, the balance between *"Free Radicals & Anti-oxidants"* is disrupted when we do not support our body. A diet high in carbs / sugars, fried food, alcohol consumption, extreme physical activity, emotional stress are all responsible for free radicals to gain the upper hand over anti-oxidants, which is also called as **"Oxidative Stress."**

4. In the fourth chapter, we had mentioned briefly about *Adipocytes* (fat storing cells). New scientific discoveries has shown that there are 3 major types, **White** adipocyte, **Brown**, and **Beige** adipocytes.
   The most important and beneficial of the three is the **Brown fat**.

   Brown fat, even though structurally smaller than white fat, is abundant with mitochondria (which incidentally also gives the cell its distinctive colour, as mitochondria is made up of a lot of iron), and the mitochondria produce energy to regulate the body temperature (especially in cold temperatures), which burns calories, control blood sugar and insulin levels and even helps in weight loss.

Brown fat in newborns, is located in their back, neck and shoulders, and during childhood and adolescence, *brown* fat scatters around the body. *Brown* fat in adults, is located around the neck, kidneys, adrenal glands, heart (aorta) and chest.

White adipocytes stores fat in various places around your body, especially around our visceral organs, and is commonly seen in obesity. It has less mitochondria and are harder to get rid of as they cannot create much ATP.

Beige fat, are *white* fat cells, which are formed while they are being converted into *brown* fat cells. *Beige* cells are regularly burning calories, to regulate our body temperature.

We have far less *brown* fat than *white* fat in our body, but people who are lean, like athletes, have more *brown* fat in their bodies than others.

We can increase the beneficial *brown* cells by lowering the body temperature (taking a cold shower or an ice bath) which activates *brown* fats to help your body burn more calories.
It also converts more *white* fats, transforming them into *beige* fat.

Eating a well-balanced diet is also found to activate *brown* fat production through a compound called **ursolic acid**.

Regular exercise as well as intermittent fasting, has been found to activate the body's thermogenic (heat creating) hormone ***irisin***, which converts *white* fat, into *beige* and *brown* adipocytes.

5. Intermittent Fasting is also an amazing tool, to produce more of, "near-perfect" copies of MtDNA and DNA.

    Autophagy and ***Mitophagy*** are processes where weak, or half dead cells, and mitochondria are recycled, stopping them from replicating further, which can in turn, help reduce the mutations (errors) that occur during MtDNA and DNA synthesis.

    This will leave our body remaining with only healthy and robust cells, which naturally, when the replication process takes place, will only have very minimal errors taking place... which in-turn means a healthier and longer lifespan for us.

6. Reduction in mitochondria numbers, or *Mitochondrial Dysfunction* has been found to be one of the supporting causes for weight gain and obesity as well.

    Imagine, if there are not enough power generators, and yet, fuel (food) is still being supplied to the body, then the body has no other option but to store all those extra fuel.

    And of course once overweight and fat deposits sets in, then *Insulin Resistance* and *Metabolic Syndrome* are not far behind.

7. A comparative study published by the *"Journal of Gerontology"* reveals that exercise can help promote mitochondrial biogenesis, a process where our body creates more mitochondria.

    Since the mitochondria are very responsive organelles, they replicate themselves to provide more help for the increased workload, if they detect an increase in energy demand.

    And also, if our mitochondria notices that our daily energy needs are minimal, if we lead a more sedentary lifestyle, our mitochondria in response, will reduce their numbers to maintain efficiency, as supporting multiple mitochondria is an ATP expensive process.

    It is important to incorporate an active lifestyle, especially as you age, so that our mitochondria multiplies and not become dysfunctional.

    But what about people who cannot exercise, due to various painful health issues such as arthritis or fibromyalgia?

    Then the best thing to do, is to practice *Intermittent Fasting*. It helps to rejuvenate the body like a wake-up call, and forces the body to be more alert and work efficiently.

8. Our body has tiny helper molecules (co-enzymes) called NAD+ (*Nicotinamide Adenine Dinucleotide*), that essentially gives a booster dose to our mitochondria, and helps in its efficient functioning. Without them, the mitochondria would be in a dormant or inactive state.

    A research study published in "EMBO *Molecular Medicine*" showed that supplementing Vitamin-B_3 which increases NAD+, resulted in *Mitochondrial Biogenesis* (new formations). NAD+ supplements are also currently available for consumers as well.

When it comes to *free radicals*...

we have so far only discussed the damage causing potential of these molecules, that contribute to ageing and disease (due to oxidative stress).

But *free radicals* are also involved in several essential biochemical processes in the body, especially in reduction reactions, and also play key roles in normal cellular functions.

Here are a few examples where *free radicals* are required -

- *Nitric Oxide* (NO) is the free radical that helps in relaxing our blood vessels (vascular relaxation), maintaining its elasticity and keeping our blood pressure under control. It is also important for neuro-transmission, and immune responses.

- Fibroblasts, are responsible for producing *Collagen* (which makes up 70% of our skin and 50% of our bones) in connective tissue. Free radicals play a role in the production of the enzyme, that causes the proper folding, and stabilization of collagen fibers.

- *Free radicals* are produced during the immune response, particularly when our WBCs like macrophages and neutrophils, engulf pathogens (phagocytosis). This process, known as respiratory burst, generates free radicals such as *superoxide anions* and *hydrogen peroxide*, which help kill, and digest microorganisms.

- Conversion of thyroid hormone from T_4 to T_3 is caused by free radicals *hydrogen peroxide* and *thyroid peroxidase*.

- ROS can act as signalling molecules that influence various cellular pathways. For instance, free radicals can activate transcription factors, which regulate genes involved in cell growth, inflammation, and survival, which is critical for cellular responses to stress, growth factors, and environmental cues.

- Mitochondria are both a source and target of free radicals, but they also rely on free radicals in normal mitochondrial function. Although excessive free radicals can lead to mitochondrial damage, moderate amounts are involved in regulating mitochondrial biogenesis (ATP production) and other functions.

- Free radicals, particularly *hydroxyl radicals*, can initiate lipid peroxidation, a process by which polyunsaturated fatty acids (PUFA) in cell membranes are oxidized. This process can serve as a regulatory mechanism in cell signalling, but excessive peroxidation leads to cellular damage.

- *Cytochrome* P450 *enzyme system* is involved in the metabolism of drugs and toxins in the liver, and uses free radicals for oxidation.

- The enzyme prothrombin is converted to thrombin through a series of reactions that are facilitated in part by free radicals, and this formation of thrombin is essential for blood clot formation and wound healing.

While free radicals are often associated with oxidative damage, they are also indispensable for a variety of essential biochemical and physiological processes, particularly those that involve redox reactions.

But only a fraction of free radicals are required for these needs, compared to the high free radical production and subsequent damage that we face through an unhealthy lifestyle.

Ageing and eventual demise of our human body is inevitable…

But when we have a clear choice to extend our life in a very healthy state, and if we have the ability to reduce the chance of occurrence, and severity of chronic diseases for ourselves, I definitely would choose it.

As we have just discussed, our mitochondria is at the center of the issue. An article published in *"Integrative Medicine"* highlights that the loss of function in our mitochondria, results in excess fatigue, wrinkles in the skin, joint aches and other common symptom of aging.

The QRS (*Quantum Resonance System*) is a machine, designed as a non-invasive, gentle and long-term therapy, for stimulating the mitochondrial function through pulsating magnetic fields, and have been found to have positive impacts on pain management as well as cell repair.

The QRS have also been found to be useful in reducing chronic pain quite quickly and effectively and increasing the energy production of all body cells and tissues.

Additionally it also improves the sleep quality, reduces inflammations, and actively stimulates the replication of RNA and DNA, among numerous other benefits.

> If we focus on, and make a habit of maintaining a healthy diet,
> and integrate daily intermittent fasting along with
> routine exercise, we might not realize it,
> but we are actually taking steady steps
> towards making a big impact
> on the molecular levels in our body.
>
> And taking care of our mitochondria is just
> one of the best ways, to ***age gracefully***.

Chapter XXI – Is Organic Food Really a Scam?

Gone are the days when those of us living in cities or developed countries, had the luxury of choosing whole, natural foods.

Today, the vast majority of food options available to the urban population are either genetically modified (GMO) or ultra-processed, to such an extent that what we consume, bears little resemblance to its original, unaltered form.
Whether it be vegetables, fruits, grains, or meat, even the 'healthier' options are often modified or subjected to heavy industrial processing.

To even remotely imagine that politicians and the governments, have our, the peoples, best interests in their hearts, in the matter of food and nutrition, is a very innocent and careless thought to have.

One would naturally assume that doctors, as trusted healthcare professionals, are the ones guiding us when it comes to food and nutrition. After all, they are the experts we turn to for advice to maintain our health, manage chronic conditions, and to prevent diseases.

However, the reality is quite different. Food trends are way more political and economically motivated than it appears.
The only voice that really matter in the present world, to any political parties or governments is the '*sound of money*' from mega-corporations.

The majority of doctors are not adequately trained in nutrition, and their understanding and guidance on food is often limited, or based on outdated or mainstream information from the researches influenced, and projected by the mega-corporations.

The extent to which food has become industrialized, means that it is no longer about nourishing the body with what nature intended.
Instead, it has become about maximizing profit, efficiency, and shelf life.

A prime example of this, is how the USA and China effectively bullied Mexico into buying their GMO crops, prioritizing financial gain over public health.

Despite Mexico's warnings about the potential health risks of these genetically modified foods, including their long-term effects on human health, both nations pushed for the sale of GMO seeds.

To top it off, these crops are designed to be sterile, meaning Mexico is forced to purchase new seeds from the USA every year, creating a perpetual financial burden.

Moreover, cross-pollination with GMOs threatens Mexico's native corn species, which is eroding its agricultural heritage and leading to increased dependence on foreign imports. This creates a cycle of food insecurity, undermining the country's sovereignty.

The situation shows us how food trends are driven by political and financial agendas, violating basic human rights.

This is not a unique case.

This pattern of exploitation extends globally, affecting nations and urban populations, where entire food systems are increasingly controlled by corporate interests rather than public welfare.

Small-scale, regenerative farming practices are being replaced by large-scale, monoculture operations, where the focus is on producing vast quantities of uniform food that can be shipped worldwide, often at the cost of human health, biodiversity, environmental health, and even animal welfare.

GMOs are increasingly prevalent in our food supply, designed to be more resistant to pests, diseases, and environmental stressors.

They are also engineered to tolerate herbicides, leading to the widespread use of chemicals like glyphosate, which has been linked to cancer and environmental harm.

For those living in cities, access to fresh, whole foods is increasingly limited to farmer's markets, which can often be out of reach for the average consumer, due to cost or location.

Even in supermarkets, an overwhelming majority of foods though labelled as 'organic' are still highly processed in some way.

Consumers are frequently bombarded with marketing tactics designed to make processed food look appealing, with phrases like *'low-fat'* or *'high-protein'* or *'natural flavours'* even when the product contains more chemicals than nutrients.

In the 1980s, over **60%** of the average food expenditure in Britain went toward whole foods or ingredients for home-cooking, like vegetables and meat, while only **25%** was spent on ready to eat or processed foods.

By the 2000s, this footing dramatically reversed, with only **25%** being spent on whole foods, and over **45%** on ultra-processed options.

This drastic change was a major contributing factor, to the rise in obesity in the UK, with rates increasing from **7%** in the 1980s to **20%** in the 2000s, and currently being around **35%**.

Even when whole foods are available, they are often subjected to extreme levels of processing. Ultra-processed foods are no longer just a convenience or occasional indulgence, they dominate the food landscape.

Fruits are juiced, canned, or turned into snack bars. Grains are refined and stripped of their fiber to create white flour and sugary cereals.

Meats are heavily processed with additives, preservatives, and flavour enhancers, often masquerading as something "natural."

In many cases, what appears on the shelf as a food product is actually a concoction of chemicals, artificial flavours, and synthetic additives designed to mimic the taste, texture, and appearance of real food.

The problem with ultra-processed food goes beyond just their lack of nutrients. They are purposely formulated to be "hyper-palatable" meaning that they are engineered to stimulate the brain's pleasure centers, that encourage overconsumption, creating a cycle of craving, overeating, and weight gain.

The most common justification for trusting such foods is…

> "the American FDA (*Food and Drug Administration*) has approved them, so why should we worry?"

Recently, a food additive just exposed a major loophole in the American FDA that was hiding in plain sight all this while. *Red Dye*-3, a petroleum-based dye, found in candies, ice cream, and cereals.

It was banned by the American FDA only in 2025, after being banned in lipsticks 35 years ago, due to its cancer causing effects on lab rats.

So why was it allowed in food for this long?

The answer lies in the different approaches to food safety.

The European government says –
'**Before you sell it, prove that it will not harm us.**'
The American government says –
'**Sell it now, we will ban it later if it hurts someone.**'

This is why *Red Dye*-3 did not enter the European food market, while Americans, and the other 60% of world countries that follow the American FDA as the golden standard, consumed it for decades, until the harm that it caused, began to show as serious symptoms.

But the even bigger issue with the American FDA, was a category created by them in 1958, called GRAS (*Generally Recognized as Safe*).

The original idea was to allow common ingredients like vinegar and salt, to not need lengthy safety tests.

This seemingly well-intentioned rule began to be exploited as a loophole.

Companies started to call any new chemical "safe" by picking their own "safety experts" and using it without telling the FDA. We had discussed about a fiber called *carrageenan* being used as such, in Chapter- 16.

Since the year 2000, around 766 new chemicals entered the American food market, but only 10 were reviewed by the FDA.

The rest were **self-certified** by the manufacturers themselves.

Food safety keeps evolving, and what is considered "safe" today, might not be tomorrow.

Nobody ever questions how bad a bottle of *Pepsi* or *Cola* is, or how much fried chicken from fast food restaurants are going to damage their health, but when it comes to vegetables or meat, everyone becomes extremely suspicious, concerned and investigative about the farming practices or pesticides used in the process.

In the same way, I have had so many patients who blindly and happily, have been taking over the counter medicines with known side-effects for years together, but when it comes to taking a multi-vitamin tablet, they would be hesitant, and start questioning for side-effects.

Poor education, forced misinformation and propaganda from mega-corporations, just like **Procter & Gamble**, still thrive to this day.

It creates a kind of anxiety and fear in the minds of the populations, leading to distrust of governments, and creates medical uncertainties that strain families. It cultivates feelings of powerlessness, which becomes a potential driving force, into making people vulnerable, and to start making ill-informed decisions in their life.

The very foods that we consume to fuel our lives are, ironically, undermining our health and well-being.
The loss of whole, naturally grown foods has started to diminish our connection to food as a life-sustaining force.

People no longer know where their food comes from or how it is grown.

The idea of a balanced, seasonal diet obtained from local agriculture is becoming an increasingly distant memory, replaced by a more artificial and convenient way of eating, taking away the true essence of our food.

Our education system, urgently in need of reform, is only worsening the challenges for future generations, especially in an era where children have access to infinite information uncensored… but lack the maturity or exposure to distinguish fact from fiction.

This is the bittersweet, yet profoundly sad world we live in.

The silver lining is that everything beneficial to us, is available all around us. We just need to learn how to look for it, and choose what's right.

Now the ironic part about most "organic" food is that, even though it is forcefully being marketed as –

Home Grown by Strong and Independent Home-makers…

…it is actually run by the very same mega-corporations that people are trying to run away from.

So unless you have a neighbour, or a local farmer who actually produces organic, home-grown vegetables and produce, you do **NOT** have to take up the headache of running behind, the very expensive and highly marketed "organic" products.

This is also the case with *Broiler Chicken*.

The most common myth circulating, is that large scale farmed *Broiler Chicken*, are the reason for PCOD, Thyroiditis, Obesity and such diseases. The argument being that they grow quickly due to being injected by growth hormones, or that they are *"lab-created"* animals.

In truth, *Broiler Chicken* are just a variety of chicken that grows very fast, compared to other varieties of chicken. Normally they used to grow around 1_{kg} in **2 months' time**.

This trait of *'fast growth'* was developed, to around 5_{kg} in **2 months**, by using the simple technique of ***Selective Breeding***, over the last 70 years.

Do you know how many kernels are present in a cob of corn?

It has an average of around **600** kernels. Would you believe that there were just around **5** kernels in a stem of corn before selective breeding?

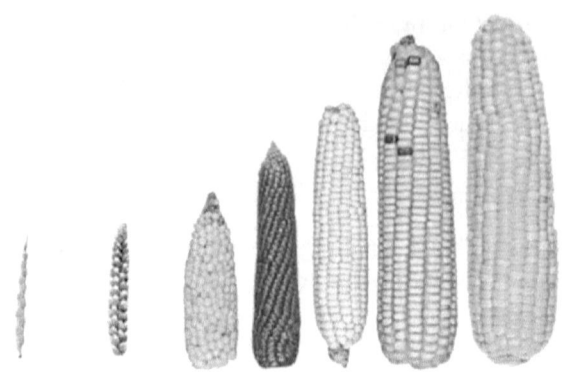

Corn Before and After Selective Breeding

Over **10,000 years** of selective breeding, helped to develop this particular trait in the corn. This same technique, has been used to develop the *Broiler Chicken* as well.
Using growth hormones will not turn out profitable for the farmers.

Now even if, in the worst case scenario, there are farmers who have the resources to inject growth hormones, we still would not have to worry, as growth hormones are highly specific to species (meaning the ones used for chicken are not effective for humans).

Furthermore, even if we consume meat that contains growth hormones, since they are protein based, it would be simply digested, and effectively become useless in the human body.
Similar to insulin used in diabetes treatment, which is a protein hormone, and so gets broken down by digestive enzymes when ingested, making it ineffective. This is why insulin must be injected.

Broiler chicken and chicken eggs are an affordable and a better choice of protein, than plant based proteins, that has helped bring physical growth, nourishment, and health to a lot of families, especially to those struggling financially.

In India, it has played one of the major helping hands, in reducing the cases of **PEM** (*protein energy malnutrition*) that caused vicious diseases such as *Kwashiorkor* and *Marasmus*.

Of course factory farming is often-times terrible... anyone with a sense of moral, would agree.

Without a doubt, most factory farmed cattle or chicken, are raised and treated in very poor living conditions, and are given carbohydrate rich feed, which causes an increase in the inflammatory *omega*-6 content in their fat and meat, especially that of poultry.

The overuse of antibiotics in poultry, can lead to the emergence of antibiotic resistant bacteria, which can be transmitted to humans through food or environment.
There is a chance for the poultry antibiotics to cause antibiotic resistance in humans, and have become a leading cause for persistent fungal infections as well.

Ultimately, when considering the balance of benefits versus potential harm, the advantages of consuming these sources of nutrition for our body, outweigh the possible drawbacks.

However, as mentioned previously, mass-scale factory farming is often-times terrible and detrimental to the well-being of the animals involved.

A change should definitely be brought about.

The solution should not be to altogether eliminate these valuable sources of nutrition from our diet, but instead, the focus should be on implementing policies and regulations that ensure the safe, and ethical farming of livestock, while at the same time, prioritizing their humane treatment and well-being.

For those fortunate enough to find and afford *pasture-raised chickens* or, even better, for those who are lucky enough to raise chicken themselves, it is worth fully embracing the benefits of both their meat and eggs, which offer a healthier and more sustainable choice.

• Is Veganism a Scam?

What is veganism?

Veganism is often times, an extreme version of the *'organic'* food craze.

It is when one avoids the consumption of all animal foods like seafood, meat, eggs, dairy products like milk, butter, cheese, ghee, yogurt, curd, paneer etc. particularly motivated by the sake of *'physical health'* and *'environmental responsibility'*.

The very first question I ask during my consultation, to those who follow a vegan diet is whether this choice of lifestyle is for the sake of their health, or due to specific religious beliefs.

If the answer is due to religious reasons, I respect their choice and explain how our body runs on various nutrients, and how important they are for the human body.

I have been able to teach almost all of my patients to take these very essential nutrients, through at least dairy products (primarily, orthodox *Hindu* and *Jain* patients of mine) for the sake of their overall health.

Orthodox followers of the "*Ahimsa*" (non-violence) philosophy often face a moral dilemma, when they must choose between their health, and their deeply held beliefs.

This does not mean that only a diet included with non-vegetarian food is going to help us for a healthy old age.

Sattvic food, and *Sattvic* diet practices, are very healthy when followed according to its principles, as it have been for centuries, in various traditional Indian communities, as discussed in earlier chapters.

But the wise, and very practical words of ***Sri Swami Vivekananda***, the renown Hindu monk, religious teacher, philosopher, author, and founder of the *Ramakrishna Mission* (Calcutta), have influenced my thoughts on food for health and beliefs...

"About vegetarian diet I have to say this - first, my Master was a vegetarian; but if he was given meat offered to the Goddess, he used to hold it up to his head. The taking of life is undoubtedly sinful; but so long as vegetable food is not made suitable to the human system through progress in chemistry, there is no other alternative but meat-eating. So long as man shall have to live a Rajasik (active) life under circumstances like the present, there is no other way except through meat-eating. It is true that the Emperor Asoka saved the lives of millions of animals, by the threat of the sword; but is not the slavery of a thousand years more dreadful than that? Taking the life of a few goats as against the inability to protect the honour of one's own wife and daughter, and to save the morsels for one's children from robbing hands - which of these is more sinful? Rather let those belonging to the upper ten, who do not earn their livelihood by manual labour, not take meat; but the forcing of vegetarianism upon those who have to earn their bread by labouring day and night is one of the causes of the loss of our national freedom. Japan is an example of what good and nourishing food can do." — *(Complete Works, 4.486-7)*

"All liking for fish and meat disappears when pure Sattva is highly developed, and these are the signs of its manifestation in a soul: sacrifice of everything for others, perfect non-attachment to lust and wealth, want of pride and egotism. The desire for animal food goes when these things are seen in a man. And where such indications are absent, and yet you find men siding with the non-killing party, know it for a certainty that here there is either hypocrisy or a show of religion." — *(Complete Works, 5.403-7)*

This is just an extract from a more detailed and wonderful conversation between the noble Swami and one of his disciples.
To read it in detail, you can refer – "***Conversations and Dialogues of Volume 5 of The Complete Works of Swami Vivekananda.***"

In most cases, vegans have chosen their path, from the 'scientific evidences' propagated by companies, as deliberate business tactics, just as **Procter & Gamble** had done. The only ones who actually suffer, are the unsuspecting victims of these marketing antics.

So far we have already discussed how fatty acids, proteins, vitamins, and minerals are all essential for our body.

One of the main argument put forth by vegans, is that non-vegetarian sources of food are primarily consumed for its *Protein* content, and that this is not necessary since proteins can be gained from pulses, legumes and nuts as well. Let us take a closer look at proteins.

- Proteins are made of building blocks called *Amino Acids* (AA). Our own body makes a few of these *amino acids*, so they are called **Non-Essential Amino Acids.**
  And then there are a few, that we cannot make, for which we have to depend on foods, so these are called *Essential Amino Acids.*
  There are around 9 known *Essential Amino Acids.*

- The best complete source for these *Essential Amino Acids* are meat, meat organs, eggs and fish. No vegetarian sources have the complete, and better bio-available proteins.

- Protein from meat sources, do not back-pack any extra 'unwanted' materials. For example, to get **20%** of proteins from pulses, you have to intake the **60%** carbohydrate that comes with it, whereas the **20%** proteins from meat sources do not bring any sugars along.

- Meat sources are nutrient dense. Which means, to get the RDA (required daily allowance) of any minerals or vitamins, you only need to eat far less amounts, compared to vegetarian sources. For example, take a look at the table below-

100 gram	Phos-phorus (mg)	Iron (mg)	Zinc (mg)	Copper (mg)	Vit-B_2 (mg)	Vit-A (IU)	Vit-C (mg)	Vit-B_6 (mg)	Vit-B_{12} (mcg)
Apple	0.6	0.1	0.05	0.04	0.02	0	7	0.03	0
Carrots	31	0.6	0.3	0.08	0.05	0	6	0.1	0
Spinach	49	2.7	0.5	0.13	0.1	2800	28	0.1	0
Red Meat	140	3.3	4.4	0.2	0.2	40	0	0.07	1.84
Liver	476	8.8	4.0	12.0	4.2	53,500	27	0.73	111.3

Notice how each mineral and vitamins content in common vegetarian sources, are just a fraction of what is available from common meat sources, or are only rich in any one, or very few of these nutrients.

And if you take a look at the table given below... in order to get the **RDA** of *Calcium* from plant sources, you will have to consume at least 1.3$_{kg}$ of spinach or 4.8$_{kg}$ of lentils a day.
But you only need 170 grams (0.17$_{kg}$) of cheese for achieving the **RDA!**

Per 100g	Calcium (mg)	Amount needed for RDA (1200 $_{mg}$)
Cheese	718	170 $_{grams}$ (about ¾ of 1 cup) = 680 $_{Calories}$
Whole Milk	117	1000 $_{grams}$ (about 4 cups) = 660 $_{Calories}$
Spinach	93	1300 $_{grams}$ (about 13 cups) = 1200 $_{Calories}$
Lentils	25	4800 $_{grams}$ (about 32 cups) = 5100 $_{Calories}$

A Short Note on RDA-
It is actually the average amount of a particular nutrient, required to only maintain, the healthy functioning, of an adult healthy body.
Which means that, if you are not in peak physical health, or if you are suffering from certain diseases, the actual requirement of certain nutrients for your body, could even be as high as 200 times more, than the mentioned RDA.
So keep this in mind as well, when we talk about RDA.

Can you imagine eating close to 5 kilograms of lentils just for the sake of the daily requirement (RDA) of calcium...

And what about all that extra load of carbohydrates (around 50% of the total content) that piggy-backs along with it?

It is never possible nor practical.

This is the case with each essential nutrient.

So, is it not logical, to eat just enough of a food item, that gives us maximum benefits?

To make things worse, the vegan lifestyle is more fatal to women.

Studies have shown that while women who consume an unhealthy conventional meal pattern, has a **50%** risk for death (directly influenced by diet related health issues) ...

And in women who follow a vegan diet, there is a drastic increase observed, as more than **85%** risk for death (directly influenced by diet related health issues).

One of the main reasons for this is found to be, deficiency of *Essential fatty acids,* and as we have mentioned in the first chapter, a **body fat percentage lower than 12%** for women can lead to multiple organs & system failure, and eventually death.

A few more popular claims by vegans include-

- Our primate relatives are vegan, so humans must be vegan as well.
- Humans were not meant to be carnivores.
- Vegan diet builds muscles in horses, cows and gorillas, and can do the same for humans.
- Eating too much protein can damage our kidneys.
- Vegans can get every nutrient from plants, without supplements.
- Drinking milk is against natural order.
- Vegan food is always healthier.
- Vegans can easily get enough healthy fat.
- Vegans never have cancer or heart disease.
- Eating vegan costs lower than eating animal products.
- Fruits are super foods, that can solve any, and all disease.

Let us briefly go through each claim.

1. Many vegans find it *'logical'* that, humans should eat like other apes (such as chimpanzee, gorilla etc.), because the DNA of humans and that of other apes are up to 99% similar, for which, the answer is already explained in detail, in Chapter- 7.

2. Some vegans claim that our lack of claws, sharp teeth and strong hydrochloric acid in our stomachs to digest meat, is proof that we are biologically programmed to only eat fruits and vegetables.

   Humans are the dominant species because of their supreme intelligence. Brute strength is not our primary survival strategy and so, neither do we have the need for long claws nor sharp teeth.

   Chapter- 15 explains how we humans have a much stronger stomach acid than that of carnivores, and even if we were to eat raw meat, it would quite easily be digested.

3. Cows, horses, and gorillas have entirely different digestive systems than humans, which is why they can thrive on grass and plants while humans struggle on a vegan diet.

   Cows (ruminants) have a four-chambered stomach full of bacteria that ferment and break down cellulose (fiber in grass) into fatty acids, which provide most of their energy. Their gut bacteria also synthesize protein from non-protein nitrogen sources.

   Gorillas (hindgut fermenters with large colons) eat a mix of leaves, fruits, and insects, but their massive gut bacteria populations help extract more protein than humans ever could from plants.

   Humans have a small cecum and a short colon, meaning we are not designed to extract high amounts of protein from plants. In fact, our digestive system is closer to carnivores than cows, or gorillas.

4. The infamous claim that eating too much protein can damage our kidneys, is mostly false. Though it is true that proteins can leak through a damaged kidney, the damage itself though, is most commonly due to high levels of blood pressure, sugar, triglycerides, uric acid, nicotine, homocysteine etc. Moreover, protein only poses a threat to an already, severely damaged kidney, with an eGFR level of 4 or 5 (discussed in later chapters).

5. Obtaining all the essential nutrients is difficult with an omnivorous diet itself, let alone a restrictive diet like the vegan diet, so the claim that vegans can get all of their nutrients from plants without supplementation, is not true.

Vitamin-B_{12} and vitamin-D are the two most common deficiencies in vegans. It is also well documented that vegans suffer from protein malabsorption, amino acid deficiencies, imbalances in *omega*-6 to *omega*-3 fatty acids, low creatinine levels, high lectin intake, mineral deficiencies in zinc, iron, selenium, calcium, iodine, etc.

For example, *L-Carnitine*, is an amino acid (building block of proteins) which play a critical role in energy metabolism, particularly in burning fat for fuel.

Even though it is classified under non-essential category (as our body can synthesize it), it is described as a "**conditionally essential amino acid**" because under certain conditions (such as metabolic disorders, aging, pregnancy, or intense physical activity) our body will not be able to produce it efficiently.

Our liver synthesizes *L-Carnitine* by using the essential amino acids *lysine* and *methionine*. Plant-based diets are typically lower in *lysine* and *methionine*, and even though legumes and nuts have these amino acids, as mentioned before, they piggy back along with large amounts of carbohydrates (sugars).

Those that include animal sources can have up to **180 mg** per day of *L-Carnitine*, whereas vegans only have an average of **12 mg** per day.

6. The argument that drinking milk goes against the "natural order" overlooks the fact that humans, in almost every way, already operate outside of the typical natural patterns.

   Humans have adapted to thrive, and are the dominant species (even though elephants and lions exist), by manipulating the environment and other organisms around us (as mentioned in Chapter- 7), including the domestication of animals for milk.

   While a significant portion of the global population (around 65%), is lactose intolerant, we can still access the nutritional benefits of milk from animals like cows, goats, and camels, by simply consuming fermented dairy products like cheese and yoghurt.

   These foods are rich in probiotics, such as *Streptococcus thermophilus*, which produce **lactase** enzymes, that help digest lactose, making the valuable nutrients from milk, and dairy products, accessible to the human body.

7. Just because something is not made from animal products, it doesn't necessarily mean that it is healthy. In fact, vegan substitutes for animal products like mock meats and dairy are harmful to the body because they're heavily processed.

   For example, the contents of vegan butter are palm fruit oil, canola oil, soybean oil, flax oil, sunflower lecithin, lactic acid, and '*naturally extracted*' food colour.

   This is the same with oats-milk, high in carbs and seed oils.
   If you have read this book up until now, I'm sure you can figure out what all harm these ingredients can do to our body.

   This myth could have taken root due to the significant feeling of rejuvenation and energy, felt during the initial months of starting a vegan diet, if they would have also avoided ultra-processed foods. But issues from nutritional deficiencies, begin to show up later on.

8. Coconuts and avocados are often hailed as excellent sources of healthy fats for vegans, but the claim that vegans can easily meet their dietary fat needs is more complex than it appears.

   While these plant-based foods provide beneficial fats, they don't necessarily supply all the essential fatty acids required for the maintenance of optimal health.

   Chapter- 8 explains the importance of EPA and DHA, two *omega*-3 fatty acids that play a critical role in maintaining brain function, cardiovascular health, and reducing inflammation.

   For vegans, the most reliable source of EPA and DHA is seaweed, which contains these essential fats.

   However, access to seaweed is limited for the majority of people, especially those who live inland, or in areas where it isn't readily available. Even when it is available, it is often not 'bio-available' for the major part of the population.

   A 2018 study in the '*Nature Microbiology*' journal found that the human gut microbiome in Japanese individuals who regularly consume seaweed had significantly different microbial profiles compared to those from populations with little to no seaweed consumption.

Seaweeds are rich in nutrients like fiber, minerals, and vitamins (such as iodine, *omega*-3 fatty acids, vitamin-B_{12}, and polysaccharides), but we require the help of particular gut microbes to completely avail its benefits.

Having the right gut bacteria with the genetic ability to break down these compounds makes it easier for our body to absorb these nutrients efficiently.

Microbial gene transfer from seaweed may be a gradual process, with populations that have consumed seaweed for thousands of years (such as Japan, Korea, China, Norway, and Iceland) being more likely to harbour these beneficial bacteria.

Alternatives like algae oil supplements can provide a vegan-friendly source of EPA and DHA, and it is essential for vegans to explore other options or consider supplementation to ensure that they're getting enough of these crucial *omega*-3s.

And so, meeting the body's requirements of various types of fat, on a vegan diet, require a more thoughtful approach beyond depending on plant-based fats alone.

9. Vegans never fall victims to cancer or heart diseases, is also just a claim and not a fact. Deficiencies of *Omega-3, Vitamin-D, and Vitamin-B_{12}* are known to contribute to cancer and heart blocks.

    Furthermore, many vegan foods are highly processed, and include GMO soy in them that's soaked with glyphosate containing herbicides, which has been shown to increase cancer risk by as much as **41%**. Vegan diets high in starches, refined grains, and sweets increase the risk of heart disease. Eating deep fried food, be it vegan or not, still contributes to heart blocks and cancer.

10. The claim that eating vegan is low-cost than eating animal products might seem true, as vegetables and fruits are typically costs lower than meat per gram.

    But going vegan is only going to raise the expenses.

    When the requirement for nutrition increases, the need for quantity and variety increases too.

Exotic vegetables and fruits, vegan alternatives for usual food produce like vegan sour cream, vegan macaroni and soy cheese, vegan ice cream, coconut milk yogurt etc. are also quite expensive.

The vegan replacements for typical animal products are actually more expensive on average than the things they replace.

11. The wrong notion that fruits are super foods, that can solve any, and all disease in our body, is not just reserved to vegans, but has somehow become the general trend, and almost everyone believes it.

The truth is that most of the fruits are not really as nutrition dense as other non-veg sources. Fruits are not as loaded in vitamins and minerals as people seem to believe.

Of course it does contain vitamins, but never to the extent, that we can solely survive on fruits and live a healthy, and disease free life.

Fruits are mostly fibers, sugars and few vitamins and phyto-nutrients, except in a few cases like avocado (contains fat as well). Fruits, when consumed in moderation, and eaten in raw form (not as juices), are be good sources of anti-oxidants, bioflavonoids, enzymes, and other active substances, that are immensely beneficial for us.

Fruits, used to contain only around **12%** sugar, but due to heavy *Selective breeding* and *Cross Breeding* processes, solely for their "***Sweetness***" trait, the sugar content has risen up to more than **50%** in current circumstances. Studies comparing the nutritional profiles of oranges reveal a significant decline in its nutritional content.

It now takes up to 8 modern oranges to match the nutrients found in just one orange from the 1920s. More specifically, protein levels in fruit have decreased by **6%**, vitamin-A by **18%**, and vitamin-B_2 by a striking **40%**, among others.

Additionally, fruits contain a sugar known as *"fructose"* which puts an excess burden on our liver, because only our liver can metabolize it. So excess fructose can become a cause of sudden fatty liver changes.

And if vegans opt to eat processed fruits or fruit juices, instead of whole fruits, then it is an even more harmful state, due to the added artificial flavouring chemicals, and extra sugars.

The overwhelming amount of fructose and other sweeteners, taken up directly to the liver in such a short period is detrimental.

Usually the majority of fructose is converted into glucose in the intestines itself to reduce the load on the liver, but this only occurs when the fruit is eaten as whole, allowing the fibers in the fruits to slow down the uptake of fructose from the intestines.

Consuming fruits during an infection in the gut, as in cases of fungal, or bacterial infections, is also not the right option in most cases, as these infections can thrive on the sugars from fruits, and will end up delaying the body's healing process (detailed in later chapters that explain diseases).

Once again, '*Veganism*' and the '***Sattvic***' way of life,
are two entirely different principles.

Being vegan, out of ***Compassion*** for animals and other
living beings is a completely valid and humane principle.

But when individuals choose to adopt a vegan lifestyle due to the ***Compulsion***, and pressure created by the influence of large corporations, which often disguise their motives under the guise of '*social and environmental responsibility*' it can be a deeply disheartening and unfortunate outcome.

It becomes even more troubling when these individuals, unknowingly, become mouthpieces for the very corporations that promote this so-called "ethical" agenda. People unwittingly aligning themselves with corporate propaganda is both troubling and saddening.

Did you know that the world's wealthiest **10%** of the population are responsible for more than **50%** of global carbon dioxide emissions. They produce more pollution in 1 hour, than an average person does in their entire life-time!

The sad part is that, un-informed vegans actually believe, that they are making a difference to help bring sustainability to our planet by avoiding egg, meat and dairy.

It's high time vegans realized, whether you eat vegetarian food or meat... Countless factories, with the very same working conditions, and with the exact same disregard to our environment, are making it possible, to bring our favourite products and food to our local supermarkets.

This situation calls for a broader awareness of what is at stake.

While urbanization and global supply chains have made food more accessible, they have also introduced a level of disconnection between people and the sources of their sustenance- *food*.

In order to reclaim control over our diets and improve our health, it is essential to return to a more conscious, sustainable approach to food.

This means supporting local and organic agriculture, choosing foods with minimal processing, and pushing for policy changes that encourage transparency in food labelling and the reduction of harmful additives.

Ultimately, we need a cultural shift a recognition that food is not just another commodity or a quick fix for hunger, but a fundamental root of our health and our future.

Only by demanding better, more wholesome food options can we hope to reverse the trend toward processed, artificial eating habits and restore our connection to the natural world around us.

Until then, we risk continuing down a path of poor health, degradation of our environmental, and loss of sovereignty over the food we eat.

Growing garden vegetables, or raising poultry in our own backyards, are practices, that must start to become normalised, in order to build a sustainable and healthy tomorrow.

For those with lack of space, or those in an urban setting, can opt for tower or vertical farming (such as aeroponic towers, food towers, hydroponic towers, geoponic towers etc.), which can be an effective way to grow food where land is limited or costly, and it is one of the best options for access to fresh, organic produce year round.

> So instead of putting the blame on meat, eggs and dairy,
> the right thing to do, is to choose our local, small scale farms,
> or turn to home gardening ourselves, instead of choosing
> highly processed foods from large scale factories,
> if we really want to make a difference.

Chapter XXII – Staple Food of The Future.

With each passing day, we witness the intensifying effects of climate change, through rise in temperatures, unpredictable weather patterns, and extreme environmental events, which not only impact ecosystems, but also resonates across the global economic structures.

Agriculture, the most climate-sensitive industry, faces unprecedented challenges as our traditional farming methods are becoming increasingly unsustainable due to water scarcity, soil degradation, and heavy reliance on chemical inputs.

As these environmental pressures mount, the affordability and availability of staple foods, are becoming more uncertain.

And the nutritional drawbacks of our current staples (rice, wheat, maize, cassava etc.) have been listed throughout the previous chapters.

Even though the current situation of the world is as such, right now, there are intense research and developments going on in the scientific world, to develop a food source that is affordable, highly nutritious, that which can be created in a short period of time, in very small spaces, with minimal requirement of water or fertilizers or even sunlight.

Now you could be wondering what crop could we possibly cultivate in such conditions…

Every kind of farm or crops that we can think of, are hundreds of acres in size, require constant attention and care for at least 4 months of a year, are heavily dependent on thousands of litres of water, and hundreds of kilos of fertilizers.

Additionally, they also require ample amount of sunlight, with a necessity of either expensive heavy machinery, or very large numbers of man-power, and are extremely dependent on the weather and climate.

All of these factors can heavily affect the crop's cost… and even if all goes well, the *'nutritional'* value of our current staple foods (rice, wheat, corn etc.) are extremely low.

The perfect food, that can replace our current staple, is *Mushroom*!

Mushrooms have the potential to be considered a significant food source in the future due to several reasons-

- *Nutritional Value*- Mushrooms are much better sources of fibers, protein, vitamins and minerals, unlike our current staples, which are mostly high in energy giving sugars.

- *Sustainability*- Mushroom cultivation is quite sustainable compared to traditional crop farming. It requires fewer resources such as water, land, and fertilizers to grow, and they can be cultivated using various substrates, including agricultural waste materials like sawdust or even coffee grounds.

  Mushrooms can be grown in controlled environments, which reduces the negative impact of large scale farming on natural ecosystems.

- *Versatility*- Mushrooms are incredibly versatile and can be incorporated into a wide range of dishes, including soups, stir-fries, salads, sandwiches, and even as meat substitutes. It's unique texture and flavour makes it a popular ingredient in cuisines worldwide.

- *Bioconversion & Waste Management*- Mushrooms have the remarkable ability to break down plant and animal waste into simpler forms, through the process of decomposition.

  This ability can be harnessed for waste management, contributing to the efforts towards environmental sustainability.

- *Cultural Acceptance*- Mushrooms are already a widely accepted and consumed food in almost all countries and cultures around the world.

  As global food preferences evolve, the familiarity and popularity of mushrooms will continue to increase, driving demand for innovative mushroom-based products and dishes.

- *Technological Advances*- Advances in cultivation techniques, genetic engineering, and food processing technologies will further enhance the efficiency, yield, diversity, and nutritional density in mushroom production. This could lead to the development of modified varieties with improved nutritional profiles, flavours, and functional traits.

- *Medicinal Properties*- Certain species of mushrooms have been used for centuries in many countries due to their potential health benefits.

  For example, varieties like Shiitake, Reishi, and Maitake mushrooms contain bioactive compounds with antioxidant, anti-inflammatory, and immune-boosting properties.

  The growing interest in functional foods and natural remedies, will only further drive the demand for mushrooms as a dietary supplement and evolve to a healthy staple.

Mushrooms embody dual extremes, some species harbour deadly toxins, like *Amanita Phalloides*, which can be fatal when ingested, yet on the other hand, other species, such as *Ganoderma Lucidum*, offer powerful medicinal benefits, aiding in immune support and even for the treatment of cancers, which highlights mushrooms' remarkable diversity.

Here are a few notable mushrooms and their potential medicinal uses -

1. ***Reishi (Ganoderma Lucidum)*** - Known as the '*Mushroom Of Immortality*' Reishi is known to support immune function, reduce stress, improve sleep, and have anti-inflammatory and antioxidant properties. It is often used to boost overall health and longevity and is used in powdered form, as capsules, or as a tea.

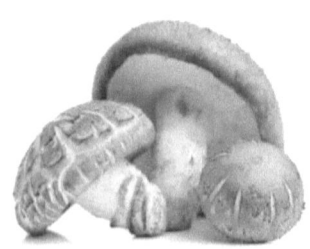

2. ***Shiitake (Lentinula Edodes)*** - Rich in polysaccharides, and compounds like lentinans, which support cardiovascular health and have anti-cancer potential.

   They are also known for their immune boosting properties, role in promoting healthy cholesterol levels, and supporting the liver function.

   They are commonly used in cooking, but are also available in supplement forms.

3. **_Maitake (Grifola Frondosa)_** - Known for their ability to support and regulate blood sugar levels. They contain beta-glucans that help modulate immune response and support overall functions of the body. They are also celebrated for their potential to enhance weight management, improve cholesterol levels, and promote healthy digestion, making them a powerful addition to a balanced diet. They are offered in various forms, including fresh, dried, as tinctures etc. for convenience.

4. **_Cordyceps (Cordyceps Sinensis)_** - 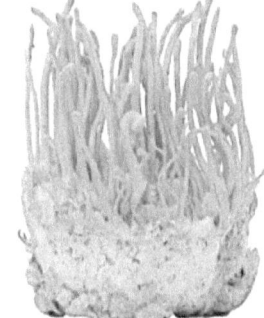 Improves our energy and endurance, supports our respiratory system, renal system and have anti-aging properties. These mushrooms are also rich in antioxidants, promote mental clarity, reduce inflammation, and supports overall well-being. They have also been found to enhance sexual function and are typically found in dried powdered form, capsules, or tinctures.

5. **_Turkey Tail (Trametes Versicolor)_** - Rich in polysaccharides such as (_Polysaccharide-K_ and _Polysaccharide Peptides_), a unique protein-bound polysaccharide, which has been used in chemo-immunotherapy for the treatment of cancer since the 1990s.

It is also known for its mild analgesic (pain relieving) and inflammation supressing properties, it is used to relieve pain and support circulation, just as the bark of the _Willow Tree_ was used (of which, its chemical compound _Salicin_ was the inspiration for the modern drug _Aspirin_).
It is available as tinctures, capsules, or as a powdered extract

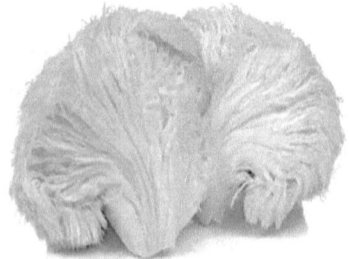

6. ***Lion's Mane (Hericium Erinaceus)*** - Reputed for its properties that stimulate NGF (nerve growth factor) production, which supports cognitive function, enhance memory, and have neuroprotective and mood uplifting effects. They are available as fresh, dried, powdered form, and capsules.

7. ***Psilocybin Mushrooms*** – They contain psychoactive compounds that are being studied for their potential to treat mental health conditions such as depression, anxiety, and PTSD.

    It is typically consumed in dried form, but its use is often controlled, and subject to legal restrictions, as research on these mushrooms are still ongoing, and they are neither widely accepted nor are they legal across the majority of countries.

8. ***Mushroom of the Gods*** *(Polyporus Umbellatus)* & ***Pouria*** *(Pouria Cocos)* - Supports digestion, and is used as a diuretic (helps in increasing urination), to reduce oedema. It is also found to be useful against issues due to mental or emotional stress, much like *Ashwagandha*, which regulates cortisol and is commonly used as dried powder or in an extracted form.

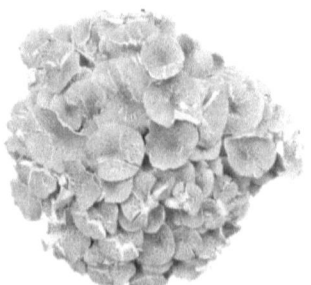

Polyporus Umbellatus

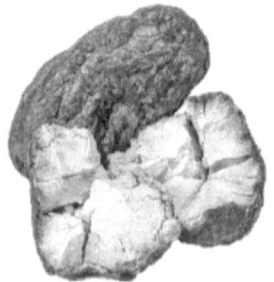

Pouria Cocos

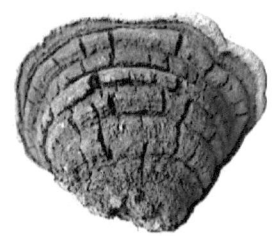

9. ***Phellinus Linteus*** - Studied and researched extensively for its potential to help with cancer treatment and overall healthy functioning of the body, this mushroom immensely supports the immune function. Phellinus Linteus also contains powerful antioxidants, reduces inflammation, and help improve liver health, promoting the healthy stimulation of bile acids, and anti-oxidants such as glutathione. It is available as an extract or in supplement forms.

10. ***Claviceps purpurea (Ergot)*** - It is a fungus that has historically been used for its effects on the nervous system. In the past, it was utilized to treat ailments such as migraines and to induce labour during childbirth. However, this mushroom is highly toxic and can cause severe side effects if consumed improperly, including hallucinations, gangrene, and even death. Due to its dangerous nature, its modern use is strictly limited to controlled pharmaceutical applications. Ergot alkaloids are now primarily used in specific medical treatments, and it is only available in regulated forms such as pharmaceutical extracts and preparations.

These are only a very few of the potentially, hundreds of species of mushrooms on this planet that can be used for its immense benefits. Each mushroom offers a unique set of benefits, and their effects can vary based on individual health conditions, and the form in which they are consumed. When using medicinal mushrooms, it's important to consult with a healthcare professional, especially if you have underlying health conditions, or are currently under any other medications.

There is still hope for our future generation and their health, as you can see, the capability to address the human species' various nutritional, environmental, economic and health-related challenges, positions mushrooms, not only as a promising staple food of the future, but also as a potent part of our healthcare as well.

Chapter XXIII – Treatment of the Future.

[i] *The most basic fact to understand is that-* "*The Body Heals Itself*"

If someone has a fractured bone, Doctors have nothing to do but wait. Wait until the fractured person's body, takes its own time, to regrow and merge, and eventually repair itself.

Of course Doctors can assist them, by covering the area in a hard cast, or by placing various types of re-enforcements for support…
but in the end, **The Body Heals Itself**.

The same goes for almost every disease known to man.
If we support our body in the right way, it will pave way for repair.

I feel the need to mention this point because, the common belief is that **Medicines,** heal the body, which is not true. **The Body Heals Itself**.

Medicines are only meant for supporting the body during emergencies.

That is why we should never, completely depend on medicines, to take care of our body.

Medicines are only a fraction of what our body requires, which will give us a little more precious time, and the essential support needed, for us to change the 'major factor' that directly influence the power of our body to heal itself, which is - *The Food We Eat*.

This is why diseases deeply influenced by diet, lie within our control.
We have the power to decide, whether the disease, should stay or not.

For example, if you take the case of Thyroiditis, the *Thyronorm* tablets, are a human made alternative to our natural thyroid hormone.

However, this is never going to solve our thyroid issue.
Of course it will give us a much needed relief, but we really need to address the exact cause of the issue in order to resolve the dysfunction.

The most common underlying issues that causes thyroid issues are -

1. Lack of raw ingredients in our body, required to naturally synthesize the thyroid hormone. Raw materials such as zinc, selenium, sodium, iodine, iron, tyrosine, vitamin-A, vitamin-D etc.

2. Conversion from T_4 to T_3, not taking place due to a sluggish bile, or an issue with our liver (wherein the conversion must take place), like fatty liver or a viral infection.

3. Uptake of the thyroid hormones into our cells, being blocked, by excess of free flowing molecules like *Cortisol* (due to excessive stress), or *Estrogen* (explained in later chapters).

4. Thyroid hormone carrier proteins like **TBG**, **TTR**, or **HSA** not being produced enough, or not produced at all, due to liver disorders, which then impairs the transport of the thyroid hormone in our body.

5. Auto-immune bodies like **Anti-TPO**, **ATG**, and **TSI** being produced in our body as a reaction, to an infection in our gut, which then does not allow our body to synthesize the thyroid hormones.

6. Nodules or abnormal growths on the thyroid gland, which obstructs its function.

In the long run, **NOT** addressing the exact cause of the issue, will only result in, the symptoms of a dysfunctional thyroid, like fatigue, weight gain, cold intolerance, joint pain, depression and much more, to hauntingly return much stronger than before.

Emergency and trauma care, on the other hand, is a different aspect altogether. Even if you are at the brink of death due to accidents, or complications of a chronic disease, or due an organ failure, there is a **40%** chance for survival, even in cases of severe injuries, compared to that of **7%** before 1960, which can be entirely credited to, the medical and technological advancements of modern medicine.

But even with the emergence of countless *Super Specialty Hospitals* throughout the world, aimed at providing a sophisticated, and symptom free life, the statistical details from leading medical journals, report that we are in fact, becoming more **unhealthy** as a species.

Here are few disheartening facts -

- The rate of **Diabetes** rose from around **211 million** in 1992 globally, to approximately **476 million** in 2017.
- **Parkinson's Disease** was reported to affect 43 out of every 100 individuals worldwide as of 2017.
- **262 million** suffering from **Asthma** in 2019, resulted in **4,61,000** deaths worldwide.
- **10 million** deaths worldwide in 2020, due to **Cancer**.

Some of the drawbacks of the current treatment systems include –

- Risk of severe *side effects*.
- *Over-reliance* on medicine.
- Potential of our body to develop *resistance* against the medicines.
- Over-emphasis on *symptomatic management*, resulting in the neglect of underlying disorders, as well as overlooking preventive care.
- *Fragmentation of care*, which means receiving treatment from multiple specialties, resulting in miscommunication, and set-backs in the overall treatment.

Hysterectomy is one such procedure, which is a befitting example for the problems that we have to face, when only the task at hand is kept in mind, with no concern on the impact of it on our body's overall system.

This surgery which is done to remove the uterus, is currently ranked the second most performed surgery done on women, with over **1.5 Million** surgeries done in the year 2016 alone.

Over 90% of hysterectomy done, were **not** life threatening and only less than 8% of those surgeries performed, were cancer related.

Life-long side effects such as –

- Back pain (due to removal of support ligaments and tendons that were attached to the uterus).
- Lowering of rib cage and pelvis joints which alters the feminine body shape (leading to body pain as well as emotional insecurities regarding their physical feminine appearance).

- Urinary incontinence (over 95% of those who undergo the surgery have reported this issue).
- Sudden mood changes and irritability due to hormonal imbalance.
- Low libido (which causes mental detachment from their partner, leading to depression and marital issues).
- Frequent fractures due to osteoporosis.
- Increase in cardiovascular diseases.
- Weight gain of over 10 kilogram within just 1 year after surgery (leading to obesity related issues such as fatty liver and thyroiditis).

These are all, some of the detrimental complications of this surgery.

Fibrosis, endometriosis, menorrhagia and dysmenorrhea or family planning are not good enough reason to simply –

"remove and throw away" this **"mere organ of reproduction."**

The uterus plays a much bigger role for the overall health of the body.

As or cases like uterine prolapse, where the uterus descends from its normal position, a procedure known as ***Sacro-hysteropexy*** is a more effective, alternative technique which involves securing the uterus back in place, offering better outcomes without the need for removal.

By focusing on preserving the uterus whenever possible, women can maintain their hormonal balance and reproductive health, and avoid unnecessary and potentially life-altering surgeries.

Proper treatment options should be explored and tailored to each individual's needs, and made known to them, ensuring that they understand the true impact of it, and have a real chance to make an informed choice.

Tonsillectomy which is the surgical removal of the tonsil nodes in the throat, is also such a commonly performed procedure.
It is usually performed to treat chronic tonsillitis and sleep apnoea.

It has been one of the most frequently conducted procedures, with over **500,000** surgeries conducted annually in the United States alone.

However, studies indicate that more than 75% of these surgeries are actually **not** medically necessary and could have been managed with alternative treatments.

The long-term side effects of tonsillectomy include an increased risk of respiratory infections due to the loss of the first line of immune defence in the throat, heightened susceptibility to allergies, and the potential for long-term changes in speech and swallowing.

Research has also linked childhood tonsillectomy to a significantly higher risk of developing respiratory diseases such as asthma, chronic bronchitis, and even pulmonary fibrosis later in life. Additionally, studies also suggest that the removal of tonsils can contribute to metabolic and autoimmune disorders, increased risk of obesity due to altered gut microbiota, and higher rates of psychological distress.

Instead of resorting to tonsillectomy as a quick fix, alternative treatments such as probiotic therapies, immunotherapy, and antibiotics offer effective and less invasive solutions.

Cholecystectomy (the surgical removal of the gall-bladder) is also such a procedure that is commonly mis-used (explained in later chapters).

Appendectomy which is the surgical removal of the appendix, a part of the large intestine (briefed in Chapter- 13), and *Thyroidectomy* (the surgical removal of the thyroid gland), can also be considered as prime examples for this issue of solely focusing on the immediate medical need, without considering its broader impact on the body's overall health.

This is why I have to insist and repeat,
that it is neither the sole dependence on *Medicine*,
nor *Super Speciality Hospitals* that give us complete health.

They might save us from imminent death,
but cannot guarantee a healthy body.

Our *Food Habits* and *Lifestyle* are
the only major factors for a healthy body.

[ii] The next basic fact that we should be aware of, is that-

"Bacteria or Viruses Cannot Cause a Disease, Unless Our Body Has Created a Comfortable Environment for Their Growth and Reproduction"

If you simply take the case of the COVID pandemic of 2020, a research published on October 2021, reports that the people who were affected the most by this infection, including deaths, were ones who had their blood vitamin-D_3 levels below $15_{ng/mL}$.

Even though it is categorized as normal to have Vitamin-D_3 levels at around $30_{ng/mL}$, the actual safe spot is around $75_{ng/mL}$.

Vitamin-D is often vastly under-estimated and overlooked, largely due to the misconception that it is *'just another vitamin'* when in fact it is a powerful, and essential hormone with major roles, in countless processes in our body.

It has a crucial role in our *Immune System* as well, and the widespread deficiency of vitamin-D in today's society, has significantly compromised the performance of our immune systems, weakening the body's ability to defend against infections like COVID. This deficiency played a key role in the rapid and deadly spread of the virus during the pandemic of 2020.

Two major antimicrobial peptides (AMPs) that are directly influenced by vitamin-D in our body are **Cathelecedin** and **Defensins**, which are crucial for initiating, and amplifying the innate immune response.

They help control infections in the early stages, by enhancing the function of TLR (toll-like receptors) which recognize various pathogens, and also through directly killing pathogens, and recruiting immune cells to the site of infection. Additionally, they stimulate the release of cytokines and chemokines, which promote inflammation and bridge the innate and adaptive immune systems.

They also provide an important defence against antibiotic-resistant pathogens, which are increasingly difficult to treat with conventional antibiotics. Their ability to act on multiple levels (e.g., antimicrobial, immunomodulatory, wound healing) makes them essential for maintaining tissue homeostasis and for our protection against infections.

Zinc, selenium, iron, magnesium, vitamin-C, vitamin-A, vitamin-E, folate, vitamin-B_6, and vitamin-B_{12} are a few of the essential nutrients that are equally vital, for *immune cell production* and *pathogen defence*.

An interesting period in my life, during the second wave of COVID, the hospital I was employed at, was completely transformed to a COVID care unit. No other cases were admitted.

And during my service, even though I witnessed truly extreme cases of COVID victims all around me, I was also able to notice, that many of their own relatives attending to them, who were in the hospital surrounded by these extreme cases the whole time, were never tested positive for COVID... not even once.

This highlights the importance of maintaining an impenetrable, and strong immune system for our body, as one of the major factors, among many others.

We can see lots of cases, of chronically ill patients, suffering from high blood sugar or fatty liver disease, for years together, and yet, have a robust and strong immunity, which saves them from secondary infections or diabetic ulcers. It mostly has to do with their strong genetics.
But these are exceptional cases, and one thing to always remember is -

Exceptions Do Not Disprove The Rule...

The rule being - The lack of nutrients in the body, as well as chronic illnesses, drastically reduces the body's immunity, and lowers our body's ability to fight off diseases.

So even though micro-organisms such as *H. Pylori* or *E. Coli* can cause gastritis, ulcers, or UTIs (urinary tract infections), the real reason that they are able to successfully form large colonies and cause damage in our body, is due to the fact, of an impaired ***Immunity***.

[iii] This brings us to one other basic fact to keep in mind, which is-
"The Starting Point Of All Diseases, Is Inflammation."

Almost all diseases known to humankind have one thing in common - ***inflammation.***

It is the very first reaction of the human body, which signals that something is going wrong, and helps to resolve the injury.

But inflammation is also the root cause of all diseases, especially when it is **chronic** (long-term), **un-addressed**, **un-treated** and **un-resolved**.

All disease can be traced back to five major inflammations in the body-

1. **Mitochondrial** inflammation -
   Diseases due to oxidative stress such as cancer.
2. **Gut layer** inflammation -
   Diseases like allergies, and auto-immune conditions.
3. **Visceral fat** inflammation -
   Leads to insulin resistance and metabolic diseases.
4. **Cellular** inflammation –
   Causes itching, pain and damage.
5. **Endothelial** inflammation –
   Causes heart blocks, varicose veins and strokes.

Now in modern medical terms, these inflammations can be translated as the work of something called as ***interleukins*** (IL), which are a part of, and a response from our immune system, which helps regulate inflammation and immune responses to certain conditions.

These interleukins are produced by various cells in our body like the macrophages, dendritic cells, and T-cells, and they can have both ***PRO***-inflammatory as well as ***ANTI***-inflammatory effects.

Pro-inflammatory interleukins, initiate an immune response from our body, towards enemies or pathogens. It activates and recruits immune cells to the site of infection or injury. **IL-1β** and **IL-6** are critical in fighting infections, but can also contribute to severe inflammation and sepsis, if overproduced.

Anti-inflammatory interleukins on the other hand, helps to prevent excessive inflammation and tissue damage. **TGF-β** (*Transforming Growth Factor-beta*) and **IL-10** and are such anti-inflammatory interleukins.

Dysregulation of interleukins can lead to autoimmune diseases, such as multiple sclerosis, SLE, and rheumatoid arthritis.
For instance, **IL-1, IL-6,** and **IL-17** are involved in these diseases and promote unregulated inflammation often leading to auto-immunity.

When it comes to treating diseases, these interleukins, can be targeted more effectively, if we know under what category they come under.

TH-1, TH-2, and **TH-17,** are the major groups of immune cells, and originate from a type of white blood cell, involved in our body's '*acquired immunity*' which has highly specific actions against diseases.

The other type of immunity is ***innate immunity***, a non-specific immune defence system, with which we are born.

- The **TH-1** (T-helper 1) cells, are involved in ***Cell-Mediated Immunity,*** or defending the body against intracellular pathogens, such as viruses and bacteria, and activates macrophages to kill, and clean infected cells.

- The **TH-2** (T-helper 2) cells, are involved in ***Humoral Immunity,*** and play a key role in allergic responses. They produce various antibodies such as IgE, which help neutralize pathogens (especially parasites), trigger histamines, and also help to recruit other immune cells involved in allergic inflammations.

- The **TH-17** (T-helper 17) cells, are involved in ***Auto-Immune Diseases,*** to protect the body against fungal and bacterial infections, particularly those involved in mucosal surfaces like the gut.
  Hyper-activity of TH-17, can attack our own body, which is auto-immune disease, leading to chronic inflammation and tissue damage.

Targeting, and regulating these specific subsets of T-helper cells, and their respective interleukins, are currently being done quite successfully through the use of specific medicines. But this only helps in successfully lowering the pain, swellings, damage and discomfort for the patient, for a short time. Targeting the root cause of the issue (which is often ignored), gives a more permanent solution for the inflammation.

When it comes to the treatment of the future…

these **Three Basic Facts** are going to dictate it.

Anything that can enhance our body's ability to heal itself, increase our immunity and that which helps reduce any inflammations, is the direction we are heading to, and have already long started.

Usually, the elite and wealthy, are the ones who enjoy the benefits of innovations, sometimes even, for many years, before it becomes affordable to the general masses.

There are countless new technology for treatment as such, that has not yet become mainstream, due to high cost.

Bear in mind, these costly machines and medicines, are still doing the very same thing that we have been discussing throughout this book. The primary role is for **NUTRIENTS.**

This begs the question, why not just eat good food for nutrients?

Why the need for costly procedures and machines?

The fact is that, all these different methods have been developed, to help the nutrients get absorbed into the body, and reach the targeted area as quick as possible, because the body, when diseased, can sometimes face issues while ingesting, digesting or during the absorption of the food.

Factors such as the presence of excessive heavy metals in the body, or parasitic, fungal, viral, bacterial infections, stress, lowered immunity and much more, can all become barriers, that prevent nutrients from the good food, from giving us its benefits.

So for a more quick and guaranteed result, extracted nutrient mixtures, specified for each individuals body requirements, are injected or infused directly into the body, and other factors that can hamper the absorption, are dealt with appropriately.

For example, I had dealt with a patient who was suffering from an extreme case of psoriasis. As we had to heal the gut, we began the treatment for the same. But since his gut was already inflamed severely, the medicines and food given, were not being properly absorbed.

Even after 3 months, we could not see any kind of improvement. We then opted to give him specific nutrients through IV infusions. We were able to notice positive results just within two weeks of starting the intra-venous infusion.

The essential nutrients, antioxidants, mitochondrial boosters etc. can be introduced into the body not only through IV infusions, but also through IM injections, suppositories, or via direct absorptions as in sub-lingual or buccal routes etc.

So even though the root cause of the issue has been identified, when it comes to the treatment, we might have to choose different methods, specific to each case.

This is the treatment of the future, with only minimal need for powerful drugs, that comes with equally powerful side-effects, and that which only focuses on the symptoms, rather than the cause.

Recently scientists have discovered a new way to destroy cancer cells.

"Molecular Jack-Hammers" a nick-name given to amino-cyanine molecules, a type of fluorescent synthetic dyes used for medical imaging, which are very good at getting attached to the fatty outer lining of cells.

These are then stimulated with near-infrared light, causing them to vibrate in sync, which breaks apart the membranes of cancer cells, with up to 99% success rate.

The Oncothermia or *Modulated Electro-Hyperthermia (mEHT)* device is gaining much popularity all over the world currently, as a treatment in combination with diet and nutrition, and also in an integrated system, along with conventional chemotherapy and radiation, due to its ability to strongly enhance the effectiveness of other treatments.

Yet another such innovation, is the *Enhanced External Counter Pulsation* or **EECP** machine. It is a natural bypass technique that encourages the growth of new blood vessels, for smooth and uninterrupted blood flow, and is an alternate for angioplasty or bypass surgery. The device puts pressure on the legs, to send more blood to the heart while it rests, and as the blood flow to the heart improves, so does the symptoms.

And as it is a non-invasive method, the patients can take the treatment as an out-patient. It increases one's ability to be physically active, without suffering symptoms like as chest pain or weakness.

A few of the other highly beneficial procedures include –

- *Automated Colon Hydrotherapy*, which cleanses the full length of our colon or large intestine in just a session of 40 Minutes, helps in the prevention and treatment of diseases that originate from inflammations of the gut (detailed in Chapter- 13).

- *Platelet Rich Plasma Therapy* (PRP) does wonders in the case of degenerative issues like osteo arthritis, degenerative inter-vertebral disc diseases, or in cases like severe hair fall, or for slow healing diabetic ulcers, and much more. This procedure has currently become mainstream, due to its success in the cosmetics industry.

- *Chelation Therapy* which involves introducing a chemical solution of EDTA, which is helpful to treat acute and chronic heavy metal poisoning, by binding to and pulling out heavy metals such as lead, cadmium, mercury etc. from the bloodstream.
  It is helpful in treating many diseases, which also includes, the reduction in formation and size of atherosclerotic plaques (heart blocks), that affect the arteries.

- *Hyperbaric Ozone Therapy* stimulates our stem cells, causing an influx of our enzymatic anti-oxidants, that supports our body in its fight against cancer, auto-immune diseases, infections, neuro-degenerative issues like Alzheimer's disease, diabetic ulcers etc.

These are just a few of the many, very successful innovations, that more than 80% of the world population are not aware of, and as always, these procedure are highly successful, when done as a supportive care, along with the primary base, of a healthy food habit.

Chapter XXIV – Diseases at Our Mercy.

In this chapter, we will briefly go through some of the very common, and a few uncommon diseases, that I come across in my clinical practice.

Even though there are many aspects to the diseases that we will be going through, I will neither be writing about the minor details of the disease, nor aspects of the disease that we have no control over.

We will only be discussing the most significant parts of the disease, and in which, we can bring about a significant improvement, through the change in our food habits.

I intend to write about the diseases as simple as possible, and will also mention what changes we can make in our food habits and diet patterns, to support our body in the healing process.

Most of the diseases have very similar root causes, and so, I would like to classify them as such.
This can help in recognising diseases for what they really are, which can then, give us a sense of power over these conditions.

But this kind of perspective, is often met with the criticism, of having a *'Reductionist'* approach, which means to describe a complex phenomenon, in terms of its simple or fundamental nature.

In truth, it is actually more logical to treat a disease at its root cause, than to simply attend to its symptoms alone, in order to try and get rid of the disease altogether.

This reminds me of a very interesting statement that I had come across-

'To get to the root cause of a disease, treat it with the mind of an Engineer, not a Doctor.'

If you took your car to a mechanic because it was emitting black smoke from the exhaust, he wouldn't simply try to mask the problem by adding a filter (which would only treat the symptom). Instead, he'd inspect the engine, check the oil, and identify the underlying cause of the issue.

By fixing the root problem, the black smoke would stop altogether.

But there must be a balance in treating both the outward symptoms, as well as the root cause of the disease.

This does not mean, that these steps are the only ones enough, to completely treat the disease in all individuals, which means that, if you are under medications or in a serious health risk, please do not try to treat yourself without the consultation, diagnosis, or professional guidance from a competent, registered Medical Doctor or Physician.

Navigating through a disease, and supporting the body throughout the healing process is a delicate balancing act, one that even when perfected after handling hundreds of such cases, can still bring a unique challenge for each individual case, in order to accomplish a positive result.

To start with, let us discuss the diseases that comes under the direct influence of **Insulin Resistance (IR)***, explained in* **Chapter- 4.**

- **24.1 – <u>Overweight & Obesity</u>**

The important thing to note about obesity, is that, a person can look lean or thin, and still be obese.
It is called **Visceral Obesity**, which is too much fat deposition in and around our vital organs, like the liver or ovaries.

It is commonly believed that having a lean body and a normal **BMI** (*Body Mass Index*) equates to being healthy. This is quite far from the truth. BMI is not reliable for health evaluation as it cannot measure the visceral fat, which is the root cause for most metabolic diseases.

	Average Indian	*Sumo Wrestlers*
Daily Caloric Intake	**2200** calories	**7000** calories
Body Mass Index	Around **24**	Around **45**
Diabetic Prevalence	**20%**	**2%**

A prime example is that of Sumo wrestlers who consume up to 7000 calories a day, which is significantly higher than the required daily intake (around 2500 calories), and have an average BMI of above 45 which is classified as 'morbidly obese' or as class-3 obesity.

Despite this, they do not typically suffer from symptoms of obesity, cardiovascular diseases, or other issues of metabolic syndrome, which are often associated with excess fat accumulation.

This is largely due to the distribution of fat in their bodies.

While they accumulate large amounts of body fat, the fat is primarily stored as *subcutaneous adipose tissue* (SAT). Sumo wrestlers' high-calorie diet, combined with intense physical training, along with adequate rest, leads to the accumulation of fat in SAT, which does not pose the same health risks as *visceral adipose tissue* (VAT).

In contrast, the average BMI of an Indian adult is around 24 which is considered within the normal weight range.

Despite this seemingly healthy BMI, India has a high prevalence of diabetes, with around 20% of the adult population affected.

While many Indians may not have excess overall weight, a significant portion of their fat is stored as VAT, which is more metabolically active and harmful than SAT. a largely sedentary lifestyle with diets high in glycaemic index, promotes fat storage in the VAT.

Waist Hip Ratio (**WHR**) on the other hand, even though mostly inaccurate for sumo wrestlers, is still a more reliable measurement to predict an early death than BMI, in normal individuals.

Researches conducted in British populations, have found that the risk of mortality (death) was lowest, for those with the lowest WHR, and it rose steadily with increase in the WHR.

It is calculated by, dividing the waist by hip circumference.

According to the *World Health Organization*, a healthy WHR is –

- 0.9 or less for men.
- 0.8 or less for women.

The most confusing part to people, is the origin, of their obesity.

Everyone has a different theory on why, their body started to put on weight, and the most commonly told reasons are, that it was due to their hypothyroidism, PCOD, pregnancy, child birth etc.

A few claims such as, COVID vaccinations or the usage of a particular skin care product, caused their obesity, is also common claim recently.

But these are all negligible factors when taking into account the role that the type of food we eat, has to play, in one ending up with obesity.
We have also debunked the infamous myth, that consuming lots of eggs and meat, causes obesity.

*'Which came first, the **Chicken** or the **Egg**?'*

*'Which came first, **Obesity** or **Metabolic Diseases**?'*

It is often confusing to most, including medical professionals, as to whether the disease caused obesity or the other way around…

as there is no argument in, the potential of both these issues becoming the causative factor for each other.

Without a doubt though, visceral obesity came first.

This then leads to other diseases, which in turn, causes even more deposition of fats in the body, leading to furthermore increase in their obesity condition.

Even though factors like genetic predisposition of obesity, and heavy doses of *Non-Steroidal Anti-Inflammatory Drugs* (NSAIDs), or prolonged stress hormones contribute to, or even accelerates this process, obesity can still be avoided, and controlled through a healthy and balanced diet and appropriate regulators (especially in the case of excessive stress).

When it comes to treating obesity, I have personally found Dr. Eric Berg's guide for body type, to be of extreme functionality.

This classification is based on the underlying issues that primarily influence a specific type of fat distribution on the body.

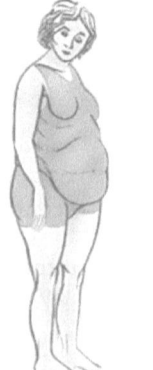 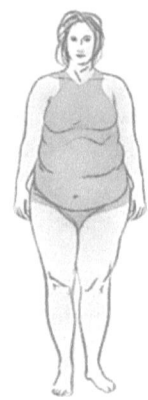 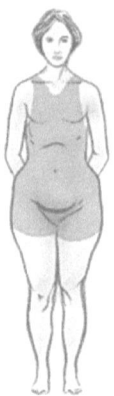 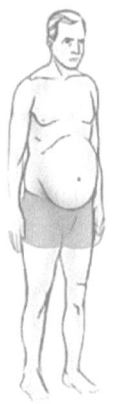

Adrenal & Pancreatic   *Thyroid Type*   *Ovarian Type*   *Liver Type*

<u>**ADRENAL**</u> - Common characteristics of the adrenal body type are sagging belly fat, high stress levels, and they often experience brain fog, crave for salty foods, and find it challenging to stay calm under stress. An imbalance of cortisol (stress hormone) is at the root of the problem so merely a healthy diet will not fully resolve this issue. Balancing stress and cortisol is the key.

THYROID - Those with the thyroid body type store fat evenly throughout their bodies instead of in one area. Slow metabolism is the primary characteristic of thyroid types, and experience digestive issues (gas, bloating, indigestion) when they consume large servings of protein. Plenty of iodine-rich foods and an OMAD (one meal a day) along with intermittent fasting plan is helpful in this type of obesity. Further details will be covered in the upcoming subtopics.

OVARIAN - Those with the ovarian body type, hold weight in their hips and below the belly button. Overactive ovaries or estrogen dominance can cause the body to accumulate fat in these areas. Those with the ovary body type are also highly sensitive to endocrine disruptors including pesticides, fungicides, and herbicides. The most important foods for balancing estrogen are cruciferous vegetables. hormone-free and non-GMO foods are also beneficial for supporting the estrogen balance. Further details will be covered in the upcoming subtopics.

LIVER - Those with the liver body type typically have a protruding belly, sometimes called a pot belly or beer belly, and may also experience skin issues like psoriasis and dermatitis. Men are most likely to have a liver body type, though women can be liver types too. There is a buildup of fat cells in their liver tissue and around other organs. It is essential to avoid alcohol and excessive protein, and instead, consume plenty of salads and low-carb vegetables with moderate proteins and healthy fats. Further details will be covered in the upcoming subtopics

PANCREATIC - Sometimes the body shape isn't enough to determine the primary body type. The pancreatic body type can have an identical body shape to the adrenal type, but the difference is the trigger. The pancreatic body type is affected by insulin resistance.

This classification though, should only be viewed as a guiding framework, as in practice, multiple issues often overlap. Successfully treating each individual typically requires a combination of approaches tailored to their unique needs. The changes that need to be included, in the diet, to treat and manage **Overweight** and **Obesity**, is explained in the sample diet charts in Chapter- 25.

- ## 24.2 – Diabetes Mellitus

The root cause for **Type-2 Diabetes Mellitus**, is *Insulin Resistance*, which is, our body rejecting the *Insulin* hormone, that leads to the presence of excessive sugar in our blood.

Type-1 Diabetes Mellitus on the other hand, occurs because the *Insulin* hormone is not produced in our body. It can be due to an auto-immune condition or due to a genetic defect. Whatever may be the cause, it may seem impossible, for a life without the *Insulin* hormone.

But as we have discussed, we can by-pass our dependence, on the sugar-insulin combination as our fuel of energy, and opt to give our body, fats to burn as fuel for energy production.

This is the most healthy and logical way to go about it, and is a total 'win' situation, with no adversities. In case you haven't noticed yet, the essence of this book is, in a way, about how we **do not** have to be totally dependent, on the inflammatory sugars and insulin!

Now other kinds of diabetes like, gestational diabetes, neonatal diabetes, LADA, MODY, brittle diabetes, secondary causes due to steroid use, endocrinopathies etc. can all be listed under either Type-1 or Type-2, according to the root cause of the issue.
So these are considered as minor details, when looking at the larger picture, and doesn't need to be necessarily addressed when choosing a healthy diet. Patients injecting *Insulin* though, as mentioned earlier, must be under the guidance of a registered Doctor or Physician.

Fasting Blood Sugar (**FBS**), Random Blood Sugar (**RBS**) and Post Prandial Blood Sugar (**PPBS**) are the usual tests done, to monitor blood sugar levels of an individual.
But these are not as reliable, because of the heavy variations, depending on the food that the individual would have had before the test, or according to their metabolism, or even stress levels.

The most reliable test to determine whether the individual is pre-diabetic or diabetic, is to conduct a serum **HbA1c**, which is the average of a person's blood glucose levels, of the past 2 to 3 months.

One other common mistake done by diabetic patients, is to check their serum *Creatinine* levels, to look for potential damage to their kidneys.

But by the time we find any alarming changes in the creatinine levels, high sugar levels would have already caused significant damage.

So, the test that can give us the accurate information on the health of our kidneys, is the **eGFR** (*estimated glomerular filtration rate*).

A small alert, to any diabetic patients following my sample diet chart is, **DO NOT** panic when you see that your FBS levels are high...
which definitely will be, when you start the diet.

During the intermittent fast, your body will start to convert the sugars, that are stored as fat in your body, back into sugars, to use them as fuels for energy production.

This is called *Gluco-neo-genesis,* and your FBS will reduce to normal levels after around 3 to 5 months of this healthy diet, when your visceral fat stores, become empty.

Patients suffering from severe low blood sugar, or Hypoglycaemia, usually get a feel of it, just before it occurs, and so all they need to do is, to have a spoonful of honey, or glucose powder or any kind of sweets, to help the body get some instant energy, just for the sake of the moment... but continue the diet as advised.

The diet itself, will help lower the *Insulin Resistance* in the long run, and effectively, help get rid of these episodes of Hypoglycaemia.

The changes that need to be included, in the diet, to treat and manage **Diabetes Mellitus**, is explained in the sample diet charts, in Chapter- 25.

- ## 24.3 – Type-3 Diabetes or Alzheimer's Disease

Recent research studies have concluded that Alzheimer's disease should also be classified as a type of diabetes, because *Insulin Resistance* and insulin-like growth factor dysfunction in the brain, is the primary cause for Alzheimer's disease.

However, **Type-3 Diabetes** is not currently, an official medical term yet.

Another classification of diabetes, *Type-3c Diabetes Mellitus* or *Pancreatogenic Diabetes*, develop due to conditions that affect the pancreas. Despite having a similar name, this is a separate condition.

Untreated diabetes can cause damage to your blood vessels over time, including vessels in our brain, and most people who have *Type-2 Diabetes Mellitus* (DMT2) do not know that they have the condition, which delays the diagnosis and treatment.

DMT2 can directly cause vascular dementia, often thought to be Alzheimer's, but it is a separate disease with diagnosis and symptoms of its own, and it is also a warning sign of what it will develop into, which is Alzheimer's disease.

According to a research, from 2016, that involved more than 100,000 people living with dementia, it was found that people who have DMT2 are up to 70% more likely to develop Alzheimer's disease or another type of dementia, such as vascular dementia.

It also showed that females with *Type-2 Diabetes Mellitus* (DMT2), had a much higher probability of developing vascular dementia than males. It was also found that more than 98% of the brains of Alzheimer's patients, on immediate inspection after death, was significantly affected by fungal infection or mold.

This indicates the importance of maintaining a healthy gut flora as well.

Symptoms of Alzheimer's can include, memory loss that affects daily living and social interactions, difficulty completing familiar tasks, misplacing things often, decreased ability to make judgments based on information, sudden changes in personality and other symptoms.

The sooner the treatment begins, the better will be the chances for improvement. How quickly an individual receive a diagnosis and start the treatment, is essential in Alzheimer's, because unlike other diseases, the brain is affected in this case, and the speed at which repair occurs in brain cells, are so slow, that it is only practical to prevent this issue rather than treat it at its extreme stages.

According to the *Alzheimer's Association*, the average life expectancy for a person with Alzheimer's is around 4 to 8 years from their diagnosis.

But the average life expectancy of those who have undergone early detection and diagnosis of Alzheimer's can live up to 20 years longer.

Prescription medications may treat cognitive symptoms of dementia, but there is an uncertainty about whether they have a noticeable impact on the symptoms of Alzheimer's disease.

Proven methods for preventing, managing and minimizing organ damage from **DMT2** and **DMT3** include, leading a healthy and well balanced life-style. The changes that need to be included, in the diet, to treat and manage **Alzheimer's** or **Type-3 Diabetes**, is explained in the sample diet charts, in Chapter- 25.

- ## 24.4 – <u>Poly-Cystic Ovarian Syndrome (PCOS)</u>

Commonly known as Diabetes of the Ovaries, it is a condition, characterized by hormonal imbalances, majorly due to inflammation from fat deposits in the ovaries, as studies have reported that more than 70% of the PCOS cases, are caused due to *Insulin Resistance*.

This disease has a wide range of negative impact on women's health, and is one of the leading cause for *Infertility* in women.

Prolonged inflammation of the ovaries in the female body, produces immature eggs in large numbers, and over time, these become cysts in the ovaries.

These cysts, itself, are almost always, neither painful nor dangerous, but causes the ovaries to become large, and secrete increased amounts of male hormones (androgens), which can cause infertility, irregular and painful menstrual cycles, hair loss, mood swings, acne, skin tags, hirsutism (excess facial hair and heavy hair growth on arms, chest and abdomen), and much more painful, and truly uncomfortable symptoms.

Even though it is visceral obesity that causes PCOS in the first place, once PCOS sets in the body, then in return, PCOS itself becomes a reason for obesity, and it becomes a never ending cycle, where one reason becomes the cause for the other and vice-versa.

Despite the name "**poly-cystic**," you don't actually need to have cysts on your ovaries, to have PCOS. The other symptoms are enough to qualify a woman with an active menstrual cycle, for being a victim of this condition, especially when high imbalance in levels of hormone occurs.

It is estimated that around 50% of girls around the age of 8 years, develop early onset of puberty in developing countries, due to estrogen mimicking compounds and increased production in estrogen, as a result of high levels of refined oils found in weening foods and infant formulas, where estrogen equivalent to 5 birth control pills per day, is consumed by children.

This sets the body up for early onset of PCOS.

It is estimated that up to 20% of women world-wide of reproductive age, suffer from poly-cystic ovarian syndrome.

The usual treatments include -

- Insulin-sensitizing medicine- *Metformin* (same drug for **DMT2**).
- Medications to block androgens, helps control acne or hair growth.
- Medications that help to induce ovulation (releasing an egg).
- Surgical procedure that help restore ovulation.
- In vitro fertilization (IVF) for those suffering with PCOS, for whom medications hasn't worked, and are struggling to get pregnant.

Even though these are all a testament to the achievements of our medical and technological advancements, yet the most effective, affordable, side-effect free option, to get rid of PCOS, is through a proper and balanced, healthy diet.

The changes that need to be included, in the diet, to treat and manage **PCOS**, is explained in the sample diet charts, in Chapter- 25.

- ## 24.5 – Male Infertility

The human species, is generally considered a group with low reproductive capacity. A fertile and young couple, for every month of intercourse, has around 20% chance of conceiving.

Conception depends on many factors, but in males, it comes down to essentially having healthy, motile sperms, with ability to fertilize the egg.

The primary symptom of male infertility, is being unable to have a biological child. But male infertility can also lead to many psychological and emotional symptoms.

When the infertility is associated with low testosterone levels, then symptoms such as tiredness, impotence, weight gain and depression are most commonly noticed.

Many biological and environmental factors can cause male infertility which include malformed sperm, low sperm count or the absence of sperm in the semen.

This can be due to diseases like diabetes or auto-immune conditions, infections (such as gonorrhoea, epididymitis, HIV), swollen veins in the testicles (varicocele), treatments (such as chemo- or radiation therapy), certain medications, testicular injury, hormonal disorders that affect the hypothalamus or pituitary glands, and in cases of genetic disorders.

Emotional stress, smoking and increased testicular temperature due to work, or choice of clothing, are common factors that aggravate the activities of the underlying diseases.

But the most common root causes are metabolic syndrome, and oxidative stress, which damages the sperm and the male reproductive organs.

One of the most overlooked issue is the damaged DNA of sperm, which can be tested through a DNA fragmentation rate (DFR) test, where it must be less than **15%**.

But an unhealthy lifestyle causes the DNA to have a fragmentation rate of more than **25%**, and chances for fertilization becomes very low.

If by chance fertilization does take place, the chances for an abnormal placenta formation is high, leading to increased risk of *Abruptio placentae* (also known as placental abruption, a serious pregnancy complication that occurs when the placenta separates from the uterine wall before delivery, leading to abortion), as studies have shown that the placental health depends majorly from the DNA of the sperm (or fathers DNA).

So even if there are normal amounts of motile sperms that may seem healthy, it is crucial to get the DFR test done in order to know the actual quality of the sperms. Many IVF treatments fail due to 'unknown causes,' often because this issue is overlooked. Proceeding with IVF without assessing the DFR, sets the stage for failure.

Physical examination , health history, semen analysis, ultra sound, MRI scans, venogram, blood tests, urinalysis, testicular biopsy, DNA fragmentation rate etc. are diagnostic tests to figure out what is the actual underlying cause of the infertility.

Varicocele has a root cause of endothelial dysfunction, just as the varicose vein disease, explained in detail in upcoming topics.

In few cases, surgeries such as vasoepididymostomy, or varicocelectomy, might be required to correct the underlying issue.

Assisted reproductive technology (ART) procedures such as IVF, are also done in extreme cases of infertility.

The changes that need to be included, in the diet, to treat and manage **Male Infertility,** is explained in the sample diet charts, in Chapter- 25.

- ## 24.6 – <u>Hyper-Triglyceridemia (HTG)</u>

Even though **hyper-cholesterolemia** or high cholesterol is most commonly considered as dangerous, it is actually **hyper-triglyceridemia** or high triglyceride levels in the blood, that are causing the various villainous damages in our body.

The good and the bad in fats or lipids are explained in detail, in the 7th and 8th chapters.

HTG is closely linked with many other medical issues, and can either be caused by, or lead to the cause of various other health conditions.

But more than 80% of the time, it is due to unhealthy eating habits. People with high HTG often develop *hyper-tension* (high blood pressure), and HTG is the third most common cause of *acute pancreatitis* as well.

HTG does not often have much outward symptoms or warning signs as such, but a few symptoms that those with HTG may experience are-

- *<u>Xanthomas</u>* - which are small yellow-red bumps that develop due to fat build-up beneath the skin, and can occur anywhere on the body, but usually appear near the eyelids, knees, feet, hands, and elbows.

- *<u>Abdominal pain</u>* - or discomfort may be a sign of acute pancreatitis, and upper abdomen pain is a common symptom. Nausea, fever, and tenderness around the abdomen may also be noticed.

- *<u>Lipemia retinalis</u>* - occur mostly when our triglyceride levels exceed $1000_{mg/dL}$, which is extremely high, and the eyes can get affected. This causes a creamy white discoloration of the retinal vessels which can severely impair the vision.

It is best to have regular check-ups and monitor the blood triglyceride levels, especially in children and teens whose parents have high triglyceride, or a history of heart problems.

Checking the triglyceride every five years starting at age nine, is a good start, especially if they have a sedentary lifestyle, or an unhealthy diet.

And for adults, who lead a sedentary lifestyle, or have unhealthy eating habits, it is better to get the triglyceride checked –

- Once every 5 years, until age 45.
- Once every 2 years, from age 45 to 65.
- Every year after the age of 65.

When we look through a lipid profile, the total cholesterol can be considered healthy even if it is high (more than $200_{mg/dL}$), as long as the TG and VLDL levels are below half of the indicated normal range. HDL and LDL (with lower triglyceride ratio) molecules are not harmful to our body.

Coronary Artery Disease (CAD), Peripheral Artery Disease (PAD), Hyper and Hypo-Thyroiditis, Chronic Kidney Disease (CKD), PCOD, Type-2 Diabetes Mellitus, stroke, and heart attacks are all potential complications of hyper-triglyceridemia.

When it comes to medications, even though *Fibrates* and *Nicotinic acids* are frequently used, *Statins* or HMG-CoA *reductase inhibitor*, are the most commonly used medicines.

Current evidence based researches all suggest that, it is more successful to treat HTG by having a sugar free diet, along with adequate doses of *omega*-3 supplementation, which helps lowers triglycerides, increase good cholesterol levels, and prevent the complications of hyper-triglyceridemia without any other side-effects.

The changes that need to be included, in the diet, to treat and manage **Hyper-triglyceridemia**, is explained in the sample diet charts, in Chapter- 25.

- ## 24.7 – <u>Non-Alcoholic Fatty Liver Disease (NAFLD)</u>

NAFLD was renamed in 2023 as MASLD – *Metabolic Dysfunction Associated Steatotic Liver Disease.*

The fatty liver disease was, around 70 years ago, exclusive to regular alcoholics, as heavy consumption of alcohol ended up damaging the liver.

But at present, this disease is now one of the most common diseases, such that, people and doctors alike, are not even bothered by it anymore.

And the largest group of victims in India are the women over 28 years of age, mostly stay at home mothers or home makers.

What caused the damage to their liver, similar to the damage caused from heavy alcohol use?

The combination of carbohydrates and refined oils.

This unholy combination causes the liver to swell and become damaged due to the fat deposits in the liver, which gets worse, and leads to serious liver scarring (***Liver Cirrhosis***).

The fat deposits in the '*sub-cutaneous adipocytes*' (located just under the skin), does not affect the liver much, as it is primarily drained through the '*systemic circulation*' (the blood flow from the heart to the body's various tissues and back), which means that it enters the bloodstream, and is in effect distributed more evenly across the body. This allows for a more efficient metabolism and minimizes the strain on the liver, because it doesn't directly interact with it.

In contrast, '*visceral fat*' (which accumulates around internal organs like the liver, ovaries and intestines), drains directly into the liver through the '*portal circulation*' (system of blood flow from digestive organs to the liver), creating a direct pathway for fat droplets to pile in the liver.

This leads to a much quicker fat buildup in the liver, and increases inflammation. Over time, this fat deposition contributes to the development of NAFLD, which in turn creates, or strengthens the existing insulin resistance.

This vicious cycle worsens insulin resistance, leading to further metabolic disturbances and increasing the risk of *type-2 diabetes*, cardio-vascular disease, and other metabolic issues.

* The decisive factor that determines whether the fat is stored in either sub-cutaneous cells or visceral cells, is explained in the sub-topic where we have discussed insulin resistance *

NAFLD, often does not show any symptoms, but when it does, it is mostly extreme fatigue, discomfort or mild pain in the upper right of the abdomen, pain in the upper right shoulder, and darkening of the skin. Patches of dark skin, especially in the folds of the neck, armpits, groin (between the legs) and under the breasts are often seen in cases of *Insulin Resistance*, and in NAFLD, which is called *Acanthosis Nigricans*.

When NAFLD progresses, and there is even more scarring in the liver, it leads to a condition called NASH (*non-alcoholic steato-hepatitis*) which shows may symptoms including, itchy skin, abdominal swelling (ascites), shortness of breath, swelling of the legs, enlarged spleen, red palms, yellowing of the skin and eyes (jaundice) and formation of spider-web like blood vessels just beneath the skin's surface.

NAFLD when left untreated, or if an individual opts to depend solely on medications, this condition can lead to other critical health issues like, severe liver scarring (which causes liver fibrosis and cirrhosis), swollen veins in the throat which can rupture and bleed, confusion, sleepiness and slurred speech, also called hepatic encephalopathy, hypersplenism (overactive spleen) which can cause low blood platelets, and can eventually pave the way for liver cancer.

Liver is responsible for producing a lot of *'carrier proteins'* that transport molecules like the thyroid hormone, oestrogen, testosterone etc. to different parts of the body. When the liver is diseased, this can impair many normal functions that depend on the liver.

It can commonly lead to diseases such as thyroiditis, adrenal dysfunction, estrogen dominance, testosterone deficiency, menstrual irregularities, infertility (due to hormonal imbalances), gynecomastia (enlarged breasts in men), low libido or low sex drive (especially in men), fatigue and muscle weakness (due to disrupted hormone balance), hirsutism (male pattern hair growth in women on the face, chest back etc).

Dysfunction of the liver also results in the impairment of the *histamine* metabolism as well, which leads to various allergic issues such as asthma, eczema, psoriasis etc. The weakened liver due to various stages of NAFLD is also exploited by viral and bacterial infections that can lead to auto-immune conditions.

The liver produces bile, which are essential for digestion, and also protects us against pathogens by disrupting their cell walls. However, conditions like fatty liver impair bile secretion, reducing its antimicrobial properties. This impairment makes the gut more open to infections, as bile's role in killing harmful bacteria becomes impaired.

As it turns out, gut bacteria also play a crucial role in the proper conjugation of bile acids (by convert primary bile acids into secondary bile acids, which are more effective at emulsifying fats and absorbing fat-soluble vitamins), which brings the process to a co-dependent circle, as the beneficial bacteria need bile, and bile requires bacteria.

Bile acids are also involved in regulating immune responses, helping to balance the body's defences against pathogens without causing an overactive inflammation.
This balance is essential in preventing auto-immune issues.

Expert studies estimate that around 32% of adults in India suffer from NAFLD (around 25% is the global prevalence), and around 7% are victims of NASH.

The changes that need to be included, in the diet, to treat and manage *Non-Alcoholic Fatty Liver Disease* **(NAFLD)** or *Metabolic Dysfunction Associated Steatotic Liver Disease* **(MASLD)**, is explained in the sample diet charts, in Chapter- 25.

- ## 24.8 – High Blood Pressure or Hypertension (HTN)

Hypertension is called as a *'Silent Killer'* because it hardly shows any symptoms, and can be dangerous if not treated. It puts us at risk for issues such as stroke and heart attack among many other issues.

Nearly 46% of adults who have hypertension don't realize it, so frequent check-ups are crucial, especially if the individual is overweight, or have symptoms such as shortness of breath, chest pains, blurry vision, anxiety, dizziness, or nausea.

When blood pressure is over $160/100_{mmHg}$ or higher, the individual may experience symptoms like headaches especially at the back of the head, fast heartbeat, and nosebleeds, which requires immediate medical care.

The World Health Organization estimates that globally, over 1.2 billion people aged 30 to 79, have HTN, and about 2 out of 3 of those, live in developing countries like India.

Around 80% of all cases of hypertension are due to *Insulin Resistance*, also called as **Primary Hypertension**.

When the body is trying rid itself of extra glucose, it also does it through fluids such as urine and sweat (this is why frequent urination is a primary symptom of diabetics).

So, to maintain the blood pressure (as there is loss of fluid), the body retains the sodium in the system, in order to raise the blood pressure and continue normal functioning of the body.

Insulin Resistance causes a drastic depletion of potassium in our body, and increases renin (an enzyme that leads to vasoconstriction).

Most of the time, the main focus and blame for HTN is given to sodium (sugar is the actual culprit), and ways to reduce salt, but what we should actually be doing is, to get rid of eating extra carbs and sugars, and balance our potassium levels. As for high renin levels, cold immersion baths are a highly effective, natural method for its regulation (do not try if physically weak or without the advice from a professional).

Negroid or African body structure and physiology, has adapted itself to retain salt in the body without much of the salt being lost through sweat or in urine, in response to the harsh desert heat that their ancestors used to live in, before migrating to various parts of the globe.

But salt is a highly used substance today, and so, people of African descent have a higher risk for hypertension.

Secondary Hypertension is a result of various other diseases and conditions, which include certain medications, viral infections, kidney disease, Conn's syndrome, drug abuse, renal vascular diseases etc.

The common complications of HTN are coronary artery disease, heart attacks, strokes, kidney diseases and failure, eye damage, vascular dementia, peripheral artery disease and complications during pregnancy.

Even though a change in lifestyle and diet is the right way to treat HTN, for the initial few months, the most effective way to keep HTN under control, is by having the conventional medications like ACE inhibitors, ARBs, calcium channel blockers, or diuretics, to lower the blood pressure, until the body adapts to the changes in the diet.

The changes that need to be included, in the diet, to treat and manage **Hypertension**, is explained in the sample diet charts, in Chapter- 25.

*Let us now discuss about a few diseases that takes origin from **Endothelial Dysfunction**, which was explained in* **Chapter- 5.**

- ## 24.9 – <u>Atherosclerosis (Thickening of Arteries)</u>

We usually mention atherosclerosis as *Heart Blocks*, but it should be more accurately mentioned as *"Hardening of the Arteries."*

Heart Block in fact, is officially recognized as an issue with the electrical signals (impulses) of our heart, where the rhythmic and methodical beat of our heart is affected.

When we talk about the commonly mentioned 'Heart Blocks' or Atherosclerosis, better described as 'hardening of the arteries' this condition occurs due to *Endothelial Dysfunction*, which was already explained on why it forms in our body.

TMAO (trimethylamine-N-oxide), a harmful metabolite of gut infections, are also presently one of the leading causes for the formation of atherosclerosis, among the other major reasons mentioned earlier.

Calcium deposition majorly contributes to the formation of these plaques as well, and a heart block consists of more than 40% of calcium deposits.

Over time, these atherosclerotic plaques can narrow or completely block the arteries and cause issues throughout the body.

But more often, the plaque actually bursts, leading to leakage of pus into the blood stream, forming into a blood clot, which travel up to very narrow blood vessels and creates a complete block, that commonly ends up into various life threatening conditions.

The complications of atherosclerosis depend on which arteries are specifically affected, for example –

- *<u>Carotid Artery Disease</u>* - is narrowing in the arteries close to our brain, which can cause a Transient Ischemic Attack (**TIA**) or commonly called, **stroke**. They may experience sudden numbness or weakness in their arms or legs, difficulty speaking or slurred speech, temporary loss of vision in one eye, or drooping muscles in the face.
- *<u>Coronary Artery Disease</u>* - is narrowing in the arteries close to the heart. The individual may experience chest pains (angina), a **heart attack** or **heart failure**.

- *Peripheral Artery Disease* - is narrowing in the arteries, in the arms or legs, where one may develop blood flow problems in the arms and legs. This can make them less sensitive to heat and cold, increasing their risk of burns or frostbite. In extreme cases, it can even cause tissue death in the fingers and toes (**Gangrene**).

- Atherosclerosis can also cause *Aneurysms* which are a serious complication that can occur anywhere in the body. Most people with aneurysms have no symptoms. Pain and throbbing in the area of an aneurysm may occur, and it is a medical emergency. If an aneurysm bursts, it can cause life-threatening bleeding inside the body.

- *Chronic kidney disease* - is narrowing in the arteries leading to the kidneys to narrow, which prevents enough oxygen-rich blood from reaching the kidneys. Slowly the cells of the kidney start to die out, and its normal function (which is filtering waste products and removing excess fluids), is impaired. This will cause the body to develop high blood pressure and kidney failure.

This is why *angiograms* can be unreliable, as they mostly assess the major blood vessels like those in the heart, neck, kidneys, legs etc. and may miss blockages forming elsewhere in the body (which has the potential to rupture, causing blood clots to travel and obstruct smaller blood vessels, leading to heart attacks or strokes).

A more reliable test for detecting hidden blockages is the **hs-CRP** test (*high-sensitivity C-reactive protein* test), which can indicate the presence of major plaque formations, even though it cannot directly indicate the location of the blockages.

The changes to be included, in the diet, to treat and manage **Atherosclerotic Plaques**, is explained in the sample diet charts, in Chapter- 25.

- ## 24.10 – Erectile Dysfunction (ED)

Erectile dysfunction (impotence) is the inability to get, and keep an erection firm enough, for sexual intercourse.

The male sexual arousal is a complex process involving the brain, nerves, hormones, emotions, muscles as well as blood vessels.

The various, common reasons for *erectile dysfunction* are -

- Diabetes.
- Tobacco use.
- Atherosclerosis.
- High cholesterol.
- Low testosterone.
- Multiple sclerosis.
- Parkinson's disease.
- High blood pressure.
- Urinary tract infections.
- Drug and alcohol abuse.
- Insomnia (sleep disorder)
- Benign prostate hypertrophy.
- Injuries to the nerves or arteries that control erections.
- Peyronie's disease (scar tissue forming inside the penis).
- Psychological conditions, such as stress, anxiety or depression.
- Surgeries or injuries that damaged the pelvic area or spinal cord.
- Medications, including anti-depressants, anti-histamines and other medications to treat high blood pressure, pain or prostate conditions.
- Certain medical treatments, such as prostate surgery or radiation therapy for cancer.

Even though *erectile dysfunction* can result due to any of these issues, the most commonly noted, up to **70%** of cases are due to –

- *Endothelial Dysfunction,* and
- *Diabetic Neuropathy...*

which in itself encompasses, most of the above mentioned, other causes.

Erectile Dysfunction not only results in an unsatisfactory sex life, but also causes extreme stress and anxiety, due to embarrassment or low self-esteem, leading to problems in the intimacy and relationship of the couple. And for those who are newly-wed, or trying for a pregnancy, this can be an even magnified issue.

Treatment options for erectile dysfunction include oral medications, vacuum pumps, therapy for psychological causes, hormone therapy, and surgical options such as penile implants.

But addressing the underlying conditions, and bringing out lifestyle changes can bring about a significant difference and improvement in symptoms along with medications.

Also note that if you experience a headache after taking **PDE5 inhibitor** medications (commonly known by a brand name **Viagra**), or similar medications for erectile dysfunction, avoid trying it again.

This side effect can indicate that blood flow is being significantly restricted, which could lead to serious cardiovascular risks, such as a stroke or heart attack.

The underlying cause may involve excessive blood pressure fluctuations, and it is essential to consult your Physician before further use.

The changes that need to be included, in the diet, to treat and manage **Erectile Dysfunction**, is explained in detail, in the sample diet charts, in Chapter- 25.

- **24.11 – <u>Deep Vein Thrombosis (DVT)</u>**

DVT occurs when a blood clot (thrombus) forms in the veins. It mostly occurs in the legs and can be very painful, along with tenderness, cramps, change in skin colour on the leg, a feeling of warmth on the affected leg, soreness and swelling in the affected area.
Sometimes there are no noticeable symptoms.

The main cause for DVT, is *Endothelial Dysfunction,* and it can also progress if one suffers from certain medical conditions, that affect how the blood clots.
DVT can also develop if the individual doesn't physically move for a long time, like when traveling long distances, or when on bed rest due to surgery, illness or an accident.

DVT can be a serious issue because blood clots in the veins can break loose, travel through the bloodstream and get lodged in the lungs, blocking blood flow, which leads to - ***Pulmonary Embolism***.
The warning signs of this issue, can include sudden shortness of breath, chest pain or discomfort that worsens when taking deep breaths or during coughs, feeling dizzy, fainting, rapid pulse, rapid breathing and coughing up blood

Birth control pills and hormone replacement therapy, can increase the blood's ability to clot. Being overweight or obese, smoking, cancer, heart failure, IBS, Crohn's disease, and ulcerative colitis are all culprits, that increases the risk of DVT.

Blood thinners are often used to treat DVT.
But a worrisome side effect of blood thinner medications, is that it could cause excessive bleeding from wounds, or during a menstrual cycle.

A few lifestyle changes that can help prevent and treat DVT include -

- When traveling, take frequent breaks to stretch the legs.

  If you're traveling by car, train or by airplane, stop every hour or so, and walk around, or perform the exercise that contract the calf muscles (explained in the next point).

- Forcing the calf muscles of the legs, to pump up blood.

  The best way to achieve this is by walking or jogging. If one cannot find time to go for a jog, they can exercise the calf muscles by first, repeatedly raising and lower the heels, while keeping their toes on the floor, while in a standing position.

  And then, repeatedly raising the toes, while keeping their heels on the floor, to pump up the stagnant blood back into circulation, and to give the hamstrings and calf muscles, a well-deserved stretch.

  This exercise can also be performed while sitting, which can be considered for those who have full time desk jobs, and do not have the time or convenience to do the exercise while standing.

- If you've had surgery or have been on bed rest, keep the legs slightly elevated, above the level of chest (periodically, such as half an hour raised, and half an hour at same level of body), and also try to move each limb (start carefully and slowly) as soon as possible.

- Do not cross the legs while sitting, which can block blood flow.

- Keep every risk factor that can lead to *Endothelial Dysfunction*, mentioned earlier, under control.

The changes that need to be included, in the diet, to treat and manage **DVT**, is explained in the sample diet charts, in Chapter- 25.

24.12 – Varicose Vein

Varicose veins are bulging, enlarged veins that appear twisted and bulging, often looking like ropes on the legs, usually with a dark blue or purple colour. The mild form of varicose veins, resembling a spider's web, are called spider veins, which are also noticed commonly.

Any vein that is close to the skin's surface, can become varicosed, but most often it affects the veins in the legs.
This is because, the veins in the lower part of the body are subjected to increased pressure, than other parts of the body.
Having to bear the whole body weight while standing and walking, makes the veins in the legs more likely to be a victim of varicose.

For some, it may not be painful, but if it does pain, it is usually as an ache or a heavy feeling in the legs.
A burning like sensation, muscle cramping, throbbing and swelling in the lower legs are also commonly noticed.

Usually the pain worsens after sitting or standing for a long time.
The area around the veins can also start to severely itch or irritate, and the formation a much darker pigmentation can be noticed, in the lower parts of the leg, or around the veins.

Veins are specially designed pipelines that carry blood. They contain tiny one-way valves, that closes to stop blood from flowing back to the legs. *Endothelial Dysfunction*, has a more destructive result in the veins of the legs, due to this reason. When these valves are damaged, blood starts to pool in the veins, causing varicose.

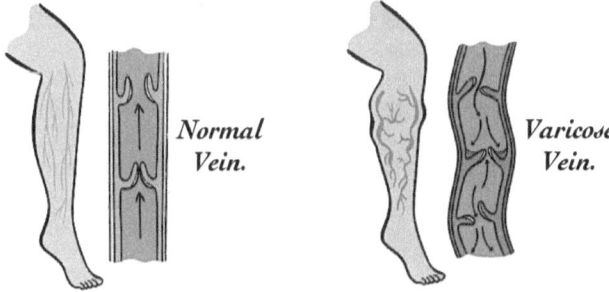

Normal Vein.   *Varicose Vein.*

Women are more likely to be victims of hormonal imbalances, and when in combination with insulin resistance, it can drastically increase their risk factor for varicose veins.

Complications of varicose veins can include swelling and painful ulcer formation on the skin near varicose veins, mostly near the ankles, which may erupt and bleed.

Usually a discoloured spot on the skin, often begins before an ulcer forms, and often times, blood clots are also formed in the veins, which aggravates the pain.

Serum homocysteine, CRP, troponin, fibrinogen, cortisol, CMV IgG, ANS analysis, renal profile, lipid profile etc. are all relevant tests that can give clues on the exact underlying issue of what is causing the varicose vein, or any diseases related to atherosclerosis for that matter.

Even though severe cases might require surgery, this will not help to stop the varicose vein from re-occurring. Only a comprehensive treatment approach which includes a balanced diet, medicines, leg raising and calf compressing exercises, along with external aids such compression stockings, is going to help treat the core issue involved in varicose veins.

The changes that need to be included, in the diet, to treat and manage **Varicose Veins**, is explained in the sample diet charts, in Chapter- 25.

Let us now discuss about a few diseases that is involved with **Fatty Liver Disease**, *which was explained in* **Chapter- 24.7**

2. 24.13 – Estrogen Dominance (ED)

Now *Estrogen Dominance* is not a disease per se, but this is a condition in the body, similar to *Insulin Resistance* or *Endothelial Dysfunction*, which stands as the root cause to so many other health issues, rising from it.

Even though I have mentioned this as an issue caused from diseases of the liver, various other issues such as –

Stress, pregnancy, ongoing hormone replacement therapy (HRT) or birth control pills, visceral obesity, PCOD, pesticides such as DDT, soy proteins (usually found in vegan protein replacements, protein bars, breakfast cereals, baby formula etc.), various infections (parasitic, fungal, viral etc.), low progesterone levels (mainly due to stress and PCOS among other causes), regular consumption of hormone injected meats (mainly red meat from commercial large scale meat factories) are all similarly responsible, either alone or in combination, for this issue.

Xeno-Estrogen which mimic the function estrogen, are also abundant around us in this modern life and is constantly finding its way into our body through micro-plastics, fragrances, makeups, pesticides, etc.

The various diseases that can arise as a result of *estrogen dominance* are -

- Thyroiditis.
- Gall-bladder stones.
- Migraine headaches.
- Uterine or ovarian Cysts.
- Uterine or ovarian Fibroids.
- Breast cancer & other cancers.
- Gynaecomastia (breast formation in males).
- Fluid accumulation in different parts of the body.

Usual symptoms of this *estrogen dominance*, are anxiety, irritability, breast tenderness, mood swings, sweet craving, joint pain, acne, fat deposits in the lower abdomen and hip, low libido, and fibroids.

Those who have severe *estrogen dominance* and have undergone menopause experience hot flashes, night sweats, vaginal dryness, increase in belly fat, cold hands and feet, and insomnia, to name a few.

One of the more severe complications of *estrogen dominance* are cancers, especially breast cancer, for which medications such *Tamoxifen*, are available, which are essentially estrogen blockers.

But as always, unless we make a difference at the root cause of the issue, the curing effects of the medications are limited.

In the case of extreme stress, when high cortisol is required in the body, it converts progesterone and as mentioned above, low progesterone causes the body to react and produce more estrogen. Detailed methods to regulate and control high cortisol is mentioned in Chapter- 10.

Aromatase is an enzyme that converts testosterone to estrogen. Including more cruciferous vegetables like cabbage, broccoli or cauliflower in the diet is helpful as these are natural aromatase inhibitors.

Make sure to also check for iodine and vitamin-D deficiencies because they play a vital role in regulating *aromatase*, and deficiencies can lead to *estrogen dominance*.

The other changes that need to be included, in the diet, to treat and manage **Estrogen Dominance**, is explained in the sample diet charts, in Chapter- 25.

3. 24.14 – **Thyroiditis (Functional)**

When it comes to functional thyroid diseases, the issues that arise are -

- During the *production* of the thyroid hormones.
- During the *conversion* of the thyroid hormones.
- During the *transport* of the thyroid hormones.
- During the *uptake* of the thyroid hormones by the cells.

A few of the common issues that can be categorized under these four broad groups are-

1. Production of thyroid hormones not taking place due to lack of raw ingredients in our body, required to naturally synthesize it, such as zinc, selenium, sodium, iodine, etc.

2. Damage to the thyroid gland, due to localized oxidative stress, from free radicals (*hydrogen peroxide* and *thyroid peroxidase*), that originally, helps in the normal conversion of iodide, into iodine form, to synthesize the thyroid hormones.

    But when there is a lack of iodine in the body, these free radicals, then damage the cells of the thyroid gland, leading to a type of *Hashimoto's thyroiditis disease*.

    The mineral selenium and glutathione, are important in helping to remove the build-up of these free radical molecules.

3. Conversion from T_4 to T_3, cannot take place in cases of thickening of the bile fluid, which is produced by the liver, commonly called as sluggish or thickened bile.

    This is caused due to lack of saturated fats and bile salts from the diet, or when there is an issue with our liver (such as fatty liver disease, or viral or bacterial infections etc), as it is responsible –

    - For the synthesis of bile.
    - Is also the site wherein the conversion of the thyroid hormone (from T_4 to T_3) majorly takes place.

4. The liver produces carrier proteins, which essentially transports the thyroid hormones, and helps in its uptake by the body.

    In cases where our liver is affected by fatty liver disease, or viral or bacterial infections, these transporter proteins such as –

    - **TBG** (*thyroxine-binding globulin*)
    - **TTR** (*transthyretin*) or **TBPA** (*thyroxine-binding prealbumin*)
    - **HSA** (*human serum albumin*) etc.

    … are not produced enough or not produced at all in the liver, and becomes responsible for a dysfunctional thyroid in our body.

5. Uptake of the thyroid hormones into our cells can be blocked, by excess of unwanted free flowing molecules such as –

    - *Cortisol* – most commonly due to excessive stress.
    - *Estrogen* – most commonly due to estrogen dominance.

    … that bond with the thyroid hormones, and then in turn, does not allow the thyroid hormones, to be efficiently taken up by the cells.

These are the common errors, that lead to thyroiditis.

The last three of these issues are almost always related to a diseased liver, directly or indirectly, and even though symptomatic treatments must be given, treating the liver should be our target point for treating the root cause of this issue.

Even though there are other factors that can cause functional thyroiditis, such as genetic factors, or as a side-effect to few psychiatric medications, or some other rare disorder, we will be only discussing here, the most common and relevant reasons, and most importantly, those causes, that we have a certain degree of control over, through changes in our diet.

The thyroid hormones affect every cell in the body, and influences factors such as our body's energy usage, controlling our body temperature, managing our heart rate, and it even plays a hand in controlling how much protein the body makes.

The common signs and symptoms of an impaired thyroid function are -

- Fatigue.
- Depression.
- Weight gain.
- Mood swings.
- Cold intolerance.
- Slowed heart rate.
- Fertility problems.
- Joint and muscle pain.
- Dry skin, thinning hair.
- Heavy or irregular menstrual periods, etc.

When thyroid issues are not treated, it can lead to complications such as,

- Goitre.
- Infertility.
- Myxoedema coma.
- Peripheral neuropathy.
- Cardio-vascular (heart) issues.
- Mental and physical birth defects, etc.

The changes that need to be included, in the diet, to treat and manage **Functional Thyroiditis**, is explained in the sample diet charts, in Chapter- 25.

4. 24.15 – Gall-Bladder Stone (Cholelithiasis)

Gall-stones are hardened, concentrated or crystallized pieces of bile that form in the gall-bladder or bile ducts.

Often, the sediment is an excess of one of the main ingredients in bile (such as *cholesterol, taurine, glycine, bilirubin* or at times, excess of *calcium*). Generally these stones won't necessarily cause any problems, but can become dangerous if it starts to travel through the biliary tract and clog it up, causing severe pain and serious complications.

Up to 75% of those diagnosed with gall-stones are women, and only 20% of those diagnosed, ever have symptoms or need treatment for the same.

Severe abdominal pain (intense, sharp, stabbing, cramping or squeezing under the right ribcage, which can radiate to the right shoulder), nausea, acidity, vomiting, fatigue, itching throughout the body, red spots on the skin, abdominal swelling and tenderness, fast heart rate, sweating, fever, yellow tint to the skin and eyes, dark urine and light-coloured stools are the common signs and symptoms associated with gall-bladder stones.

If a gall-stone blocks the flow of bile, it can cause inflammations and could even lead to bacterial infections.

When severe, it can also cause complications like pancreatitis, hepatitis, jaundice, infections in the bloodstream, low blood pressure etc.

Not enough of raw ingredients for bile such as cholesterol, taurine or glycine, lack of vitamin-C (which helps convert cholesterol to bile), high levels of the hormones estrogen, progesterone, cortisol or insulin, gut infections, fatty liver, regular consumption of excess fried foods or sweets, antacid medications etc. are some of the most common reasons for the formation of gall-bladder stones.

An abdominal ultrasound scan is a reliable and quick test to detect the gall-bladder stones, but other tests may be required if we are not able to locate the gall-stones.

Removing the whole gall-bladder (**cholecystectomy**) has become one of the most common surgeries world-wide, even at times when not necessary, as they are largely unregulated on the exact criteria of when to do so. The common belief is that the gall-bladder is of no significance to overall health and so, even non-emergency cases are admitted for cholecystectomy.

In fact, the gall-bladder is a significant organ for our health as it fixes the bile to its proper consistency, by concentrating the bile up to **20 times** more, after the liver has produced, and secreted it.
This consistency helps in the absorption of fat soluble vitamins, long chain fatty acids, and even in the conversion of the thyroid hormones.

Removing the gall-bladder puts these processes in danger, and up to **40%** of the side effects of **cholecystectomy**, like bloating, nausea, regurgitation, anal leakage of bile or mucous (with foul odour), constipation, diarrhoea etc. are present life-long after the surgery.

To maintain a healthy bile consistency, saturated fats (such as butter or coconut oil), amino acids such as taurine and glycine (abundant in meat) that form bile salts (***taurocholic*** and ***glycocholic*** acids), are needed to be part of the diet, so that the consistency of the bile do not turn to sludge, or form into stones.

If in case one has undergone cholecystectomy, be mindful while eating and stop as soon as hunger has stopped (do not overfill), and consuming diluted ACV (apple cider vinegar) just before meals, has been found to help in reducing the symptoms to a great extent. Gall-stones less than 6_{mm} in size, are sometimes found to be excreted through the stools.

The changes that need to be included, in the diet, to treat and manage **Gall-Bladder Stone** or **Cholelithiasis**, is explained in the sample diet charts, in Chapter- 25.

5. 24.16 – <u>Hyper-uricemia & Gouty Arthritis</u>

Uric acid, is usually considered as a metabolic waste in our body, but in actuality, it is a potent anti-oxidant, that actually helps our body to battle free-radicals (detailed in Chapter- 5).

But if there is an excessive amount of uric acid in our body, (known as *Hyper-uricemia*), it clumps together and forms into sharp crystals, which can settle in our joints and cause **gout**, a painful form of arthritis, and can also build up in our kidneys and form kidney stones. Hyper-uricemia is very common, and it is estimated that **1 in 5** individuals has the issue.

Usually, hyper-uricemia is blamed on the excess consumption of red meat and proteins, but we must understand that the root cause of this issue, is due to various other causes, which, if not treated, will not resolve this issue.

Hyper-uricemia occurs commonly due to three underlying issues -

1. Liver is responsible for excreting the uric acid out from our system, after its beneficial use. But in cases of a diseased liver, as in fatty liver disease, or viral infections, the liver is not able to efficiently excrete the uric acid, causing it's stagnation, leading to hyper-uricemia.

2. Foods and drinks with high fructose sugar content, triggers a bio-chemical pathway in the liver, leading to hyper-uricemia, due to over-production of uric acid.

3. E.coli bacterial infection, releases a type of toxin called ***Shiga-toxin***, to which our body responds by producing excess of an enzyme called *Xanthine Oxidase* (**XO**), to neutralize the toxin.

    But the issue is that, **XO**, incidentally, is also the molecule responsible for producing *uric acid* from the ***Purines*** (from either purine rich food, or from breakdown of DNA from dying cells).

    And since **XO** has more affinity towards the purines, it reacts and produces more uric acid, rather than neutralizing the *Shiga-toxin*.

    Through this issue, hyper-uricemia can occur due to the excessive production of uric acid.

The symptoms of a gout attack, is usually felt in smaller joints, and include those such as intense pain, discoloration or redness, stiffness, swelling, and warmth.

A feeling like the joint is "on fire" and extreme tenderness are also commonly noticed. And in cases of a kidney stone, pain in your lower back or side, nausea or vomiting caused by the pain, fever or chills, blood in the urine, pain while urinating, unable to urinate, a feeling for the need to urinate more often, urine that has a foul odour, or looks cloudy, are the usually noted symptoms.

I recommend my patients to avoid high purine foods, only if they suffer from cases of pain and gout attacks.

If they do not suffer from any symptoms of high uric acid levels, then I advise them to follow the *Insulin Resistance Diet Chart*, so that their liver inflammation subsides as soon as possible, which brings the uric acid levels under control.

Omega-3 fatty acids act wonderfully to block **NLRP3** which activates inflammation and pain due to the high uric acid levels in the body. Vitamin-C have been found to help flush excess uric acid in certain cases. In cases of an E.coli infection, appropriate antibiotics with a suitable diet, will target the issue at the root cause.

Even in cases of pain, one can contentedly consume eggs and dairy products, because they are very low in purines, and it also helps to fulfil the protein requirements of the body.

The changes that need to be included, in the diet, to treat and manage **Gout** and **Hyper-uricemia**, is explained in the sample diet charts, in Chapter- 25.

- **24.17 – Gut Related Disorders**

Let us now discuss about a few diseases that takes its origin from a bacterial, viral, fungal or parasitic infection of our gut, which was explained in **Chapter- 13**.

The common gut related disorders are –
- Auto-immune disorders.
- Digestive disorders.
- Mental disorders.
- Allergies.

Auto-immune Disorders include diseases such as –
- Uveitis.
- Vitiligo.
- Rosacea.
- IgA nephropathy.
- Multiple sclerosis.
- Myasthenia gravis.
- Sjogren's syndrome.
- Ankylosing spondylitis.
- Diabetes Mellitus Type-1.
- Rheumatoid arthritis (RA).
- Immune thrombocytopenia (ITP).
- Thyroiditis (Hashimoto's & Graves').
- Systemic Lupus Erythematosus (SLE).

Digestive Disorders can be roughly classified as –
- **Auto-Immune -**
    - Irritable Bowel Disease (IBD) such as (Crohn's disease & Ulcerative colitis)
- **Functional -**
    - Halitosis.
    - Hyper-acidity.
    - Hypochlorhydria (hypo-acidity).
    - Gastroesophageal reflux disease (GERD).
    - Irritable Bowel Syndrome (constipation, diarrhoea or both).

Mental Disorders include diseases such as –
- Autism.
- Schizophrenia.
- Attention Deficit Hyperactivity Disorder (ADHD).

Allergic Disorders include diseases with elevated levels of serum IgE –
- Asthma.
- Eczema.
- Sinusitis.
- Psoriasis.
- Urticaria.
- Dermatitis.
- Scleroderma.
- Few cases of Fibromyalgia & Rheumatoid Arthritis.

There are many more disorders that can be classified under these broad groups, and they require extreme care during treatment.

Most of these disorders are not as straight-forward as I have written them. They can have multiple sources of origin, and multiple sites of injury or complications, which are highly unique to each individual case.

Symptomatic treatment is as important, as treating the root cause in cases of these disorders, as some of these diseases can cause extreme discomfort or pain.

Even though gut infections, or gut dysbiosis is the potential root cause in up to **70%** of the cases, liver toxicity or infections due to heavy metal presence, and oxidative stress resulting from the gut or liver toxicity.

Viral infections, commonly by EBV (*Epstein Barr virus*), herpes virus, entero-virus, or CMV (*cytomegalo-virus*), which can be suspected in cases where there is high lymphocyte, and low monocyte counts in the blood work, are the root cause for around **20%** of the cases.

Severe vitamin-D deficiency has also found to be the root cause in around **10%** of these conditions.

Treatment can become complicated when a combination of these root causes present themselves with varying blood work, and a not so straight forward symptoms are present in the patient.

So it is essential that -

Treatments should ONLY be done, with the consultation, diagnosis, supervision and guidance from an expert and registered Medical Doctor or physician.

And so, I will describe in short, a few of these diseases that I routinely handle, in the same way that I have mentioned the other diseases.

But do keep in mind that these diseases are a little more complex for anyone, who do not have any prior experience treating these conditions.

Let us begin discussing about the **Disorders Of The Gut**...

... by first going through the *Functional Digestive Disorders*, as more often than not, I have found that this is truly the main villain, that leads to all other categories of Disorders Of The Gut.

- **24.18 – <u>Chronic Gastritis</u>**

Simply put, it is the inflammation in the mucosal lining of our stomach, which protects the stomach, from the acids and micro-organisms that pass through it every day.

Gastritis happens when our immune system detects a threat to this barrier, and triggers inflammation in the tissues to help fight infections and promote healing.

Gastritis can be sudden and temporary (**Acute**), or may persist long-term (**Chronic**). It can also be erosive, which means that the gastric issue is damaging our stomach lining, leaving wounds or ulcers, often from too much stomach acid, bile, alcohol, or certain drugs.

Non-erosive gastritis does not cause ulcers, but may cause irritation, and reddening of the stomach lining.

A specific form of non-erosive gastritis, called ***Atrophic Gastritis***, can cause our stomach lining to shrink and waste away, and become the cause for severe indigestion.

One very important classification of gastritis, when it comes to its treatment, is whether the gastritis is of **Hyper**-acidic or **Hypo**-acidic nature. We will discuss this in more detail, under the upcoming sub-headings with the same names.

Gastritis may not cause any noticeable symptoms, until it is so severe, that when our stomach lining is worn down enough, and our body is not able to defend itself against its own acids and enzymes anymore, and symptoms such as burping, bloating, indigestion, sour eruptions, chest burns, gastric as well as mouth ulcers, loss of appetite, nausea, stomach aches, regurgitations and vomiting are often noticed.

Infections, especially viral and bacterial ones are among the most common causes of gastritis, but less commonly, parasitic and fungal infections are also found to be reasons for this issue.

The Dominant Role of H. Pylori Bacterial Infection in Gastritis-

Helicobacter Pylori is uniquely adapted bacteria, that is able to survive the acidic environment of the stomach, primarily by producing an enzyme called *urease*.

Urease enzyme breaks down *urea*, a compound found in the stomach, into *ammonia* and *carbon-dioxide*.

The ammonia neutralizes stomach acid, creating a more alkaline environment that allows the H. pylori bacteria to thrive.

The heavy metal *Nickel*, is a vital component for this bacteria, that helps in the production of urease enzyme.

Many factors play a role in creating this heavy metal toxicity in our body which includes smoking, or eating food with high nickel content such as cocoa, chocolate, soya beans, oats, nuts, almonds, unpolished grains and legumes, to name a few, and other environmental pollutants as well.

It is vital to take this into account when dealing with persistent or chronic H. pylori bacterial infections and gastritis.

In addition to urease production, H. pylori employs other virulence factors to establish infection. It has *flagella* that enable it to move through the mucus layer of the stomach lining, and it secretes various toxins, such as **Cag-A** (*Cytotoxin-associated gene A*) and another known as **Vac-A** (*Vacuolating cytotoxin A*), which disrupts the cellular signalling pathways, and effectively creates inflammation, and induces *vacuole formations* in the gastric epithelial cells, leading to cell injury and *apoptosis*. These factors contribute to the chronic inflammation characteristic of gastritis.

(*Helicobacter Pylorus*)

The bacterium's presence leads to chronic inflammation by disrupting the protective mucus layer of the stomach lining and stimulates an immune response. This immune response can cause further damage to the stomach lining and worsen the inflammation, leading to symptoms such as abdominal pain, nausea, and bloating.

Over time, persistent inflammation results in the development of peptic ulcers and, in severe cases, even leads to gastric cancers.

Depending on the site of infections and subsequent inflammation, H. pylori is often times the cause for both **hyper-** and **hypo-** acidity, discussed further under each sub-headings.

Severe cases of *acne vulgaris* (commonly found on the face, upper arms, trunk, and back) have also recently been found to be primarily caused due to H. pylori infection, leading to an increase in sebum production, which then highly increases the chances for clogged pores and causes a **secondary** bacterial infection (commonly by *Cutibacterium acnes* - formerly named as *Propioni-bacterium acnes*).

Chronic gastritis is a common issue, with research suggesting that, as much as half of the world-wide population are victims of chronic gastritis associated with a widespread, long-term bacterial (H. pylori) infection. Even though gastritis itself isn't contagious, the infections that cause it are contagious, especially in crowded living conditions or when in close contact with an infected individual.

Poor sanitation and hygiene is also a common risk factor and the bacterium is transmitted primarily through *oral-oral* or *faecal-oral* routes, so this can be prevented by practicing good hygiene, such as handwashing after going to the washroom, before handling food, and by stopping the habit of nail-biting.

Several other risk factors are associated with this infection includes alcohol consumption, high nickel content in the body, low vitamin-D levels, chronic stress, radiation therapy, chemotherapy, bile stones or a sluggish bile, and certain prescription drugs can cause either acute or chronic gastritis, depending on how much and how often it is used.

Overuse of NSAIDs such as *aspirin* and *ibuprofen*, and recreational drugs, like cocaine, are also found to cause gastritis.

Addressing these risk factors and treating H. pylori infections with appropriate antibiotics and acid-reducing medications are crucial for managing gastritis and preventing complications.

Complications of gastritis include peptic ulcer disease, gastro-intestinal bleeding, anaemia, gastric outlet obstruction due to scar formation, indigestion, vitamin and mineral deficiencies due to malabsorption, gastro-intestinal perforation (a hole in the stomach), auto-immune diseases (triggered from secondary infections), allergies and even stomach cancer.

Endoscopies, blood tests, stool tests, H. pylori breath test, X-rays, or biopsies may be taken by your physician, to diagnose the type of gastritis that you are suffering from.

Treating long-term or persistent gastritis, require specific and appropriate antibiotics, along with a healthy and balanced diet.

The changes that need to be included, in the diet, to treat and manage chronic **Gastritis**, is explained in the sample diet charts, in Chapter- 25.

- **24.19 – <u>Hypo-chlorhydria (Hypo-Acidity)</u>**

Hydrochloric-acid (HCl) plays a vital role in digestion and immunity.

It helps break down food, especially tough proteins, which allows for the absorption of essential nutrients, and it helps control viruses and bacteria that might otherwise infect our stomach and body.

Hypo-chlorhydria means low stomach acid.

If you have hypo-chlorhydria, you'll have trouble digesting food properly, especially protein.
Over time you can develop serious nutritional deficiencies.
You'll also be prone to infections, which can cause further damage to your digestive system and immune system and trigger an auto-immune response from your body leading to allergies or auto-immune diseases.

Often-times gastritis or digestive issues are attributed to
hyper- chlorhydria (excessive acid), mostly because the majority of the population, are not actually even aware of a condition called **hypo**-acidity.

And since the usual symptoms like acid reflux, heartburn and stomach aches are noticed in both *Hyper* and *Hypo*-acidity...
Doctors often prescribe medication to suppress the stomach acid, which only worsens the case of *Hypo*-acidity.

The most significant causes of *Hypo*-acidity include-

- <u>*Atrophic gastritis*</u>- It is when the cells that secrete stomach juices, shrinks and stop working. Atrophic gastritis is the end result of chronic inflammation of the stomach (gastritis).

    Chronic gastritis can be caused by a variety of things, including bacterial infection (H. Pylori), alcoholism and autoimmune diseases or chronic diseases.

- ***H. pylori infection*** - This common bacterial infection affects more than half of the global population, but usually causes no symptoms. But in individuals with lowered immunity, it can take over, spread and eventually decrease production of stomach acid.

  In the case of hypo-acidity, the infection is seen in the ***corpus region*** of the stomach, where the '**D-cells**' are located.

  D – cells (*secretes somatostatin*).

  Parietal cells (*secretes HCl acid*).

  These cells secrete ***somatostatin***, a vital hormone which sends signals to hinder and stop the release of stomach acids (normally, to stop acid production when the food is done digesting).

  When these cells are inflamed due to the infection, it causes, over secretion of ***somatostatin***, leading to prevention of the normal secretion of our stomach acid, hence hypo-acidity.

  Ironically, low stomach acid can also allow for H. pylori to take over.

- ***Acid-reducing medications*** - Chronic use of antacids, H_2 receptor blockers, and especially PPIs (*proton pump inhibitors*) can cause low stomach acid. PPIs were originally approved only for short-term use, but they are now commonly overprescribed and used to treat chronic symptoms such as GERD and heartburn.

  Eventually, they can cause the acid-secreting glands in the stomach to stop working.

- ***Malfunctioning vagal nerve*** - In cases of Vitamin-B_1 and B_{12} deficiency or prolonged diabetes, the vagal nerve is damaged causing lowered production of stomach acid.

Other contributing causes also include advanced age, chronic stress, low zinc, low vitamin-D levels, and those who have undergone stomach surgery (such as gastric bypass surgery).

Immediate symptoms of *Hypo*-acidity are bloating, abdominal pain, gas formation, headache, diarrhoea, constipation, presence of undigested food in faeces, acid reflux and heart burn.

Prolonged *Hypo*-acidity can produce symptoms of nutritional deficiencies, including brittle fingernails, hair loss, paleness, fatigue, weakness, numbness in hands and feet, memory loss, osteoporosis, anaemia, allergies, ulcers, auto-immune disorders and migraines.

Dry skin is a common symptom of *hypo*-acidity and protein indigestion issues, leading to a deficiency in filaggrin (a protein), which in turn impairs the skin's barrier function and its ability to retain moisture, leading to **dry skin**.

To diagnose *Hypo*-acidity, healthcare providers use a variety of tests, but there are a few tests you can try at home, which offer a relatively simple and inexpensive way of finding out your acid state.

I recommend that if you do get a positive result from an at-home test, you should follow up with a professional healthcare provider.

The Baking Soda Test-

- The theory behind this do-at-home test, is that baking soda (alkaline) combined with stomach acid produces carbon dioxide (CO_2), which will cause you to burp.
- For the test, you'll have to drink a quarter (¼) glass (around 50 ml) of normal or cold water, combined with a quarter (¼) teaspoon of baking soda, on an empty stomach.
- Then time how long it takes you to burp.
- If you burp within 3 minutes after drinking, there is an increase in acid production in your stomach or you are ***Hyper-acidic**.*
- If a burp takes 5 minutes or more, then production of acid in the stomach is below normal level or you are ***Hypo-acidic**.*
- Note that if the burp is within 3 minutes, make sure that it is a strong, loud burp, and not a weak, feeble one, to avoid a 'false-positive' result.

Medical tests to diagnose stomach acid include-

- **_The Heidelberg pH Test_**- For this test, you'll swallow a small capsule with a radio transmitter that measures the pH levels in your stomach. After taking a baseline measurement, you'll drink a baking soda solution to neutralize your stomach acid.
  Then the test measures how long it takes your stomach to return to baseline acid levels. This shows healthcare providers how well your stomach secretes acid.

- **_The Smart-Pill Test_**- It is another wireless transmitter that you swallow. Unlike the Heidelberg test, which measures pH levels, this test measures gastric acid levels.

- **_The Gastric String Test_**- This test involves swallowing a capsule attached to a string, and then pulling it out by the string after 10 minutes. The string is tested with pH paper.
  Normal stomach acid has a pH level of 1 to 2, which is highly acidic, with zero being the most acidic level on the scale. If you have _Hypo-chlorhydria_, your stomach acid would be in the range of 3 to 5.
  Above 5 is a severe condition called **_Achlorhydria_**, means you have a severe issue with secretion of hydrochloric acid.

If you suffer from _Hypo_-acidity, over the counter HCl (Hydrochloric Acid) supplements are a good option, but they are not safe for everyone, so you should talk to your healthcare provider first, before self-prescribing it.

HCl supplements (_Betaine Hydrochloride_) are often combined with the enzyme pepsin, so that these supplements can help digestion. Sometimes, the stomach acid levels gradually return to normal levels, where you must discontinue taking them to prevent _Hyper_-acidity.

But one of the best alternatives, in terms of efficiency and convenience, is an easy home remedy which is to drink ACV (_apple cider vinegar_).
Drink 1 tablespoon of ACV diluted with quarter (¼) glass (around 50 ml) of normal water, around 5 minutes before every meal.

Apple cider vinegar could cause tooth-wear and degradation due to its acidic nature, so be careful not to get it on your teeth while drinking. It is best to use a straw while drinking ACV.

One other trick to provide symptomatic relief from *Hypo*-acidity is, by squeezing lime and ginger juice along with the meals you eat, so that it helps in digesting the food that have been just consumed.

But from my experience, stubborn cases of *Hypo*-acidity might require ACV or HCl capsules along with digestive enzyme supplements for better results.

And even more stubborn cases of *Hypo*-acidity require a complete soup based diet, during meals, and buttermilk with infused ginger, during snack times.

It is also better to follow these few simple tips to tackle *Hypo*-acidity -

- Drink diluted ACV or HCl, at least **5 mins prior** to large meals.
- Eat **proteins at beginning of the meal**, to stimulate acid production.
- Eat smaller mouthfuls, and **chew thoroughly** to give the digestive system its best chance to break the food down, as chewing stimulates the release of so many enzymes that aids it.
- Eat **probiotic foods**, including yogurt and sauerkraut, to help boost the beneficial gut bacteria and keep harmful bacteria in check.
- If you're a vegetarian, **fortify your vegetarian diet**. Many of the deficiencies associated with low stomach acid, including protein, iron, calcium and vitamin-B_{12}, are most abundant in animal-sourced foods, such as meat, fish and dairy products. Make sure you're supplementing these nutrients.
- **Drink fluids later**, up to at least 30 minutes after you've finished your meal, which gives your stomach more time to produce acid and metabolize proteins.
- Drink regularly, **water boiled and infused** with black cumin seeds, ginger, fennel seeds, cardamom, cloves, and turmeric which are effective natural anti-inflammatory and anti-biotics.
- Finish your last meal **2 to 3 hours before bedtime**, and give your body time to digest before lying down.

Now as in all other cases, only when we address the underlying causes of the issue will we be able to get a more stable result or cure.

If it is due to an infection, or due to nutritional deficiencies or heavy metal toxicity, or any other cause, get on track with the right steps to solve the problem, with the proper course of anti-biotics or nutritional supplements, with guidance from a registered physician.

The changes that need to be included, in the diet, to treat and manage *Hypo*-**acidity**, is explained in the sample diet charts, in Chapter- 25.

24.20 – **Hyper-chlorhydria (Hyper-Acidity)**

Hyper-acidity is brought on by the over-production of stomach acid, which is characterised by heartburn, that causes pain or burning sensation in the lower chest cavity, due to the stomach acid flowing back into the food pipe. The most common cause for acidity is due to the effects from the infection of H. Pylori bacteria.

In hyper-acidity, the infection is seen in the **antral region** of the stomach, where the '**G-cells**' are located. These cells secrete *gastrin*, a hormone which sends signals to activate the parietal cells, which when stimulated causes the release of stomach acids such as HCl. When these cells are inflamed due to the infection, it causes the over secretion of *gastrin*, leading to over secretion of acid, causing hyper-acidity.

Parietal cells *(secretes HCl acid)*.

G – cells *(secretes gastrin)*.

Antral Region

The risk of acidity increases in individuals who are obese, or under chronic stress, those with low levels of vitamin-D, eat very spicy food, drink excessive amounts of alcohol, frequently use NSAIDs (*non-steroidal anti-inflammatory drugs*), those approaching menopause or is pregnant, have diseases like *Zollinger-Ellison* syndrome, asthma, diabetes, peptic ulcers, hiatal hernia, and even those with a sluggish bile or gall-bladder stones, to name a few.

Symptoms of *Hyper*-acidity heartburn, nausea, difficulty in swallowing, constipation, indigestion, burning sensation, pain in the stomach and throat, restlessness and bad breath.

When left untreated, acidity could become more severe and lead to complications such as GERD (*Gastro Esophageal Reflux Disease*), gastric ulcers, esophageal or peptic strictures, esophageal cancers, etc.

Commonly used methods for diagnosis of acidity are upper GI endoscopy and biopsy or EGD (*esophago-gastro-duodenoscopy*), MRI, esophageal manometry, esophageal pH monitoring etc.

Conventional treatment for acidity include-

- Antacids (medications that neutralise stomach acid, commonly *magnesium carbonate, magnesium trisilicate* and *aluminium hydroxide*), available in tablet and liquid form. Some antacids add *'alginate'* compounds which help soothe the oesophageal lining from the effects of stomach acid.

- H_2 receptor blockers (*famotidine* and *nizatidine*) are also commonly used medicines which work by lowering the amount of stomach acid secreted by glands in the stomach's lining, which helps reduce heartburn sensations.

- PPI (*proton pump inhibitor*) medications lessen the amount of acid the stomach produces, and acid reflux is frequently treated with these. The strongest type of medication currently available for managing stomach acid is proton-pump inhibitors.

    Omeprazole, esomeprazole, lansoprazole are all PPIs, available without the need for prescription from a registered medical doctor. PPIs come in tablet or pill form which are ingested orally 30 minutes prior to the morning meal.

Even though these can be effective in managing acid-related conditions, prolonged use of these medicines, or depending solely on these medications without any other changes in lifestyle (that which caused the triggering of the acidity), can become reasons for side effects such as-

- *Antacids*: Constipation, diarrhoea, stomach cramps, nausea, and even rebound acid hyper-secretion (which means even more acid being secreted).

- H_2 *receptor blockers*: Headaches, dizziness, fatigue, diarrhoea or constipation, rashes, mental confusions.

- *Proton Pump Inhibitors*: Risk of bone fractures, kidney issues, nutritional deficiencies, infections, nausea and vomiting, diarrhoea or constipation, abdominal pain, headaches.

Home remedies for *Hyper*-acidity –

- Eating half a banana or 2 to 3 slices of ripe papaya after meals.
- Drinking 1 glass of lukewarm water after meals, in mouthful sips.
- Drinking a glass of cold milk (without sugar), or tender coconut water, or buttermilk or watermelon juice after meals.
- Drinking regularly, water boiled and infused with black cumin seeds, ginger, fennel seeds, cardamom, cloves, and turmeric.

It is also better to follow these few simple tips to tackle acidity –

- Avoid late meals.
- Avoid over spicy foods.
- Avoid tight-fitting clothing.
- Refrain from eating large meals.
- Maintain an ideal and healthy weight.
- Avoid smoking and consumption of alcohol drinks.
- Elevate the head of the bed (or use more than 1 pillow).
- Do not lie down immediately after a meal, and do not sleep on the stomach (position).

As in all other cases, only when we address the underlying causes of the issue will we be able to get a more stable result or cure.

If it is due to an infection, or nutritional deficiencies, or heavy metal toxicity or any other cause, get on track with the right steps to solve the problem, with the proper course of anti-biotics or nutritional supplements, with guidance from a registered physician.

The changes that need to be included, in the diet, to treat and manage ***Hyper*-acidity**, is explained in the sample diet charts, in Chapter- 25.

- ## 24.21 – <u>Gastroesophageal reflux disease (GERD)</u>

Your stomach contents are supposed to travel downwards.
When acid from inside your stomach flows back upwards, into your esophagus and throat, it's called **acid reflux**.

This reflux can irritate and cause inflammation the tissues inside the esophagus. Almost everyone would have experienced an occasional episode of acid reflux.

Chronic acid reflux or GERD (having reflux at least twice a week, for several weeks) can really affect the quality of life, and it can also do real damage to the tissues of our food pipe.

For acid to travel back into the esophagus, it needs to get past the valve, called the **LES** (*lower esophageal sphincter*), at the bottom of the esophagus which keeps food from coming back up.

The LES is a circular muscle that opens when you swallow, or to let gas bubbles out when you're burping or have hiccups.

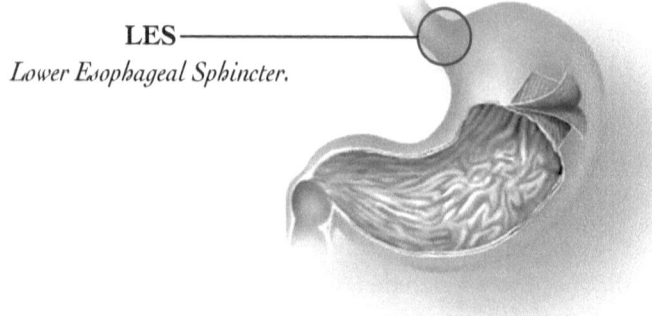

LES —
Lower Esophageal Sphincter.

When LES weakens or relaxes enough to let acid pass, **reflux** occurs.

Many things can contribute to weakening the LES, either temporarily or permanently. The occasional 'acid reflux' turns into chronic GERD, when these factors overlap or persist for a long time.

Common causes of GERD include –

- *Gastritis*- The most common cause for GERD is gastritis, be it Hyper or Hypo-acidity, and relieving gastritis often solves the persisting GERD issue as well.

- *Hiatal Hernia*- Occurs when the top of stomach pushes up through the hole in the diaphragm where the esophagus passes through. It squeezes in next to the esophagus, compressing them both, and trapping acid. It also moves the LES above the diaphragm, where it loses some of its muscular support.
Hiatal hernias are quite common, especially as one gets older, occurring gradually, and worsening over time.

- *Pregnancy*- Causes temporary acid reflux. The pressure and volume in the abdomen can push, stretch and weaken the muscles of the diaphragm, which supports the LES. Pregnancy hormone *relaxin*, which relaxes the abdomen muscles to stretch and accommodate the foetus, also causes the LES to relax. High levels of *estrogen* and *progesterone* also causes the LES to relax.

- *Obesity*- It increases the pressure and volume in the abdomen, which affects the LES similarly to how pregnancy does. Obesity also tends to last longer than pregnancy, which can weaken the muscles more permanently, and is also a common contributing factor to developing a hiatal hernia. Since fat tissue secretes *estrogen*, obesity also raises the *estrogen* levels and causes the LES to relax.

- *Smoking*- Tobacco or other kinds (sheesha, vaping etc.) of smoke relaxes the LES, whether it is primary or second-hand smoke. It also triggers coughing, which causes the LES to stay open for longer periods. Smoking and chronic coughing weakens the diaphragm muscles and contribute to developing a hiatal hernia, and it also slows down digestion and causes the stomach to produce more acid.

Other less common causes of GERD include birth defects, connective tissue diseases, surgery in the chest, certain medications like calcium channel blockers (for high blood pressure), *theophylline* (a common asthma medication), hormone therapy medications for menopause, *benzodiazepines* (a type of sedative), tricyclic antidepressants, and NSAIDs (non-steroidal anti-inflammatory drugs like aspirin and ibuprofen), to name a few.

Symptoms of acid reflux and GERD may include –

- *__Backwash__*- When food or liquids backwashes from your stomach into your throat after eating, typically with a sour tase of acid. It is also called regurgitation.
- *__A burning feeling__*- Acid actually dissolves or burns the tissues in your esophagus. If it feels like it's in your chest, it's called heartburn. If it feels closer to your stomach, it is usually called as indigestion.
- *__Non-cardiac Chest Pain__*- Esophagus pain triggers the same nerves as heart-related pain does, so it might feel like that.
- *__Nausea__*- Acid overflow or backwash often feel uneasy and makes one lose their appetite. Although you may have eaten a while ago, it may feel like there's still more food to digest.
- *__Sore Throat__*- Reflux into the throat often happens at night and constant damage makes one feel like there's a lump in their throat, or like it's hard to swallow.
- *__Asthma Symptoms__*- GERD can trigger asthma-like symptoms, like chronic coughing, wheezing and shortness of breath. If acid particles gets into the airways, it can cause unwanted contractions.

GERD symptoms may be worsen –

- After a large meal.
- After bending over.
- At night or while lying down.
- After smoking or drinking alcohol.

Possible complications include, intestinal metaplasia (a precancerous condition), *Barret's* esophagus, LPR (*laryngo-pharyngeal reflux*), asthma, asphyxiation, esophageal strictures, which can cause difficulty in swallowing, eating and drinking.

GERD is diagnosed through evaluation of the symptoms and tests may include an esophagram (a type of X-ray), upper endoscopy, esophageal pH test, esophageal manometry etc.

Treatments for GERD include almost the same medications as in gastritis and in case of surgery, '**fundoplication**' is the most common surgery for GERD.

A recent procedure also uses a device called LINX, which is implanted during surgery, where a ring of tiny magnets help keep the junction between the stomach and esophagus closed.

During an acid reflux attack, it is helpful to –

- Stand up, so the reflux goes back down to the stomach.
- Take a sip of water, not a lot. Small sips helps wash the acid down.
- Loosen the waistband, take off belt or change pants if it is tight.
- Consume an over-the-counter antacid.

The changes that need to be included, in the diet, to treat and manage **GERD**, is explained in the sample diet charts, in Chapter- 25.

- ## 24.22 – <u>Migraine & Epilepsy</u>

Migraine is felt as a severe throbbing or pulsing headache on one side of the head, or felt in the eyes (retinal or ocular migraine).

The headache phase of a migraine usually lasts at least **four hours**, but it can also last for days (as in *'status migrainosus'* which is when the pain lasts for more than **72 hours** or **3 days**), and can be triggered by, or worsen with stress, physical activity, bright lights, loud noises, strong odours etc.

Studies estimate that around **25%** of people in India suffer from migraines, which are extremely disruptive and can interfere with the daily routine of an individual.

Up to **80%** of people with migraines have a biological relative who suffers from the same, which could indicate infection spread among close members, along with a genetic factor.

There are several types of migraines, but the most common and relevant ones are –

- Gastric mediated migraine.
- Menstrual migraine.

Every patient experiences migraine differently, and will have unique combinations of triggers, as well as site and intensity of pain, ranging from mild to severe.

A dull, throbbing, pulsing or pounding pain can start on one side of the head and shift to the opposite side, or may also occur around the eyes or temple, and sometimes, around the face, sinuses, jaw or neck.

Migraines can occur with or without an *'**aura**'* which is a phase before the headache begins, where the patient knows that the migraine is going to set in.

Other symptoms include mood changes, difficulty in concentrating, sleeping trouble, fatigue, nausea and vomiting, dizziness, increased hunger and thirst, frequent urination, muscle weakness, vision changes, ringing in the ears (tinnitus), numbness and tingling etc.

Stress, hormonal changes during menstrual cycle, certain medications, changes in sleep pattern, changes in weather condition, physical activity (over exertion), addictive substances like caffeine or tobacco, missing a meal, exposure to bright lights, loud noises and strong odours are the various, most commonly noticed, triggers of migraines.

The usual things that give temporary relief to those suffering from a migraine attack, vary from voluntary or involuntary vomiting, resting in a dark and cool room with no other sounds, applying a cold or luke warm cloth to the forehead or behind the neck, massaging the scalp, applying pressure to the temples in a circular motion, applying tight tourniquets around the head, and sometimes meditation is effective too.

Usually, taking medications (painkillers or anti-emetics etc.) at the first sign of a migraine, stops or reduce migraine symptoms like pain, nausea, sensitivity and more.

But it is advised to be cautious when taking over-the-counter pain relievers, as their over-use could potentially cause analgesic-rebound headaches or a dependency issues.

Taking supplements of vitamin-B_2, magnesium, or anti-oxidants such as co-enzyme Q_{10} have also been found to reduce the headaches.

Blood tests, CT and MRI scans, EEG, are done to rule out any other causes like **tumours** or **cancers** that could be a potential triggering factor of the headache.

Gastric mediated migraines occur when the **trigeminal ganglion** is over stimulated and causes it to release excess of **CGRPs** (*calcitonin gene receptor peptide*), which causes inflammation, *vasodilation* (widening of blood vessels), and transmits pain to the trigeminal nerve branches (which are situated in the face).

The trigeminal nerve is responsible for sensory (feeling of touch, pain, and temperature) and motor functions (such as blinking, biting and chewing) in the head and neck, such as the eyes, scalp, forehead, sinus, cheek, jaws, lips, teeth, gums, and nose etc.

This is why migraine is triggered directly from its branches, by bright lights, loud noises, strong odours, sinusitis or sinus infections etc. and indirectly, through acid fluctuations, caused by indigestion, stress, H. pylori infection, sluggish bile, gall-bladder stones etc.

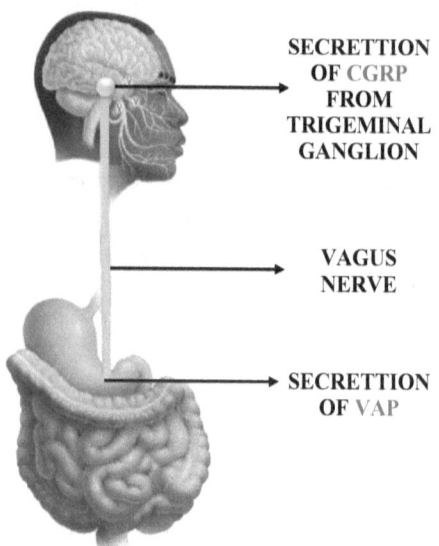

Acid fluctuations, trigger the vagal nerve, which causes the vagus nerve endings in the stomach and intestines to secrete **VAP** (*vaso-active peptides*), which in turn stimulates the trigeminal ganglion (causing release of CGRP), and becomes the indirect cause for migraine.

Studies have attributed ***histamine*** production from triggering of the afore mentioned nerves, to be a cause for migraine as well.

Over **50%** of cases of ***epilepsy***, have been found, to be just extreme cases of this very same cause of migraine, with exaggerated symptoms.

In many individuals, in response to the vasodilation effect of CGRP, the body releases several potent vasoconstricting neurotransmitters such as *tyramine*, **GABA** (*gamma-aminobutyric acid*), *serotonin* and *dopamine* (in large doses), which backfires in most cases, as this alternating effect of vaso-**constrictors** and vaso-**dilators**, has been found to be the reason for the throbbing or pulsing nature of migraines.

Gastric mediated migraines can be reversed by treating the root cause of the gastric issue as mentioned in previous sub-headings.

<u>Estrogen mediated migraines</u> or migraines felt during, or around the time of a menstrual period, is due to the **sudden drop in estrogen level**, which are potent vasodilators (causes widening of blood vessels), that maintains the relaxed state of blood vessels normally.

This sudden drop in estrogen levels, along with a genetic predisposition in the affected woman, as well as insufficient nutritional vasodilators in their body due to unhealthy eating habits, together when combined, causes a severe vasoconstriction (narrowing) in the blood vessels, and inflammation of where the migraine pain is felt.

Cod liver oil, or *omega*-3 supplements, L-arginine and magnesium glycinate supplements have been found to help relieve the pain to a drastic extent when consumed at the time of the feeling of migraine pain.

Mix of pomegranate and beetroot juice without sugar (helps produce *nitric oxide* leading to vasodilation), have also been found to be a very helpful home remedy.

The changes that need to be included, in the diet, to treat and manage **Migraine & Epilepsy**, is explained in the sample diet charts, in Chapter- 25.

24.23 – IBS (Irritable Bowel Syndrome)

Irritable bowel syndrome (IBS) is a common disorder that affects the stomach and intestines, but doesn't cause visible changes in the bowel (intestinal) tissue.

Only a small number of people with IBS have severe symptoms. Some people can control their symptoms by managing diet, lifestyle and stress. More-severe symptoms can be treated with medication.

It is estimated that about **10%** of adults in the India have IBS, but only about **7%** of those affected by this disease, visit a physician and receive a diagnosis.

Symptoms of IBS vary, but they are mostly chronic and include cramping, abdominal pain, bloating, flatulence, burping, either diarrhoea or constipation, or in some cases, alternation between both constipation and diarrhoea in the same individual.

Other symptoms that are often noticed are sensation of incomplete evacuation, increased gas or mucus in the stool, disformed stool (for example, shaped like beads, pellets, or at times, a thin strand like structure), and depression (due to poor production of serotonin).

Bristol Stool Form Chart -

Type 1	Type 2	Type 3	Type 4	Type 5	Type 6	Type 7
Separate hard lumps, like nuts, hard to pass.	Sausage shaped but lumpy.	Like a sausage with cracks.	Like a sausage, smooth and soft.	Soft blobs with clear cut edges.	Fluffy pieces with ragged edges, a mushy stool.	Watery, no solid pieces. Entirely liquid.

Indicate Constipation.   *Ideal Stools.*   *Indicate Diarrhoea.*

Extreme weight loss, rectal bleeding, iron deficiency anaemia, vomiting, pain that isn't relieved by passing gas or a bowel movement, may indicate a more serious condition, along with IBS.

Many people with IBS also have other chronic pain conditions such as fibromyalgia, chronic fatigue and chronic pelvic inflammation and pain. It is better to undergo treatment under the guidance of professionals during these changes.

Even though extreme stress and dysfunction of nerves in the digestive system are possible causes for IBS, the most important cause are, infections and change in gut microbes such as gastritis, GERD, indigestion, SIBO, IBS, IBD, intestinal motility disorders (as in pelvic floor dysfunction or gastroparesis), bowel obstructions (by faecal matter, tumours, scar tissue, strictures, stenosis, hernias etc).

IBS symptoms can worsen or be triggered when the patient eat or drink certain foods or beverages, which are specific to each individual, and can include wheat, dairy products, citrus fruits, beans, cabbage, milk and carbonated drinks. Stress is a common triggering factor as well, and those with IBS experience worse, or more frequent symptoms during periods of increased stress.

Bloating is a feeling of tightness, pressure or fullness in the stomach which may or may not be accompanied by a visibly distended (swollen) abdomen. The feeling can range from mildly uncomfortable to intensely painful. It usually goes away after a while, but for some people, it is a recurring problem.

Bloating even though commonly occurs due to a digestive issue, it can also be triggered due to hormonal fluctuations or imbalances, as in perimenopause and normal menstrual cycles.
Estrogen causes water retention, which in addition to increase in volume of uterus just before menstruation, can cause bloating.

Estrogen and progesterone can each cause intestinal gas by either slowing or speeding intestinal motility. Estrogen receptors in the gastro intestinal tract also affects the visceral sensitivity, leading to bloating.

Sometimes a bloated stomach can indicate a more serious medical condition, like ascites (fluid in abdominal cavity, due to issues such as liver disease or kidney failure), pancreatic insufficiency (where digestive enzymes are not produced enough, leading to indigestion), and cancer (ovarian, uterine, colon, pancreatic, stomach or mesenteric etc).

Around **25%** of otherwise healthy people, complain of occasional bloating. Out of those, around **75%** describe their symptoms as moderate to severe, and the rest say that they experience it regularly.

Among those diagnosed with IBS, bloating is noticed in, as much as **90%** of cases. Over **75%** of women experience bloating, around the time of their menstrual period. And in total, only **50%** of people who experience bloating also report a distended abdomen.

Home remedies to debloat the stomach in a day or two are, diluted apple cider vinegar, antacids, probiotics, magnesium supplements, diluted baking soda, fiber laxatives, drinking water or herbal tea (with ginger, peppermint, turmeric and fennel), which can aid digestion and could possibly be a simple solution for the bloating.

In cases of persistent bloating, with other symptoms such as fever or vomiting, you should seek professional medical attention.

There isn't any one test that can diagnose IBS, instead, it is determined depending on the symptoms, and few tests, to confirm a diagnosis.

Questions on frequency of bowel movement, or pain related to it, shape and form of stool, stress factor etc. gives clues to the present issue.

Most lab tests (like blood and stool tests, hydrogen breath test, colonoscopy, endoscopy etc.) are done to rule out other symptoms that could suggest various, more serious disorders like polyps, celiac disease, IBD or even cancerous growths.

The usual medications to provide symptomatic relief, include medications that reduce intestinal spasms, antidepressants, laxatives, anti-diarrhoeal etc.

It is, at the same time, important to add probiotics, and treat the root cause of the issue with specific medications along with an appropriate, personalised healthy diet.

Specific triggering food varies for each individual, and so it is advisable to ask the patient to avoid the particular food trigger, even if it generally could be a healthy choice.

The changes that need to be included, in the diet, to treat and manage **IBS**, is explained in the sample diet charts, in Chapter- 25.

24.24 – **Constipation**

Having fewer than three bowel evacuations a week is, technically, the definition of constipation.

Even though the normal frequency of how often a person evacuates, varies widely from person to person (several times a day to just 1 or 2 times a week), I have found that it is best to have a regular evacuation of at least once a day, to be healthy for a person.

This is because even though having comfortable bowel movements on alternate days, is actually considered normal, there is a high chance of the individual having other health issues that they might not relate to their delayed evacuation, but scientifically is very much connected to issues like sinusitis, allergies, chronic or acute lower back pain etc.

And more importantly, the longer one stays before they evacuate stool, the more difficult it becomes for the stool to pass through. It is also defined as constipation if the stools are dry and hard, or if the bowel movements are painful, and if the stools are difficult to pass, or if the person has a feeling that they haven't fully emptied their bowels.

According to a recent Indian survey, nearly **17%** of India's adult population suffers from constipation due to various root causes.

Constipation can occur when the colon (large intestine) absorbs too much water from the stool, which dries it out, making it hard in consistency and difficult to push out of the body.

It can also occur when stool is not formed to its proper consistency, or if there is not enough serotonin hormone produced, which initiates and sustains the *peristaltic movement* (rhythmic, wave-like motion that pushes out the stool), both of which, is the work that should be done by our friendly gut microbiomes.

The main causes of constipation are –

- Intestinal Methanogenic Bacterial Overgrowth.
- Reduced Serotonin Production.
- Reduced Cortisol Production.
- Bile-acid Malabsorption.
- Parasitic Infection.

IMO (intestinal methanogenic overgrowth) symptomsm –

- Primarily caused by archaea.
- Abdominal pain or discomfort.
- Bloating and belching.
- Joint and muscle pain.
- Anxiety and fatigue.
- Skin conditions.
- Constipation.
- Malnutrition.
- Heart burn.
- Leaky gut.
- Nausea.

Common lifestyle causes of constipation include, not eating enough fiber, dehydration, not enough exercise, stress, changes in the regular routine of the person (such as traveling, or not sleeping on time), resisting the urge to evacuate a bowel movement, certain medications such as in strong pain killers, NSAIDs, iron pills, antidepressants, antacids, antihistamines, etc.

Health conditions that can cause constipation include, pregnancy, thyroiditis, diabetes, hypercalcemia, uraemia, colorectal cancer, IBS, diverticulitis, defect in the coordination of the pelvic floor muscles, paralytic ileus or *Ogilvie* syndrome, stroke, *Parkinson's* disease, multiple sclerosis, spinal cord injury, fistula, haemorrhoids etc.

Apart from a detailed medical history, examining the rectum and other vital signs to diagnose constipation, blood, urine and stool tests, MRI, colonoscopy etc. are also commonly used.

You can manage most cases of mild to moderate constipation at home. One simple home remedy, is to have a glass of lukewarm milk or water with 3 tbsp ghee or coconut oil, after dinner.

Having a glass of lemonade with salt (no sugar), twice a day is also found to be helpful.

Gel forming soluble fibers like psyllium husk are also helpful to bulk up the stool and relieve constipation.

Magnesium citrate (up to 500 mg/day) is also highly beneficial.

The rectum is pulled and folded by a muscle known as the ***Puborectalis*** muscle, and the *full squatting position*, allows the proper unfolding of the rectum (resulting in an almost straight passage), which helps in complete, and better evacuation of faecal matter.
Few cases of constipation can be overcome by this simple practice (full squat) while evacuating.

Surgery is rarely needed to treat constipation, but may be unavoidable in extreme cases of structural problems like intestinal obstruction or strictures, anal fissures, rectal prolapse etc.

The changes that need to be included, in the diet, to treat and manage **Constipation**, is explained in the sample diet charts, in Chapter- 25.

- **24.25 – <u>Diarrhoea</u>**

Diarrhoea means having a loose or watery stool.

It is quite common and mostly mild (only a few washroom trips a day) and goes away within a few days. Sometimes, though, it is a sign of a serious underlying condition. It can cause the person to lose too much fluid, or prevent their body from absorbing nutrients.

- *Acute diarrhoea* is loose and watery stool that lasts 1 to 2 days, and usually goes away without any treatment.
- *Persistent diarrhoea* lasts about 2 to 4 weeks.
- *Chronic diarrhoea* lasts more than 4 weeks or comes and goes regularly over a long period and is a serious issue.

It is a relatively common issue that affects people of all ages. Most adults get acute diarrhoea at least once a year, while children tend to get it at least twice a year.

Infections (bacterial, viral, parasites etc), food intolerance (like lactose, gluten etc), food poisoning, IBS, IBD, surgery, medications are among other causes for diarrhoea.

The main sign of diarrhoea is loose or watery stool, commonly along with bloating, stomach pain and cramps, nausea, vomiting, fever, headache, dry skin, fatigue, dehydration, and in severe cases, blood and mucus can be noticed in the stool as well.

Dehydration is one of the biggest concerns with diarrhoea, mainly among those vulnerable such as infants, elders (55 years and above), and those with severely compromised immune systems.

Without treatment, dehydration can lead to kidney failure, stroke, heart attack or even death.

Common causes of Diarrhoea and the possible Associated Symptoms -

	Causative Disease	Investigations
Functional Diseases	1. **Hypoacidity**	Baking Soda Test
	2. **SIBO- Types** • SIBO (Hydrogen) _Symptoms_- Watery diarrhoea, depression, Anxiety. • SIBO (Hydrogen Sulfide) _Symptoms_- Fibromyalgia, body sensitivity, foul odour flatulence.	Hydrogen Breath Test (HBT)
	3. **IBS Types -** • IBS (SIFO) _Symptoms_- Tongue coating, fever, diarrhoea, vomiting.	Stool mapping
	• IBS (SIPO) _Symptoms_- Anal itching, skin rashes, low ferritin.	CBC Ferritin
	• IBS (Post infection) _Symptoms_- Chronic diarrhoea.	Anti-CDTB, Anti-Vinculin
	4. **Fructose intolerance** _Symptoms_- Low blood sugar, chronic fatigue.	HBT Liver Biopsy
Auto-immune	5. **Ulcerative colitis** _Symptoms_- Weight loss, fatigue.	Calprotectin Test Elevated ESR, CRP
	6. **Crohn's disease** _Symptoms_- Rectal bleeding & mucous discharge, weight loss, stool incontinence.	Calprotectin Test Elevated ESR, CRP, Low Hb
	7. **Ileitis** _Symptoms_- Fever, weight loss.	Colonoscopy, Yersinia Serology Stool culture.
	8. **Celiac disease** _Symptoms_- Nausea, vomiting.	TTG- IgA, Intestinal biopsy, DGP- IgG

	9. **Intestinal TB** *Symptoms*- Night sweats, weight loss, vomiting, anaemia.	Elevated ESR, CRP T-spot TB
	10. **Clostridium difficile colitis** *Symptoms*- Nausea, fever, severe cramping.	Faecal Examination, NAAD
	11. **Acute gastro-enteritis** *Symptoms*- Nausea, vomiting, belching.	Anti-CDTB Anti-Vinculin
Infectious diseases	12. **Post-infectious diarrhoea** *Symptoms*- Persistence of abdominal discomfort.	Stool culture
	13. **Lactose intolerance** *Symptoms*- Bloating and gas within 30 mins of consuming dairy (especially milk).	Hydrogen Breath Test, Lactose Breath Test.
	14. **Histamine intolerance** *Symptoms*- Vomiting, flushing, dizziness, fatigue, migraine, cramps, difficulty breathing.	Serum Histamine
	15. **Bile acid malabsorption** *Symptoms*- Faecal incontinence, sense of urgency.	Faecal Bile Acid Test, Serum C4 test
	16. **Digestive enzyme insufficiency** *Symptoms*- Weight loss, anorexia.	Cholecystokinin Stimulating Test

<u>SIBO (small intestinal bacterial overgrowth)</u> **symptoms:**

- Caused by bacteria.
- Abdominal discomfort.
- Bloating and belching.
- Constipation (less often).
- Diarrhoea.
- Weight loss.
- Malnutrition.
- Nausea.
- IBD and IBS.

Methane Dominant SIBO	Causes mostly constipation.
Hydrogen Dominant SIBO	Causes mostly diarrhoea.
Hydrogen Sulfide Dominant SIBO	Mostly diarrhoea, with body aches and food sensitivities.

You can often get rid of acute diarrhoea through remedies you can make at home. The main thing to get done is to drink plenty of electrolyte balanced fluids which include tender coconut water, bone broths, buttermilk etc.

Electrolytes are substances that help with important processes, like maintaining the balance of fluids in your body, so it is advised to drink these, instead of plain water. The ORS (*oral rehydration solution*) available in pharmacies are also recommended.

Usually, over-the-counter medicines, like *bismuth subsalicylate* often give quick relief from diarrhoea, but a visit to the physician is mandatory if it doesn't improve, or other severe symptoms are noticed.

Your physician may recommend antibiotics or antiparasitic, medications for underlying conditions like IBD or IBS etc.
Probiotics are also highly recommended, and **Saccharomyces Boulardii** is a wonderful species that help alleviate diarrhoea. Pickles, curd, sourcrouts and kefir are good natural sources.

Diarrhoea can commonly cause the anus to feel sore, itchy or like it's burning, and may hurt while evacuating stool. Sitting in lukewarm water in the bathtub, or trying a sitz bath, can help relieve this discomfort. Pat and dry the anus, instead of rubbing it when you get out of the water, and applying aloe vera based moisturizer, petroleum jelly or a haemorrhoid cream to the anus, can keep it from getting too inflamed and tender.

The changes that need to be included, in the diet, to treat and manage **Diarrhoea**, is explained in the sample diet charts, in Chapter- 25.

- ## 24.26 – Urinary Tract Infection (UTI)

UTI is when there is an infection in any one, or all of the main areas of the urinary system (*kidneys, ureter, urinary bladder* and *urethra*).

It is a common issue, especially in women, and studies estimate that more than half of the women population world-wide, will have a urinary tract infection at some point during their lives.

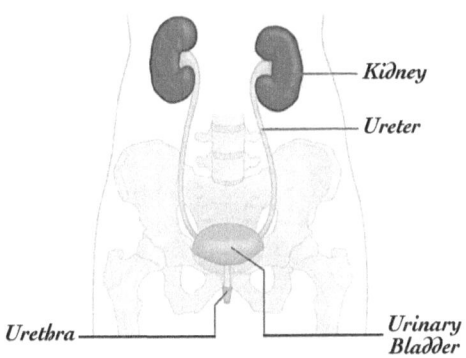

UTI causes inflammation, which leads to pain in the flanks, abdomen, pelvic area or lower back, a feeling of pressure in the lower part of the pelvis, cloudy and foul smelling urine, urinary incontinence, frequent urination, pain when urinating, blood in the urine etc.

Other indirect UTI symptoms may include, feeling extremely tired or fatigued, fever, chills, nausea and vomiting, mental changes or confusion.

The leading cause for UTI, of more than **90%** cases, is due to a micro-organism called *E. coli*. This bacteria typically exist in the large intestines, and enter through the urethra and causes infection.

This is why there are more cases of UTI in women, as their urethra is short and closer to the anus, where *E. coli* bacteria thrive.

Urinalysis, urine culture, ultra sound, CT scan, and cystoscopy can be utilised while diagnosing a UTI. The usual treatment is to have specific anti-biotics against the infection.

But the most common issue with UTI is that this infection has become more persistent, and recurring in more than half of those, who already have had episodes of the infection.

Recurrent UTIs that don't respond to antibiotics can happen for a few reasons which include –

- *<u>Antibiotic Resistance</u>*, caused due to **incomplete** eradication of the infectious bacteria.
- *<u>Chronic Colonization</u>*, due to improper hygiene, or underlying health issues such as diabetes and nutritional deficiencies, or due to hormonal changes, which can change the vaginal pH and flora, all of which, can lead to UTIs.
- *<u>Biofilm Formation</u>*, where clusters of bacteria that attach to the walls of the urinary tract creates biofilms, which act as a protective shield, and are resistant to antibiotics, which then allow the bacteria to evade the medication.

Addressing recurrent UTIs requires an approach that takes into account the metabolic, nutritional and gut health of the individual.

Probiotics, cranberry extract, D-mannose, along with a balanced diet is found to be effective in raising the body's own immune responses, and help in subduing UTIs.

Practicing good hygiene, regularly changing the 'period products' during menstrual cycles, avoiding the use of deodorants on vagina, drinking enough amounts of fluids, urinating when the urge begins (do not withhold), urinating and washing genitals after intercourse, wearing loose-fitting clothing (cotton underwear) to prevent moisture from accumulating around the urethra, are all positive habits that can help prevent frequent, and easy occurrence of UTIs.

The changes that need to be included, in the diet, to treat and manage **Urinary Tract Infection**, is explained in the sample diet charts, in Chapter- 25.

24.27 – Halitosis

Halitosis is the medical term for bad breath.

Everyone gets bad breath, especially after eating garlic, onions or other strong foods. But bad breath that doesn't go away (chronic halitosis) could mean that the person has an oral health issue, or a different condition that's affecting their body.
Finding the root cause of halitosis is the first step in treating the issue.

Halitosis is a widespread condition, affecting approximately 1 out of 4 people around the globe. One research study, which combined the findings of 13 medical journal articles, found that halitosis affects about **31.8%** of the global population.

The main halitosis symptom is foul-smelling breath that doesn't go away. The odour may be strong enough for other people to notice.

- **Poor oral hygiene**, (not brushing or flossing regularly) causes cavities and gum disease due bacterial infections.
- **Diabetes** which has an increased risk to cause gingivitis.
- *Gingivitis* or **'gum disease'** where inflammation of gums can cause redness, swelling and bleeding, usually caused by plaque (a hardened structure that evolves from a sticky biofilm, produced by harmful bacteria on the teeth to protect themselves).
- *Periodontitis* and **'trench mouth'** which are advanced forms of gum disease that can involve intense pain, bleeding, fever and fatigue.
- *Tonsilloliths* also called tonsil stones, are formed due to food particles that sediment in the tonsils, at the back of the throat, that hardens into calcium deposits, and are often foul smelling.
- Head and neck **cancers**.
- Liver or kidney disease.
- *Scurvy*, a deficiency disease of vitamin-C.
- **Infections** of nose, throat or lung as in pneumonia.
- **Dry mouth** (due to smoking, fasting or *Sjogren's* syndrome).

But the most common cause for persistent and chronic halitosis is gastritis, GERD, and other infections of the gut, which can only be solved by repairing the gut flora.

A common symptom that accompanies this kind of halitosis is white coated tongue, or an 'oral thrush' which is fungal infection of the mouth, or fungal infection from the gut, that has spread to the mouth.

Chewing gum and 'breath mints' can only cover up the problem, so halitosis treatment depends on the root cause of the issue. If due to poor oral hygiene, a dental cleaning and improved oral hygiene at home will help. In extreme cases, it is better to get the guidance of a dentist.

If the halitosis is due to vitamin-C deficiencies, then have citrus fruits or related supplements.

If due to gastritis, IBS or other infections of the gut, get it treated with appropriate medicines and changes in diet.

In cases of tonsilloliths, regular gargling with luke-warm salt-water, or staying for a week on a fruit diet, or practicing intermittent fasting, is found to be highly effective, where the tonsil stones are spontaneously dislodged and excreted.

The changes that need to be included, in the diet, to treat and manage **Halitosis**, is explained in the sample diet charts, in Chapter- 25.

*Let us next discuss about a few **Auto-Immune Disorders** due to an **imbalanced gut microbiota**.*

24.28 – IBD (Crohn's Disease & Ulcerative Colitis)

Inflammatory bowel disease (IBD) refers to diseases that cause chronic inflammation in an individual's gastro-intestinal (GI) tract.

Its symptoms may come on suddenly (flares) and cause intense stomach cramps and diarrhoea, among other issues.

IBD can affect more than the gut, as it can challenge their overall physical health, emotional well-being and even mental health. Experts estimate that **2.7 lakh** people in India have IBD as of 2019.

Crohn's disease and ulcerative colitis are the main types of IBD.

Crohn's disease (CD), causes *ulcers* in the GI tract and can affect any part of it, from the mouth to the anus, but is typically developed in the small intestine and the upper part of the large intestine. It is a TH-1 issue (explained in Chapter- 23).

Ulcerative colitis (UD), causes swelling (*cobblestone appearance*) and ulcers in the large intestine. It usually starts in the rectum and can spread to all of parts of the colon. It is in most cases, a TH-2 disorder.

IBD symptoms may be mild or severe, and you can't always predict when it occurs, as they come and go. Common IBD symptoms include lower abdominal pain, blood or mucous in stools, severe diarrhoea, fatigue, and weight loss.

IBD happens when immune system cells in the GIT mistakenly attack healthy tissue, causing inflammation that leads to Crohn's disease and ulcerative colitis.

Antibiotics, NSAIDs, smoking, stress, alcohol, gluten or lactose intolerance, fast food, etc. are all possible causes for altering the gut microbiomes which leads to this auto-immunity.

Complete blood count (CBC), stool tests, GGT, ALP, p-ANCA, endoscopy, colonoscopy, capsule endoscopy, MRI and CT scan, etc. are the usual tests done to diagnose IBD.

In most cases, a positive results of stool lactoferrin and calprotectin levels are enough to diagnose IBD (inflammatory bowel disease), and differentiate it from IBS (irritable bowel syndrome).

IBD causes other medical conditions in the GIT and beyond, which may become medical emergencies or serious illnesses, including colon cancer (higher risk in cases of UC), perforated bowel, toxic megacolon, anal fistula and stenosis, anaemia, blood clots, eye pain and irritation, kidney stones, mouth ulcers, liver diseases, malnutrition, swollen joints, skin sores and rashes, osteoporosis, and can even lead to the formation of heart blocks (atherosclerosis).

Antibiotics, anti-diarrhoea medication, corticosteroids, immune-modulators and immune-suppressants are the usual medications available for conventional treatment. Colectomy surgery is also preferred when years of medications are not able to curb the symptoms.

Targeting biofilms formed by the bacteria is one of the most important tasks in IBD. The issue with it though, is that there is no test yet, that can identify these biofilms, which protect the pathogens and trigger inflammatory responses from the body.

But research has proven that over 80% of the cases with presence of faecal calprotectin levels, have these formations. *N-acetyl cysteine* (NAC) and vitamin-C complex, are potent disruptors of biofilms, which aid in the treatment of IBD.

The changes that need to be included, in the diet, to treat and manage **IBD (Crohn's Disease & Ulcerative Colitis)**, is explained in the sample diet charts, in Chapter- 25.

24.29 – **Ankylosing Spondylitis (AS)**

Also called as *axial spondylarthritis*, it mostly affects the joints where the base of the spine meets the pelvis. Even though un-common, AS can affect other joints, including the knees, hips and shoulder joints.

As discussed earlier, *ankylosing spondylitis* occurs due to an infected gut flora (commonly due to **Klebsiella pneumoniae**). But there is a speciality in this case, because the auto-immunity in AS occurs, as a confirmed result, of the combination of a mutated gene, as well as an infected gut.

There are more than 60 mutated genes that might cause AS, the most common examples being the *human leukocyte antigen*- B27 or B51 (**HLA-B27** and **HLA-B51**) gene. More than **90%** of people who have *ankylosing spondylitis*, also have a mutated HLA-B27 gene.

This mutated gene is actually a blessing, and gives these individuals '*Super Immunity*' which means, that they have superior immunity than that of normal individuals.

It has been observed that these individuals with the super-immunity gene mutation, lead an almost normal, symptom-less lives even when affected by the deadly **HIV virus** that causes AIDS.
Unfortunately though, when in combination with certain infections of the gut, it can cause these super immune bodies, to turn against the own body, and cause inflammation in the joints leading to stiffness and pain.

Each person with *ankylosing spondylitis* experiences a unique combination of symptoms, but the most common issue is lower back pain due to *sacroiliitis* (painful inflammation in your sacroiliac joints).

Pain in the hips, buttocks, neck, abdomen, are also common. Stiffness or trouble moving the hips and lower back (especially first thing in the morning or after rest, or in the same position for a long time), fatigue, shortness of breath, low appetite, unexplained weight loss, diarrhoea, skin rashes and vision problems are also usually noted symptoms.

Bamboo spine, or fused vertebrae (joined bones in the spine with no flexibility) is the most common complication of *ankylosing spondylitis*.

Higher risk of spinal fractures, kyphosis (forward curve in the spine), osteoporosis, eye and vision issues like uveitis or light sensitivity, heart issues and nerve damage are also usual complications of AS.

Blood tests to check for the mutated HLA-B27 gene and ANA test, X-rays, MRI scans, etc. are usual diagnostic procedures for detecting and confirming *ankylosing spondylitis*.

Various medications and even surgical interventions are available for the treatment of AS, but unless the root cause is targeted, and the needed lifestyle changes brough into action, the success rate of these treatments and the quality of life for the patient, will always remain low.

And as the root cause of this issue lies in gut flora infection and a leaky gut, (explained in Chapter-13), or an infected liver, the treatment should coincide with a dietary habit that supports the liver, friendly gut flora and prevent indigestion or gastritis.

The changes that need to be included, in the diet, to treat and manage **Ankylosing Spondylitis**, is explained in the sample diet charts, in Chapter- 25.

- **24.30 – Ig-A nephropathy (Berger's Disease)**

IgA is an antibody, a protein in the immune system, that protect us from bacteria and viruses.

But in rare cases, the IgA builds up in the kidneys and causes inflammation, and damages the glomeruli or nephrons, which are kidney tissues. This causes the kidneys to leak blood (*haematuria*), and protein (*proteinuria*), into the urine.

Eventually, the nephrons may scar, causing kidney disease, and as the scarring progresses, it causes ESRD (*end-stage renal disease*).

This process can happen quickly, over the course of months, or can take as long as 20 years after the initial diagnosis.

If the ESRD stage has commenced, the kidneys cannot work well, and the patient may need dialysis (machine that helps filter the blood), or a kidney transplant.

About 1 in 4 adults, and 1 in every 20 children, with IgA nephropathy, eventually develop ESRD (*end-stage renal disease*).

The IgA forms masses, or clusters, called immune complexes, with substances that the body considers '**foreign**' (which are mostly undigested food, or protein, like galactose, lactose, gluten, or any other substance, or micro-organisms). The immune complexes get stuck in the glomeruli, causes inflammation and damage, resulting in kidney disease.

At first, there may be no symptoms, and it could be years or even decades before signs appear.

The most common symptoms are visible blood in the urine (haematuria), flank pain (at the sides of the back), ankle swelling (edema), hypertension (increased blood pressure), proteinuria (too much protein in the urine, causes foamy urine), cold or other respiratory infections etc.

Acute kidney failure, chronic kidney failure, nephrotic syndrome, hypertension, cardio-vascular problems, IgA vasculitis are common complications of the issue.

Serum IgA, eGFR (*estimated glomerular filtration rate*), urinalysis (to check presence of blood in the urine), blood tests (lipid profile, creatinine), urine protein test, physical exam (monitor BP, check for signs of swelling) are the various tests used to diagnose, and monitor the health of the individual during the disease. A kidney biopsy procedure is also done to confirm a diagnosis of IgA nephropathy.

Blood pressure regulators, diuretics (to remove extra fluid or edema in the body), steroids to control the immune system, etc. are the most commonly used medications.

But as the root cause of the issue lies in gut flora infection and a leaky gut, (explained in Chapter- 13), or an infected liver, the treatment should coincide with a dietary habit that supports the liver, friendly gut flora and prevent indigestion or gastritis.

The changes that need to be included, in the diet, to treat and manage **Ig-A Nephropathy**, is explained in the sample diet charts, in Chapter- 25.

- **24.31 – <u>Systemic Lupus Erythematosus (SLE)</u>**

Lupus is a condition that causes inflammation throughout the body including the skin, blood, joints, kidneys, brain, heart, lungs, eyes etc. Systemic lupus erythematosus (SLE) is the most common type of lupus, which means that the patient has lupus throughout your body.

Other types include –
- **Cutaneous** lupus erythematous (only affects the skin),
- **Drug-induced** lupus (triggered by any medicine, often temporary),
- **Neonatal** lupus (babies are sometimes born with lupus).

Lupus causes symptoms throughout the body, depending on which organs or systems it affects. Everyone experiences a different combination and severity of symptoms, and it usually has severe flare ups (that often affects daily routine), and then subsides.

Symptoms usually develop gradually, with one or two signs of lupus appearing first, and then more of the symptoms appearing later on, such as joint and muscle pain, chest pain (when taking deep breaths), headaches, fever, hair loss, mouth ulcers, fatigue, shortness of breath, swollen glands, rashes (commonly across the face also called as butterfly rash), swelling in the arms, legs or face, and blood clots, are some of the other usual symptoms.

Lupus can also lead to other health conditions including, photosensitivity (sensitivity to sunlight), dry eyes, confusions and depression (or other mental health conditions), seizures, anaemia, osteoporosis, heart issues, kidney disease, *Raynaud's* syndrome etc.

A healthcare provider will diagnose lupus with physical examinations, blood tests, urinalysis, ANA (anti-nuclear antibody) test, biopsy of skin or kidney tissue and other various diagnostic methods depending on the various presenting symptoms.

Frequently used medications to control symptoms of lupus are –
- Disease-modifying anti-rheumatic drug (DMARD).
- Immuno-suppressants.
- Corticosteroids.
- NSAIDs.

However, unless the root cause of the issue is figured out, and the needed lifestyle changes brough into action, the success rate of these treatments and the quality of life for the patient, will always remain consistently low.

As the root cause of this issue lies in gut flora infection and a leaky gut, (explained in detail in Chapter-13), or an infected liver, the treatment should coincide with a dietary habit that supports the liver, friendly gut flora, and prevent indigestion or gastritis.

The changes that need to be included, in the diet, to treat and manage **Systemic Lupus Erythematosus**, is explained in the sample diet charts, in Chapter- 25.

- ## 24.32 – **Rheumatoid Arthritis (RA)**

Rheumatoid arthritis occurs in the joints on both sides of the body, which makes it different from other types of arthritis.

The individual may have symptoms of pain and inflammation in the fingers, hands, wrists, knees, ankles, feet, toes, skin, eyes, mouth, lungs or even the heart during *rheumatoid arthritis*.

Uncontrolled inflammation damages the cartilage, which normally acts as a 'shock absorber' in the joints, and over time, it can deform the joints, and eventually cause the bone itself to erode, which can lead up to the fusion of the joint, and cause joint deformities.

Rheumatoid arthritis is estimated to affect approximately **1%** of the **Indian** population, and is the most common form of autoimmune inflammatory arthritis. It is found to be **twice as common** in women.

Rheumatoid arthritis affects everyone differently. In some people, joint symptoms develop over several years. Whereas in others, there is rapid progression. Flare-ups and remission periods are also common in RA.

Symptoms of *rheumatoid arthritis* include pain, swelling, stiffness and tenderness in more than one joint (usually the same joints on both sides of the body), especially in the morning or after sitting for long periods. Fatigue, weakness and fever are also noticed.

People suffering from *rheumatoid arthritis* are at a higher risk of developing cardio-vascular disorders.

People born with variations in the human leukocyte antigen (HLA) genes (as in ankylosing spondylitis, Chapter- 24.28) are more likely to develop *rheumatoid arthritis*.

The general diagnostic criteria for *rheumatoid arthritis* are -

- Inflammatory arthritis in two or more joints,
- Elevated levels of RF (*Rheumatoid Factor*),
- Elevated levels of CCP (*Cyclic Citrullinated Peptides*) antibodies,
- Elevated levels of ESR (*Erythrocyte Sedimentation Rate*),
- Elevated levels of CRP (*C-Reactive Protein*),
- X-rays, ultra-sound and MRI scans are also helpful in supporting the diagnosis.

Around **80%** of people suffering from rheumatoid arthritis, are under the **'sero-positive RA'** category, as their blood work, tests positive for RA (*rheumatoid factor*), and about **70%** of those suffering from *sero-positive rheumatoid arthritis*, are also found to have antibodies to a protein by-product known as CCP (*cyclic citrullinated peptide*).

This can indicate that a gut infection is responsible for triggering the auto-immunity, in over **90%** cases of *sero-positive rheumatoid arthritis*, majorly due to the overgrowth of **Prevotella Copri** bacteria, but can also be caused due to various species of fungi and parasites as well.

Additionally, around **10%** of *sero-positive rheumatoid arthritis* cases may be linked to oral infections, majorly caused by the by **Porphyromonas Gingivalis**, a bacterium commonly associated with periodontal disease, which produces enzymes that modify proteins, leading to the formation of citrullinated peptides, which the immune system may then target, subsequently contributing to the development of RA.

This is why the traditional practice of **'*coconut oil pulling*'** (swishing oil around the mouth like one would when using mouthwash, but for a longer period of time), used to prove fruitful in few cases of *rheumatoid arthritis*, as the **'*lauric acid*'** compound from coconut oil, reduces inflammation and gets rid of harmful oral bacteria.

Around **30% of total** rheumatoid arthritis cases, are under the 'sero-negative RA' category, which is when, blood tests do not show antibodies, but the inflammatory markers in the body are typically high, which most commonly indicates a viral origin to the condition, and the most commonly found viruses are EBV (*Epstein-bar virus*) or CMV (*Cytomegalo-virus*) infections.

A much smaller percentage of the total rheumatoid arthritis cases have also been linked to be triggered from mere vitamin-D deficiency alone, as it alters the way body responds to various inflammations, that further lead to the production of inflammatory cytokines and auto-immune bodies that contribute to joint damage and pain.

NSAIDs, corticosteroids, JAK (*janus-kinase*) inhibitors, DMARDs (*disease modifying anti-rheumatic drugs*), and biologics (biologic response agents), are the commonly used drugs for treating the symptoms of RA, along with surgeries to correct a deformity that might occur.

However, unless the root cause of the issue is figured out, and the needed lifestyle changes brough into action, the success rate of these treatments and the quality of life for the patient, will always be low. The treatment should coincide with a dietary habit that supports the liver, friendly gut flora and prevent indigestion or gastritis.

The changes that need to be included, in the diet, to treat and manage **Rheumatoid Arthritis**, is explained in the sample diet charts, in Chapter- 25.

- ## 24.33 – **Immune Thrombocytopenia (ITP)**

ITP is a condition that causes low platelet count, which prevents the blood from clotting, and can cause the body to bruise easily, or over bleed when a cut or injury is present. It can sometimes even cause spontaneous bleeding without any external cuts.

80% of all cases are *'Primary*-ITP' caused when the immune system attacks our platelets. *'Secondary*-ITP' is when it is caused by other underlying conditions like chronic infections or blood cancers. People with HIV infections, H. pylori, hepatitis-C and EBV infections have an increased risk of developing ITP.

ITP that goes away within three months, is called *Acute*-ITP, and it affects more children than adults. *Persistent*-ITP, is that which lasts between 3 and 12 months, and if it lasts for more than a year, it is known as *Chronic*-ITP.

ITP may not show symptoms, but it can appear slowly or quickly. Commonly noticed symptoms are, *petechiae* (red or purple tiny dots on lower legs that resemble a rash), *purpura* (is when petechiae join together, forming red, purple or brown spots on the skin, due to small blood vessels under the skin leaking blood), *bruises* (blood pools under your skin), *hematoma* (large bruise), swollen and bleeding gums, blood in stool and urine, menorrhagia (heavy menstrual periods), nosebleeds, fatigue etc.

When suffering from ITP, it is best to avoid contact sports like football, basketball, hockey etc. where there are high chances for injury or bruises.

A complete blood count (CBC), and peripheral blood smear tests, are done in order to diagnose the condition. To find the root cause, test for various infections and to rule out cancerous growths, are done as well.

Common treatments of ITP include **corticosteroids** medications (which block the antibodies that destroy platelets), **thrombopoietin receptor agonists** (boosts platelet production), **immunosuppressants**, treating underlying infections, and having a **platelet transfusion**.

In some cases, surgeons decide to remove the spleen through surgery. This is not very helpful though, as even though it may help with ITP, it puts the patient more at risk for infections.

Unless the root cause of the issue is figured out, and the needed lifestyle changes brough into action, the success rate of these treatments and the quality of life for the patient, will always be low, as the risk of severe internal or external bleeding always looms about.

As the most common root cause of this issue lies in gut flora infection and a leaky gut, (explained in Chapter- 13), and infections or toxicity of the liver, the treatment should coincide with a dietary habit that supports the liver, supports the growth of friendly gut flora, and prevent indigestion or gastritis.

The changes that need to be included, in the diet, to treat and manage **Immune Thrombocytopenia**, is explained in the sample diet charts, in Chapter- 25.

- ## 24.34 – <u>Thyroiditis (Hashimoto's & Graves')</u>

When it comes to auto-immune thyroid diseases, the issues that can arise, are mainly the body's reaction to an infected and imbalanced gut flora, where auto-immune bodies such as –

- **ATG** (*anti-thyro globulin*)
- **Anti-TPO** (*anti-thyro peroxidase*)
- **TSI** (*thyroid stimulating immuno-globulin*)

… are produced in our body which then, impedes the thyroid synthesizing function. Often times, these anti-bodies are also responsible for the growth of nodules or abnormal growths on the thyroid gland, which can sometimes even turn out to be cancerous.

Hashimoto's or ***Lymphocytic*** thyroiditis is a condition that causes **hypo-thyroidism** or an underactive thyroid function. It is estimated that around **42 Million** people in India, suffer from this condition.

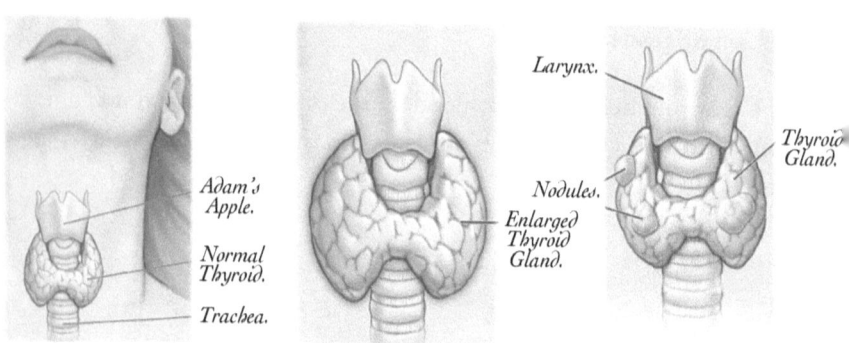

Graves' disease is the most common form of **hyper-thyroidism**, where there is an excess of thyroid function, meaning that the thyroid gland makes too much thyroid hormone. *Graves'* disease affects **16.7%** of India's adult population, according to population research.

1 in 3 people suffering from *Graves'* disease, suffer from 'thyroid eye disease' or orbitopathy or ophthalmopathy, with symptoms like gritty, irritated eyes, swelling of the tissues around the eyes (puffy eyes), bulging eyes, light sensitivity, pressure and pain in the eyes, blurred vision or double vision etc.

Common associated symptoms of thyroiditis-

Hashimoto's Thyroiditis	*Graves' Thyroiditis*
Weight gain.	Weight loss.
Often decreased appetite.	Increased appetite.
Slow heart rate (bradycardia).	Rapid heartbeat (palpitations).
Constipation.	Diarrhoea or frequent bowels.
Dry skin.	Thin, warm and moist skin.
Feeling cold.	Heat intolerance, excess sweating.
Joint stiffness, and muscle pain.	Muscle weakness.
Puffy eyes and face.	Enlarged thyroid gland (goiter).
Fatigue, lethargy, sleepy.	Difficulty sleeping, insomnia.
Dry, brittle hair, slow hair growth, or hair loss.	Hair loss and change in hair texture (brittle).
Low or depressed mood.	Feeling shaky or nervous.
Memory problems or difficulty concentrating.	Brain fog, memory and concentrating issues.
Heavy or irregular periods.	Menstrual irregularities.
Decreased libido (sex drive).	Decreased libido (sex drive).
Infertility (male and female).	Infertility (male and female).

The thyroid gland sometimes become enlarged, causing a condition called Goiter, which makes the front of the neck look swollen.
It doesn't usually hurt, but can create a feeling of fullness in the throat and lower neck.

Rarely, patients with *Graves'* disease, have also been noticed to develop a lumpy, reddish thickening of the skin on their shins known as 'pretibial myxoedema' (*Graves'* dermopathy), which is usually painless and mild, but can be painful in few cases.

The thyroid hormones affect every cell in the body, and influences factors such as our body's energy usage, controlling our body temperature, managing our heart rate, and even plays a hand in controlling how much protein the body makes. Its functions affects every organ in the body, including the precious heart and brain.

A thyroid profile test (TSH, free T_4, T_3) helps to diagnose whether it is *Hypo-* or *Hyper-* thyroidism, and antibody tests such as Anti-TPO and ATG confirms *Hashimoto's* thyroiditis.

The TSI antibody (also known as **TRAb** - *thyrotropin receptor antibodies*) helps confirm *Graves'* disease, along with radioactive iodine uptake scan, and Doppler ultrasound for all cases.
Thyroid ultrasound scan is done to check the size of the thyroid gland, and to make sure that there aren't any thyroid nodules or growths.

Untreated or undertreated auto-immune thyroiditis disease can lead to issues and complications such as osteoporosis (causes frequent bone fractures), heart conditions (stroke, heart attack), thyroid storm or thyrotoxic crisis (a medical emergency with high fever and palpitations), damage to optic nerve (causing vision loss), hyper-triglyceridemia, peripheral neuropathy, hypertension, depression, myxoedema coma (due to severe hypothyroidism), swelling or edema (face, tongue, lower legs or ankles), hypothermia (body temperature below 35° Celsius), and slowed breathing, or difficulty in breathing.

Untreated hypothyroidism during pregnancy can affect the foetus' growth and brain development, and increase the risk of miscarriage, premature birth, still-birth, pre-eclampsia (dangerous rise in blood pressure in late pregnancy), congestive heart failure, and is also found to be a cause for infant hyperthyroidism.

Various medications and surgical interventions are available for the treatment of thyroiditis, but unless the root cause is figured out, and the needed lifestyle changes brough into action, the success rate of these treatments and the quality of life for the patient, will always remain low.

Parasitic infections are one of such persistent underlying causes, that are often overlooked. These infections can vary greatly in severity, from mild cases that go unnoticed to serious, life threatening conditions.
The impact of a parasitic infection depends on the type of parasite, the individual's health, the effectiveness of treatment, and how quickly the infection is detected.

Direct contact with infected soil, faecal to oral route, mother to child infection during pregnancy or childbirth, infections through pets and animals, insect bites, and sexual contact are the various ways for parasite transmission.
The most common route for transmission of various parasites though, are through contaminated food and water, especially raw or undercooked meat (usually fish, pork, and beef).

It is often argued that the Japanese are healthy despite eating raw fish, like 'sushi.' Japanese culinary practices are built on centuries of experience with handling raw fish. The fish used in sushi and sashimi are often frozen at temperatures around -20°C before serving, for at least 24 hours, to kill parasites.
The Japanese also consume vinegar prior to meals, in order to increase the stomach acid production, which helps neutralize pathogens.

In addition to freezing, other common practices to prevent parasitic infections from raw seafood include careful sourcing, cleaning, and preparation. The use of wasabi and other strong condiments (like pickled ginger) in sushi, also mildly serves the purpose of being anti-microbial, even though its role is more about flavour and tradition.

Moreover, a healthy body is naturally equipped to eliminate most parasites, but this ability can be compromised by poor lifestyle choices. Regular consumption of ultra-processed foods, fast foods, and diets low in essential nutrients like vitamin-D and zinc weakens the immune system, making it harder for the body to fight off parasites. Without proper nourishment, the body's natural defences are unable to function optimally, leaving us vulnerable to the harmful effects of parasites.

The treatment for parasitic infections depends on the type of parasite and the severity of the infection. Parasitic infections are treated with antiprotozoals, anthelmintics, or antimalarial medications.

A deworming course is best done every six months, but severe infections may require a higher dosage for longer durations. In such cases, it is crucial to deworm all household members to prevent reinfection. Additionally, clean and sun-dry inner-wear, bedsheets, and pillow covers to eliminate any parasite eggs.

In severe cases of parasitic infections such as *leishmaniasis* or *echinococcosis*, surgery may be required to remove cysts or affected tissue

The changes that need to be included, in the diet, to treat and manage **Auto-Immune Thyroiditis (Hashimoto's & Graves' Disease)**, is explained in the sample diet charts, in Chapter- 25.

- **24.35 – <u>Multiple Sclerosis (MS)</u>**

An auto-immune condition that affects the brain and spinal cord, where the immune system mistakenly attacks **myelin cells**, which are the protective covers (sheaths) that surround brain, nerves and spinal cord.

This damage interrupts messages (signals) that our nerves send throughout the body to perform functions like vision, sensation and movement.

India has witnessed shift from being low MS risk zone to moderate, with the prevalence rate increased from 2 individuals, to around 9 individuals affected, per 100,000 of the population.

MS affects individuals in various patterns such as-

- CIS (*<u>clinically isolated syndrome</u>*) where a sudden attack or inflammation of the myelin sheaths occur once, and then re-occurrence is rarely seen.

- RRMS (*<u>relapsing-remitting multiple sclerosis</u>*), which is the most common way that MS begins, and around 85% of people diagnosed with MS have this type, where there are regular flare-ups or attacks of new or old symptoms, along with periods of remission, where there are no symptoms noticeable.

- SPMS (*<u>secondary progressive multiple sclerosis</u>*), is an advanced form of MS, where the nerve damage accumulates and symptoms gradually worsen. Flare-ups are not as common as in RRMS, and periods of remission are even more rare.

- PPMS (*<u>primary progressive multiple sclerosis</u>*), are cases where, multiple sclerosis symptoms start off slowly, and gradually worsen over time, without any periods of remission.

Three rare MS variants include-

- *Tumefactive*-MS where there are demyelination of large areas in the brain, which may appear similar to tumours.
- *Balo's concentric*-MS is when there are lesions (myelin damage) that appear in concentric rings (in the shape of a target) when viewed on an MRI scanning report.
- *Marburg variant*-MS is a rare and aggressive form, characterized by rapid progression, which may result in death when left untreated.

Early signs and symptoms of MS include changes to the vision (optic neuritis, double vision, vision loss), muscle weakness, numbness or abnormal sensations usually affecting one side of the face or body, or below the waist.

Common symptoms of MS include fatigue, clumsiness, dizziness, urinary incontinence, loss of balance and coordination, difficulty with cognitive function (thinking, concentration, memory, learning and judgment), mood changes, muscle stiffness, spasms and tremors etc. to name a few, which vary for each person, and may fluctuate in severity from one day to the next. It is rare to experience all of the symptoms at the same time.

The immune system protects the myelin sheath from things that can harm it, like bacteria or viruses. But during MS, the immune system mistakes healthy myelin (and sometimes, the nerve cells below the myelin) as a threat to the body, and attacks it, which causes demyelination.

Even if the immune system doesn't directly attack the myelin sheath, the myelin is constantly degraded in the body due to the action of free radicals. But one of the body's major natural anti-oxidant *'Glutathione'* plays a pivotal role in preventing this damage.
Recent studies have shown that gut dysbiosis, with a dominant bacteria named *Desulfo-vibrionaceae*, prevents glutathione formation.

This bacteria digests *sulfur*, and prevents the formation of *'cysteine'* which is one of the three amino-acids that make up glutathione.

So **no** cysteine means **no** glutathione formation as well, which leads to the unchecked damage of the myelin sheath by free radicals.

In many auto-immune cases just as in MS, there is also the issue of a compromised liver function due to toxicity or infections, which prevent the formation of glutathione (synthesized in the liver by combining its amino-acid precursors which are glutamine, cysteine, and glycine).

Selenium deficiency is also found to be a major issue in the deficiency of glutathione peroxidase, as it is essential in its formation.

While oral glutathione supplementation is commonly used, it proves largely ineffective because the compound is broken down back into its constituent precursors or amino acids during digestion, which must then be re-assembled in the liver to form glutathione.

This process becomes further complicated in the presence of chronic infections like EBV (*Epstein-Barr virus*) and CMV (*Cytomegalo-virus*), which can cause persistent liver inflammation and damage, thereby creating a cycle of continuous oxidative stress, and reduced glutathione production.

The body's attempt to replenish glutathione levels, is thus, in vain, which then further extends the toxicity and dysfunction.

To break this cycle and to restore the body's glutathione levels effectively, intravenous (IV) nutrient therapy is often required, as it bypasses the digestive breakdown, and delivers the necessary nutrients directly to the bloodstream, allowing for more efficient liver detoxification and immune system support.

Blood test, stool and urine tests, OCT (*optical coherence tomography*), MRI (*magnetic resonance imaging*) scans, EP (*evoked potential*) test, lumbar puncture for analysis of the spinal fluid, along with physical and neurological examination may be required to diagnose cases of multiple sclerosis, as most symptoms can look like or happen with several other common conditions or diseases.

Various symptomatic medications are available to treat MS including stem cell transplant, but often times, regardless of treatment, MS can lead to disability and make it difficult to do routine work without assistance, over time.

But as the root cause of the issue lies in gut flora infection and a leaky gut, (explained in Chapter- 13), or an infected liver, the treatment should coincide with a dietary habit that supports the liver, and the beneficial gut flora and which prevents indigestion or gastritis.

The changes that need to be included, in the diet, to treat and manage **Multiple Sclerosis**, is explained in the sample diet charts, in Chapter- 25.

- **24.36 – <u>Type-1 Diabetes Mellitus (DMT1)</u>**

DMT1 is often a chronic life-long autoimmune disease that prevents the pancreas from making insulin.

Synthetic insulin is the go-to treatment considered, to tackle DMT1, but the much easier and healthy way to tackle it, is through depending on fats and ketones for energy.

DMT1 occurs when our immune system attacks and destroys cells in the pancreas, which make insulin.

This destruction can happen over months or years, ultimately resulting in a total arrest of production of insulin.

DMT1 is diagnosed through blood glucose tests (FBS, RBS and PPBS), HbA1c (glycosylated haemoglobin), and an antibody test (usually ANA profile). Urinalysis, basic metabolic panel, and arterial blood gas tests, are done to check for ketoacidosis.

Symptoms of DMT1 include excessive thirst and hunger, frequent urination, unexplained weight loss, fatigue, blurred vision, slow healing injuries, and vaginal yeast infections.

One of the severe complication of DMT1 is diabetes-related ketoacidosis (DKA), which show symptoms like fruity-smelling breath, nausea and vomiting, stomach-ache, rapid breathing, confusion, drowsiness, and loss of consciousness.

The only known efficient conventional treatment and medicine for DMT1 is synthetic insulin, which work at different speeds, and lasts in the body for different lengths of time, based on the patients weight, age, physical activity level, their blood sugar level at any given time, the type of foods they consume etc.

Usually, a base level of insulin is administered (called a basal rate), and on top of it, specific amounts of insulin are also given, for when they eat, or to correct spikes in blood sugar levels (due to various factors, like those mentioned before).

Insulin dosages are changed throughout the life of the patient based on various factors and by regular blood sugar monitoring, by the use of blood glucose meter or CGM (*continuous glucose monitoring*) device.

Multiple daily injections, disposable pre-filled insulin pens, insulin pumps (devices that deliver insulin continuously and on demand, which mimics the action of pancreas), and rapid-acting inhaled insulin (much like an asthma inhaler, quickly absorbed than other types) are all various methods for administering insulin into the body.

The major side effect of DMT1 treatment by insulin, is low blood sugar or hypoglycaemia, which occurs when too much insulin is administered, disproportionate, to the food intake or to the level of physical activity.

Blood sugar below 70 mg/dL usually causes shaking or trembling, sweating and chills, dizziness or light-headedness, faster heart rate, headache, hunger, nausea, nervousness or irritability, pale skin, restless sleep, and weakness.

Hypoglycaemia also occurs in DMT1 as a result of the body not being able to efficiently convert the blood sugar into energy. But this issue, as mentioned in Chapter- 4, occurs when the body is only given a choice of sugars, from the diet, for the body's energy needs. It would not have happened, if the body was offered a different option as well, to create energy, like that from ketones, which are converted from true fats.

> Hypoglycaemia can sometimes be life-threatening and needs to be attended to right away.

Patients suffering from hypoglycaemia, usually feels it, just before it occurs, and so all they need to do is, to have a spoonful of honey, powdered glucose or any kind of sweets, to help the body get a shot of instant energy, just for the sake of the moment.

But continue the diet as advised (this method though, might not work for those suffering from advanced stages of DMT1, with extremely damaged pancreas and a total lack or deficiency of insulin).

The diet, in the long run, will help the body become more efficient in the conversion of healthy amount of ketones from fats, and with a steady and effective energy production from these ketone bodies, the person will eventually get rid of episodes of hypoglycaemia.

Blood sugar levels that are even below 50 mg/dL would thus, not matter, as the body will be able to rely on another source of fuel for energy.

Scientists are working on ways to prevent or slow down the progression of DMT1 through research into pancreatic islet transplantation, an experimental treatment. This procedure aims to replace destroyed islets with new ones from an organ donor, that make and release insulin.

Stem cell therapy, which involves using stem cells with the potential to differentiate into insulin-producing cells, is an area making amazing breakthroughs as well. Stem cell research aims to create a renewable source of islet cells by coaxing stem cells to become functioning pancreatic islets, providing a long-term solution without relying on human donors.

Close to **50%** of people with DMT1, develop serious complications over their lifetime, such as eyes issues (diabetic retinopathy, macular edema, cataracts and glaucoma), and foot problems (like ulcers and infections that can lead to gangrene and need for amputation).

Heart diseases, high blood pressure, kidney diseases (nephropathy), oral health issues (cavities and persistent infections), nerve damage (diabetic neuropathy), skin issues (dry skin, bacterial and fungal infections and diabetes-related dermopathy), stroke etc. are also typical complications that seriously affect the quality of life.

To manage and live with DMT1, it is of utmost importance to learn and understand how different foods, exercise and illnesses affects the body, and how we can successfully by-pass the sole dependence on the sugar-insulin combination for energy.

And since the root cause of the issue commonly lies in gut flora infection and a leaky gut, (explained in Chapter- 13), or an infected liver, the treatment should coincide with a dietary habit that supports the liver, friendly gut flora and prevent indigestion or gastritis, and various other auto-immune triggers. The changes that need to be included, in the diet, to treat and manage **Type-1 Diabetes Mellitus**, is explained in the sample diet charts, in Chapter- 25.

- **24.37 – Sjögren's Syndrome**

Sjögren's syndrome is an auto-immune disorder, that damages glands in the body which produce and control moisture, causing the glands to produce less moisture than usual, leading to chronic dryness and pain throughout the body, especially the eyes and mouth.

The lacrimal gland (tears), salivary glands, nose, throat, digestive system and vagina are all possible targets of this disease.

The most common symptom of Sjögren's syndrome is, unusual dryness or itching in eyes, *xerostomia* (dry mouth, mouth ulcers, thickened saliva, vaginal dryness, dry skin, dry throat with regular coughing, nose and frequent nose-bleeds.

In addition to dryness, other symptoms like joint pain, muscle pain or muscle weakness, swollen lymph nodes, fatigue, dysphagia (trouble swallowing), brain fog, loss of taste, tooth decay, skin rashes, gastritis, heart burn, neuropathy, indigestion, and light sensitivity are noticed.

Sjögren's syndrome can cause complications, such as oral and eye infections, abnormal liver or kidney functions, lymphomas (cancerous tumours in the lymph nodes), lung issues that may be mistaken for pneumonia, neurological issues that lead to weakness or numbness.

Common symptomatic treatments for dryness include –

- *Artificial tears,* prescription drops or lubricants to keep eyes moist.
- *Punctual Plugs* (dry eye surgery) where a few, or all tear ducts are surgically closed, to keep natural tears in the eyes for a longer period.
- *Saliva producer* supplements or medicines.
- Special mouthwash or dental care products.
- Vaginal moisturizers or *lubricants*.
- *Hormone therapy* if vaginal dryness is due to hormonal imbalances.

Immune-suppressants like DMARDs (disease-modifying antirheumatic drugs), anti-inflammatory drugs like corticosteroids, pain-killers such as NSAIDs are also the most commonly prescribed drugs to manage the symptoms of Sjögren's syndrome.

The root cause of the issue lies in the infection of the gut flora, and a leaky gut, (explained in Chapter- 13), or liver toxicity or infection, and the common viral infections that can trigger the auto-immune response of the body during Sjögren's syndrome include hepatitis-C, CMV (*Cytomegalo-virus*), HTLV (*human T-lymphotropic virus*-1), EBV (*Epstein-Barr virus*), COVID-19 etc.

The treatment for Sjögren's syndrome should coincide with a dietary habit that supports the liver, growth of friendly gut flora and prevent indigestion or gastritis. The changes that need to be included, in the diet, to treat and manage **Sjögren's Syndrome**, is explained in the sample diet charts, in Chapter- 25.

24.38 – Vitiligo

Vitiligo is an auto-immune condition that causes the skin to lose its colour or pigment, which makes the skin appear lighter than its natural skin tone, or turn white, and white or silver discolouration in areas that is covered by hair.

Areas of skin that lose pigment are called macules (less than 1 cm), or patches if larger than that. The condition occurs when the immune system, or attack of free radicals, destroys melanocytes, cells that produce melanin, the chemical that gives skin its colour, or pigmentation.

Vitiligo occurs in over **1%** of the world population.

Types of vitiligo include –

- *Generalized* - most common, with macules on various parts of body.
- *Segmental* - only affects one side or area, such as the hands or face.
- *Mucosal* - affects mucous membranes of the mouth or genitals.
- *Focal* - rare type, macules develop in small area and don't spread.
- *Universal* - rare type affecting more than 80% of the skin.
- *Trichome* - causes a bullseye appearance, with alternating coloured, and colourless concentric areas.

Vitiligo can sometimes be mistaken for other similar conditions such as *tinea versicolor* due to a type of yeast infection, or ***pityriasis alba*** where red, and scaly areas of skin is noticed, which later fades into a scaly, lighter patch of skin.

Studies indicate that about 30% of vitiligo cases have a genetic influence along with triggers.

Anti-TPO and ATG (auto-immune thyroid antibodies) have been found to be major associated factors for vitiligo as well.

Reduction in SOD (*superoxide dismutase*) anti-oxidant due to copper and zinc deficiency, is also noticed in vitiligo where high rates of *free radical* damage is known.

Even though it is a painless condition, vitiligo can usually cause the skin to quickly burn, instead of tanning, as it is sensitive to sunlight than the rest of the skin. Abnormalities in the retina and iris of the eyes, also occur but usually vision isn't affected.

People with vitiligo usually undergo emotional challenges as they may feel embarrassed about the way their skin looks, and develop low self-esteem, which leads to anxiety and depression. Visiting a mental health professional for counselling is beneficial in such cases.

Common treatments for vitiligo include oral and topical medications, light therapy, depigmentation therapy and surgery.

There isn't a specific medication to stop vitiligo from affecting the skin but there are medications that can slow the speed of pigmentation loss, help melanocytes regrow or bring colour back to the skin.

Research has shown high doses of daily vitamin-D supplementation to have yielded up to **75%** improvement in 14 out of the 16 individuals, the research was conducted on.

As the root cause of the issue commonly lies in gut flora infection and a leaky gut, (explained in Chapter- 13), or liver infections, the treatment should coincide with a dietary habit that supports the liver, friendly gut flora and prevents indigestion or gastritis, and auto-immune triggers.

But even after bringing balance to the gut flora, melanocyte regrowth usually occurs quite slowly, and could even end up taking several years before visible changes, in most individuals.

The changes that need to be included, in the diet, to treat and manage **Vitiligo**, is explained in the sample diet charts, in Chapter- 25.

- **24.39 – <u>Fibromyalgia</u>**

Fibromyalgia is a condition that causes pain and tenderness throughout the body, and have episodes of flare-ups, when the symptoms are severe.

Fibromyalgia does not cause inflammation or produce auto-antibodies that destroy healthy cells. In few cases, low-grade inflammation and production of pro-inflammatory proteins called cytokines are noticed. But anti-inflammatory medication and immune suppressing drugs are not very effective in reducing the symptoms in most of these cases.

Recent research suggests that fibromyalgia is related to the nervous system, and an imbalance in chemicals like serotonin and norepinephrine, are causes for fibromyalgia. So even though it is not a typical auto-immune disorder, it still is a disorder due to an infected gut.

There is a significant correlation between constipation type of IBS (irritable bowel syndrome), and fibromyalgia. Both conditions frequently coexist, with studies showing that a high percentage of fibromyalgia patients also experience gastrointestinal issues, particularly constipation.

The exact mechanisms linking these two conditions are still being explored, but several factors contribute to their overlap.

Commonly noticed symptoms and associated conditions in fibromyalgia are muscle pain or tenderness, fatigue, face and jaw pain, headaches and migraines, digestive issues such as diarrhoea and constipation, bladder control issues, memory problems, brain fog, anxiety, depression, sleeplessness (insomnia) and other sleep disorders.

Emotional stress, changes in daily routine or diet, hormone changes (as in during menstrual cycles), not getting enough sleep, catching a cold, weather or temperature changes, are all likely triggering factors, for a fibromyalgia flare-up.

As of now, there is no specific test that can diagnose fibromyalgia. Usually, it is diagnosed through various questions to the patient regarding their symptoms, and by ruling out the possibilities of other similar diseases (differential diagnosis), through various blood works and scans according to the various presenting symptoms.

Conventionally, pain killers and anti-depressants are the go to medicines, to relieve the symptoms of this issue.

More integrated approaches such as inclusion of exercises (like stretches or strength training), sleep therapy, cognitive behavioural therapy and stress management therapy, are all supportive steps to tackle the issue.

But until the root cause of the issue is addressed, which is gut flora infection and a leaky gut, explained in Chapter- 13, or an infected liver, the other steps to manage and treat the disease are going to prove futile, and will not completely help the individual.
All treatments and medications must coincide with a dietary habit that supports friendly gut flora and prevents indigestion or gastritis.

The changes that need to be included, in the diet, to treat and manage **Fibromyalgia**, is explained in the sample diet charts, in Chapter- 25.

- **24.40 – <u>Prostatitis</u>**

Prostatitis is inflammation of the prostate gland (that is present only in males, just like uterus is for females), which is situated next to the urinary bladder, and the urethra (tube that carry urine and semen out of the body), runs through the center of the prostate gland.

Prostate helps pump the semen while ejaculating, and the seminal fluid produced from the prostate gland, is essential for nourishing and protecting sperm.

Prostatitis is when the tissue in and around this gland, becomes swollen, tender and irritated. The various types of prostatitis are classified as –

- Acute bacterial prostatitis.
- Chronic bacterial prostatitis.
- CPPS (*chronic pelvic pain syndrome*)
- Non-bacterial prostatitis (asymptomatic inflammatory prostatitis)

More than **2 million** males world-wide has symptoms, with up to **50%** of all males having symptoms of prostatitis at some point in their lives.

It is the most common urinary tract issue in males under 50 years of age, and the third most common in males over 50 years of age.

People with non-bacterial prostatitis may not have any symptoms.

The other three types of prostatitis share symptoms, such as pain in the lower abdomen, genitals or perineum (often radiating to the lower back), frequent urge to urinate, painful urination and ejaculation, having a urine stream that stops and starts or that is not in control, blood in urine or semen, pain during sexual intercourse, and erectile dysfunction.

Acute bacterial prostatitis often causes flu-like symptoms, such as fever and body aches.

Pelvic floor muscle weakness or damage, pelvic nerve irritation or inflammation, UTI, stress, and gut infections that leads to auto-immune factors, are the notable causes of prostatitis.

Usual causes of bacterial infection in the prostate gland include, low immunity due metabolic diseases or nutritional deficiencies, bladder infections or bladder stones, STIs (sexually transmitted diseases), and injury to the pelvic area.

Less common reasons, are having a prostate biopsy, prostate stones, and use of urethral catheter (to drain blocked urine).

Concentration levels of the mineral Zinc in-

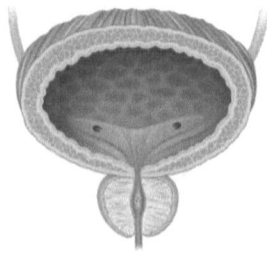
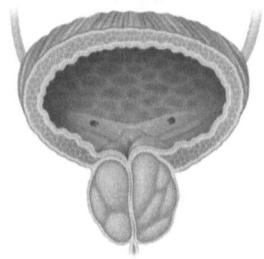

Normal Prostate
Zinc (744$_{mcg}$)

Enlarged Prostate
Zinc (470$_{mcg}$)

The relationship between the mineral zinc and prostate health is often overlooked, but just as iodine is vital for thyroid health, zinc is essential for the prostate.

Zinc concentrations in the prostate are significantly higher than in blood, with normal levels at **744 mcg**. This level has been seen to be drastically reduced to **470 mcg** in cases of prostatitis, and reduced even further in cases of prostate cancer where the average has been found to be around **273 mcg**, a drastic contrast when compared to the normal levels.

Zinc also acts as a natural DHT (dihydrotestosterone) blocker, which helps regulate testosterone levels. Excessive DHT, can cause issues such as prostate enlargement, hair loss, and other related issues. Although zinc is not the sole nutrient required for prostate health, its high concentration in the prostate emphasizes its critical function in supporting prostate tissue and maintaining a balanced hormonal level.

Prostatitis is often benign (not cancerous), known as BPH (benign prostate hyperplasia), but in cases of prostatitis due to auto-immune conditions, where there is a presence of elevated levels of PSA (prostate specific antigen) in the body, there is a much higher risk of the individual to develop prostate cancer.

The tests for prostatitis, include digital rectal exam, urinalysis, blood test for PSA and other inflammatory markers or infections, cystoscopy, transrectal ultrasound and urodynamic tests.

Conventionally, antibiotics, pain killers and anti-inflammatory medicines are useful in relieving the symptoms of this issue.
More integrated approaches such as inclusion of exercises (like *Kegel* exercise to strengthen the pelvic floor muscles), sitz bath, and stress management therapy, are all supportive steps to tackle the issue.

But the root cause of the issue needs to be addressed, to completely help the individual. The changes that need to be included, in the diet, to treat and manage **Prostatitis**, is explained in the sample diet charts, in Chapter- 25.

- ## 24.41 – <u>Myasthenia Gravis (MG)</u>

Myasthenia gravis is basically a neuro-muscular disease, which causes weakness in the *skeletal muscle* (those which are attached to the bones and helps us move our limbs and other body parts).

Typically, the muscle weakness gets worse after physical activity, and improves after rest. Patients feel strongest at the start of the day, and weakest at the end of the day.

MG affects about 20 out of every 100,000 people around the world. The actual number may be higher, as some people with mild cases may not know that they have the condition.

Neonatal myasthenia, is when the foetus gets auto-immune antibodies from the mother who has myasthenia gravis. An infant may have a weak cry, or weak sucking reflex at birth, usually temporary, the symptoms go away after around three months. ***Congenital myasthenia*** isn't an autoimmune condition, it is a genetic fault that causes it.

There are two subtypes of auto-immune myasthenia –

- *<u>Ocular</u>* - The muscles that move the eyes and eyelids weaken, and droop (ptosis), causing difficulty to keep the eyes open. Some people have double vision.

- *<u>Generalized</u>* - Muscle weakness affects the eye, and other muscles in the face, neck, arms, legs and throat, affecting the ability to move the eyes or blink, make facial expressions, chew, swallow or talk, raise arms up or lift objects, or walk upstairs or get up from a chair.

1 in 5 people with MG experience a myasthenic crisis or severe respiratory muscle weakness, causing shortness of breath, which affects the normal breathing. It is an emergency situation that require professional emergency care.

MG affects communication between the nerves and muscles.

- Nerves send signals to muscles, across a synapse or area called the neuromuscular junction. To communicate, nerves release a molecule called *acetylcholine*.

- Muscles have acetylcholine receptors, which receives the signal, and triggers the muscle fiber to contract.

Nerves signal the muscles effortlessly, but during MG, antibodies destroy the receptor sites, blocking nerve-muscle communication, which becomes sluggish or doesn't work at all.

There are five main stages of myasthenia gravis –

- **Class I**: Muscle weakness only affects the eyes (ocular muscle).
- **Class II**: Muscle weakness is mild.
- **Class III**: Muscle weakness is moderate.
- **Class IV**: Muscle weakness is severe.
- **Class V**: Severe muscle weakness that affects regular breathing, which may require intubation or mechanical ventilation.

Blood tests for myasthenia gravis have shown unusually high levels of –

- *Acetylcholine receptor antibodies* in **85%** of people.
- *Muscle-specific kinase* (MuSK) *antibodies* in about **6%** people.

Inflammation or tumours in the thymus gland (a gland that helps protect the immune system), are ruled out through CT and MRI scans.

An EMG (electromyography) measures the electrical activity of muscles and nerves, and helps to detect any communication problems between the nerves and muscles.

Medications commonly used to control the symptoms of MG are –

- *Cholinesterase inhibitors* (anticholinesterase), that boost signals between nerves and muscles to improve muscle strength.
- *Immunosuppressants*, like corticosteroids decrease inflammation and reduce the body's production of abnormal antibodies.
- *Monoclonal antibodies* are biologically engineered proteins, administered through intra-venous (IV) or sub-cutaneous infusions, that helps to suppress an overactive immune system.
- *Plasma exchange* (plasmapheresis), much like a kidney dialysis, where an IV connected to a machine removes harmful antibodies from the blood plasma and replaces them with donor plasma or a plasma solution.

In few cases, **thymectomy** (surgery to remove the thymus gland), is also considered an option for treatment, as studies suggest, that certain immune system cells in the thymus gland, have trouble identifying what's a threat to your body (like bacteria or viruses), versus healthy components, that may trigger symptoms.

The thymus gland is a small organ next to the thyroid gland, which makes white blood cells that fight infections, and is most active during childhood. After puberty, it slowly decrease in size and is replaced by fat. Removal of the thymus gland in children could lead to infections, autoimmune conditions, allergies and an increased risk of cancer.

The primary function of the thymus gland is to train special WBCs (white blood cells) called as T-lymphocytes or T-cells, which originates from the bone marrow and travels to the thymus. The lymphocytes mature, and become specialized T-cells in the thymus. After the T-cells have matured, they help the immune system fight disease and infection.

Two-thirds of people with MG have overactive thymic cells (thymic hyperplasia), and about 1 in 10 people have thymus gland tumours called thymomas, which have chances to be cancerous. Issues with the thymus, could lead to creation of auto-immune antibodies.

The treatment for myasthenia gravis should coincide with a dietary habit that supports the liver, growth of friendly gut flora and prevent indigestion or gastritis.

The changes that need to be included, in the diet, to treat and manage **Myasthenia Gravis**, is explained in the sample diet charts, in Chapter- 25.

Let us discuss about **Mental Disorders** *due to an **imbalanced gut microbiota**.*

- ## 24.42 – **Depression**

Depression is a disorder that can cause one to feel sad, irritable or hopeless. Everyone feels sad or low sometimes, but these feelings usually goes away after a short time.

Depression (or clinical depression) is different. It can cause severe symptoms that affect how a person feels, thinks, and handles daily activities, such as sleeping, eating, or working. In severe cases, depression can lead to thoughts of suicide.

Depression can affect anyone regardless of age, gender, race or ethnicity, income, culture, or education, and even though there are genetic, biological, environmental, and psychological factors that play a role in the disorder, more than **70%** of these issues can be traced to some sort of underlying physical condition.

The rest are due to emotional or mental stress, from exposure to traumatic experiences, or due to strained relationships with family or friends, or due to the pressure and responsibilities of life. Commonly, both of these root issues can be seen in the same individual.

Physical issues known to cause symptoms of depression include gastritis, IBS, IBD, anaemia, auto-immune & metabolic disorders, concussion, epilepsy, thyroiditis, nutrition deficiencies, and hormonal imbalances (even those during puberty, menstrual cycles or menopause).

Women are diagnosed with depression more often than men, because men may be less likely to recognize, talk about, and seek help for their negative feelings, and are at a greater risk of their depression being undiagnosed and untreated.

To be diagnosed with depression, a person must have symptoms most of the day, nearly every day, for at least two weeks.

Mood changes, sadness, increased irritability, lack of interest in fun activities, low energy levels or general tiredness, negative self-talk or low self-esteem, eating more or less than usual, or not eating at all, trouble sleeping or sleeping too much, difficulty concentrating, remembering, or making decisions, isolating from family and friends, inability to meet responsibilities, or ignoring other important roles, problems with sexual desire and performance, suicidal tendencies, and substance (alcohol or drugs) abuse are symptoms to be noted.

Serotonin is one of the major hormones that regulate the mood. So much so that it is known as the *'Happy Hormone.'* It was thought to be created solely from the brain, until recently, where it was found to be primarily secreted in the gut (over **90%** of total amount in body), by the influence of friendly gut microbiome.

The primary role of serotonin is to induce the peristaltic movement (the rhythmic, wave-like motion of the intestines, that pushes out the stool), and the mood uplifting part, is secondary. This is why depression is found in gastric issues, IBS, IBD and other auto-immune conditions which affect the gut, as there is a malfunction in serotonin synthesis or transport. Deficiencies of vitamin-B_1 which is a precursor, and vitamin-D which is an activator of serotonin, also leads to depression.

During the dark, cold winter months, when sunlight is scarce, many people experience the various symptoms of depression also known as *Cabin Fever*. This is because reduced sunlight leads to lower levels of vitamin-D, which as mentioned before, plays a crucial role in serotonin synthesis, by helping in the activation of the serotonin hormone.

When exposure to sunlight is minimal, serotonin production declines, making individuals more vulnerable to depression. This link between vitamin-D deficiency and mood disorders is especially evident in environments where sunlight is limited, and this is evident in prisons where isolation is used as a disciplinary action.

Inmates who misbehave are often sent to solitary confinement, where they are deprived from, not only contact from other people, but also from sunlight and the positive effects of natural light as well. Over time, this deprivation can mentally break individuals, leaving them with long-lasting psychological damage due to the combined effects of isolation, lack of sunlight, and disrupted serotonin regulation.

Post-partem depression (PPD) is a common condition that affects many new mothers, is also majorly due to severe nutritional deficiencies. Nutrients like EPA, DHA, magnesium, and choline are crucial for brain health, and a lack of these can significantly impact the mothers mental well-being after childbirth.

EPA and DHA, *omega*-3 fatty acids found in fish and algae, play a critical role in reducing inflammation and supporting healthy brain function. Magnesium helps regulate mood, and choline is vital for neurotransmitter synthesis, all of which are essential for preventing or managing PPD.

Additionally, a common genetic mutation, the MTHFR gene mutation, that affects up to **44%** of women and impairs the body's ability to process folic acid. This deficiency can lead to elevated homocysteine levels, which can increase the risk of mood disorders like postpartum depression. Together, these factors can significantly contribute to the development of PPD, highlighting the importance of proper nutrition during pregnancy and maternal health.

A detailed evaluation, as well as blood works, and further tests related to the presenting signs and symptoms of other underlying issues, are all procedures that help with identifying, and treating the cause of the depression. The changes that need to be included, in the diet, to manage **Depression**, is explained in the sample diet charts, in Chapter- 25.

- **24.43 – <u>Autism Spectrum Disorder (ASD)</u>**

ASD, is a neuro-developmental disorder, where the structure of the brain is normal at birth, but there are issues with the signalling, or an interference from harmful neuro-toxic metabolites (such as ammonia, D-lactic acid etc.), from altered gut microbes which dysregulate the gut's communication with the brain, and alters the cognitive development, and additionally impair memory. Genetics do play a role in autism, but are rare and have only been identified in around **15%** of the cases.

A person suffering from autism may behave, interact and learn in ways, that are different from other people and usually, have trouble with social interactions. They can find difficulty in using, and understanding nonverbal communication, like eye contact, gestures and facial expressions. Delayed or absent language development, difficulty in understanding and forming relationships, repetitive motor behaviours (like flapping arms, body rocking, repetitive speech etc.), and a demand for routines, are also commonly noticed traits.

ASD varies widely in its severity and impairment of day-to-day activities. The symptoms of some people aren't always easily recognized, especially in women, who cope better in social situations than men, because they learn to hide the signs of autism, and show fewer signs of repetitive behaviours, to fit into society, by copying people who don't have ASD.

High-functioning autism isn't an official medical diagnosis, but this term is used to describe a mild form of autism, that require lower levels of support, and the affected individuals can speak, read, write and handle basic life skills. It is also commonly called as *Asperger syndrome*.

The behavioural signs of autism characteristics typically surface between the ages of 1 and 3 years old, and symptoms range from mild to severely disabling, with every person being unique.

Delay in cognitive milestones of infants and children, especially when seen along with symptoms of an infected digestive system, should be considered as signs of possible ASD, and must be professionally evaluated for the same.

Feeding issues, poor sleep, gastro-intestinal problems, epilepsy, ADHD, anxiety, depression, OCD (obsessive-compulsive disorder) are the commonly noticed issues in ASD.

In the case of ADHD (attention deficit hyperactivity disorder), it has been widely regarded as being part of the autism spectrum, but the majority cases of ADHD are misdiagnosed, and in fact, the misdiagnosed individuals wouldn't be actually suffering from ADHD, but would just be individuals with a different neurological or character type.

Children who are hyper-active, and impulsive are usually labelled as suffering from ADHD just because they might not be "obedient" enough for the typical class-room.

But when they are placed in an environment that doesn't overwhelm them with excessive information overload, or that require long hours of sedentary classroom work, or places where the stimuli are not limited to the artificial input from screens... these individuals are shown to thrive and develop just like their peers.

In such settings, they do not require special care or medication.

Lots of the most successful people in the world have ADHD, and the solution lies in identifying, and choosing the method for learning, that they are best suited for.

There is currently no specific autism test yet, and healthcare providers perform specialized evaluations including *Developmental surveillance, Developmental screening,* and *Formal evaluation,* to diagnose ASD.

Autism treatment include behavioural interventions or therapies, which teach individualized new skills, to address the core deficits of autism, and reduce the specific symptoms unique to each case.
Medications for gastrointestinal issues, seizures and sleep disturbances are also commonly administered.

Early intensive treatments especially before the age of 7 years, is found to have the best results, as the level of neuro-toxicity in the body decreases, normal cognitive function can resume with healthy growth and development, of the brain and body.

And as the root cause of the issue lies in gut flora infection and a leaky gut, (explained in Chapter- 13), the treatment should coincide with a dietary habit that supports friendly gut flora and which prevents indigestion or gastritis.

The changes that need to be included, in the diet, to treat and manage **Autism Spectrum Disorder (ASD)**, is explained in the sample diet charts, in Chapter- 25.

*Let us discuss about a few **Allergic Disorders**, with **elevated levels of serum IgE**, due to an imbalanced gut microbiota.*

- ## 24.44 – Dermatitis & Eczema

Dermatitis, is inflammation of the skin, which leads to irritation and rashes, and is caused by an overactive immune system, infections, genetic issues, allergies, or a combination of it all.
Common symptoms are dry skin, redness and pruritus (itching).

The types of dermatitis are categorized by the cause and location of the inflammation of skin on the body, which include, but are not limited to –

- Atopic dermatitis (also known as *Eczema*).
- Contact dermatitis.
- Dyshidrotic dermatitis.
- Periorificial dermatitis.
- Neuro-dermatitis.
- Nummular dermatitis.
- Stasis dermatitis.
- Seborrheic dermatitis.

Dermatitis can appear anywhere on the body, as in *atopic dermatitis*, but, in teens and adults, it is typically on the hands, inner elbows, neck, knees, ankles, feet and around the eyes.

Seborrheic dermatitis is when the scalp, face and ears are affected, and *periorificial dermatitis* is commonly found around the eyes, mouth, nostrils and sometimes the genitals.

Additional symptoms of dermatitis can include, dry or cracked skin, scratch marks (excoriations), thick leathery patch of skin (lichenification), pain at the site of itching etc.

Gut parasites are the most common underlying cause (**40%**), followed by hypo-acidity (**30%**), fungal infections (**20%**), and heavy metal toxicity (**10%**), all of which contribute to an overactive immune response.

Dermatitis is often caused by a combination of immune system hyperaction, genetics, environmental triggers, and is often accompanied by depression, anxiety, sleeplessness, asthma, and other allergies.
Stress is also a major causative and aggravative factor, for dermatitis, as in for all other diseases.

To diagnose dermatitis, it is important to understand what caused it, so a detailed evaluation is necessary, starting from questioning what might have triggered the itching, to several lab investigations and tests, that include allergy tests, blood tests to reveal vitamin and mineral deficiencies, or problems with the internal organs.
Imaging tests such as X-ray or MRIs, and skin biopsies, help reveal conditions that extend beneath the skin, like cancer.

Treatment for dermatitis is unique to each person and varies based on what caused it, and could include anti-histamines, topical or oral steroids, immune-suppressants, topical creams, lotion or ointment for the skin, that contain hydrocortisone, or aloe vera and menthol extracts if using natural or plant based ointments.

Moisturizing the skin using natural oils or creams, keeping away from irritants (such as certain fabric clothes or detergents), and taking cold or warm showers (depends on each individual) are various steps to treat dermatitis at home while ongoing treatments for the condition.

The changes that need to be included, in the diet, to treat and manage **Dermatitis & Eczema**, is explained in the sample diet charts, in Chapter- 25.

- **24.45 – Psoriasis**

Psoriasis is an auto-immune condition that causes inflammation in the skin. Psoriasis and dermatitis can look similar, as both conditions involve patches of red skin, with flakes of skin on the top and around the reddish skin. However, in psoriasis, the scales are often thicker and the edges of those scales are well-defined, which are called plaques, whereas in dermatitis and eczema, there is a rash of dry and bumpy skin, and it typically causes more intense itching than psoriasis.

There are several types of psoriasis, including –

- *Plaque psoriasis* - Most common type, about 90% of all cases.
- *Inverse psoriasis* - Appears on skin folds, thin plaques without scales.
- *Guttate psoriasis* - Small, red, drop-shaped scaly spots, often in kids.
- *Nail psoriasis* - Skin discoloration, pitting on fingernails and toenails.
- *Pustular psoriasis* - Has small, pus-filled bumps on top of plaques.
- *Sebo-psoriasis* - A cross between psoriasis and seborrheic dermatitis.
- *Psoriatic-arthritis* - Causes inflammation and damage to the joints.
- *Erythrodermic psoriasis* - Severe type, affects large area, commonly more than 90% of the skin.

It usually takes up to 30 days for new skin cells to grow and replace old skin cells, but due to the over-reactive immune system, this time reduces from 30 days to around just about 4 days, which causes multiple layers of skin to form, creating scales and skin plaques.

This is caused by the activation of IL-17 by either gut or liver toxicity, and infections. An outbreak of psoriasis, or a flare up, commonly occurs due to triggers, which are different for each person, and can include emotional stress, infections, skin injury like cuts, scrapes or surgery, certain medications, and changes in body temperature or climate etc.

To diagnose psoriasis, a detailed evaluation starting with questioning, lab investigations and tests that include allergy tests, blood tests to reveal vitamin and mineral deficiencies or other issues with the internal organs, imaging tests such as X-ray or MRIs, and skin biopsies are used to figure out the underlying issue.

Common treatments to manage psoriasis include steroid creams, moisturizers for dry skin, medication to slow skin cell production, vitamin-D_3 ointments, vitamin-A or retinoid creams.

Lights at specific wavelengths can decrease skin inflammation, and help slow down skin cell production, and so various improved methods of light therapy, are also used to treat psoriasis.

PUVA, retinoid drugs, immune therapy medications, and other powerful medications are also used to treat severe forms of psoriasis, but these medications bring along severe side-effects, such as damage to the liver and kidneys.

It is of utmost importance, to bring dietary changes in the patients routine, to treat psoriasis, as the root cause of the issue, in **60%** of cases, lies in gut flora infection and a leaky gut, explained in Chapter- 13. Around **30%** of cases are due to oxidative stress and toxicity of the liver due to virus or heavy metals, and around **10%** cases are due to severe deficiency of vitamin-D in the body

The various medications should coincide with a dietary habit that supports friendly gut flora and prevents indigestion or gastritis. The changes that need to be included, in the diet, to treat and manage **Psoriasis**, is explained in the sample diet charts, in Chapter- 25.

- **24.46 – <u>Sinusitis</u>**

Sinuses are structures inside the face that are normally filled with air. Bacterial, viral or fungal infections, and allergies can irritate them, and cause inflammation, or swelling, of the tissue, lining the sinuses, causing them to get blocked, and filled with fluid.

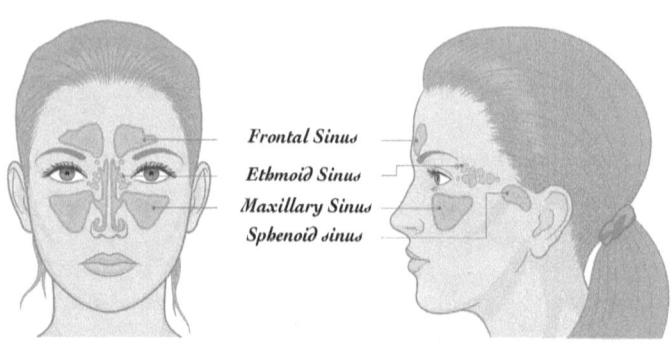

Frontal Sinus
Ethmoid Sinus
Maxillary Sinus
Sphenoid sinus

Sinusitis is also sometimes called *rhinosinusitis*, as viruses, like the ones that cause the common cold, cause most cases of sinusitis. Bacteria can cause sinusitis, or they can infect, after a virus has infected the sinus cavity (secondary infection). If the person has a runny and stuffy nose, with facial pain that doesn't go away after ten days, they could be having bacterial sinusitis.

Sinus infections caused by fungus, are usually more serious than other forms of sinusitis. They are more likely to happen if the person has a weakened immune system.

Colds, allergies and sinus infections, all have similar symptoms and can be difficult to tell apart. The ***common cold*** typically builds, peaks and slowly disappears, and lasts for a few days to a week.

Nasal allergies cause sneezing, itchy nose and eyes, congestion, runny nose and postnasal drip (mucus in your throat). They usually don't cause the facial pain that sinus infections do.

Common symptoms of a *sinus infection* include, postnasal drip (mucus dripping down the throat), runny nose with thick yellow or green mucus, stuffy nose, facial pressure (more around the nose, eyes and forehead), pressure or pain in the teeth, ear pressure or pain, fever, halitosis, cough, headache, and fatigue.

Streptococcus pneumoniae, Haemophilus influenza, and *Moraxella catarrhalis* bacteria are commonly seen in sinusitis. Allergies, asthma, nasal polyps, blockage due to a deviated septum (line of tissue that divides your nose), weakened immune system due to illnesses like HIV or cancer, or from certain medications, or due to nutritional deficiencies, are all the various common risk factors, and root causes for sinusitis.

Sinusitis often goes away on its own, but rarely, the infections can increase to life threatening levels, if the bacteria or fungi spread to the brain, eyes or nearby bones.

Sinusitis itself isn't contagious, but the viruses and bacteria that can cause it, are contagious.

We had discussed in detail, in Chapter- 13, about a type of special, beneficial sugar, EPS (exopolysaccharides) that form in our body, through the work of our friendly gut-microbiomes.

Fungal **β-glucans** are such, natural sugars found in the cell walls of fungi, yeast, and some bacteria. They have gained significant attention for their immune-modulating properties, particularly in supporting the body's defence against infections.

In recent studies, fungal β-glucans have been found beneficial in the treatment of sinusitis and other fungal-related infections. Their main mechanism involves activating key immune cells such as macrophages, neutrophils, and natural killer (NK) cells, enhancing the body's ability to detect and fight off pathogens.

For sinusitis, especially chronic or fungal-induced cases, β-glucans help reduce inflammation and strengthen mucosal immunity of the sinuses. By promoting a more balanced immune response, they can help prevent excessive inflammation while still supporting effective pathogen clearance. Additionally, β-glucans have antioxidant properties, which further aid in reducing tissue damage and promote healing in the sinuses.

Apart from their direct antimicrobial support, β-glucans also act as prebiotics, nourishing beneficial gut microbes that indirectly boost immune function. They are generally well-tolerated and can be consumed through supplements or certain medicines.

Blood work to test allergy or other infections, nasal endoscopy, nasal swabs, X-rays and CT scans, are commonly used to diagnose a sinusitis, when suspected through symptoms.

Anti-histamines, decongestants, nasal saline rinses, intranasal steroid sprays, antibiotics, leukotriene antagonists, surgery for structural issues (polyps or deviated septum), are conventional treatments for sinusitis.

Go to the nearest emergency room or seek medical attention right away, if the symptoms of a serious infection, including high fever (over 103^0 F), confusion, or other mental changes, vision changes (especially if pain or swelling around eyes), and seizures are noticed.

As the root cause of this issue in most cases, lies in gut infection and low immunity, the various medications should coincide with a dietary habit that supports friendly gut flora, and prevents indigestion or gastritis. The changes that need to be included, in the diet, to treat and manage **Sinusitis**, is explained in the sample diet charts, in Chapter- 25.

- **24.47 – <u>Bronchial Asthma (BA)</u>**

Normally when we breathe, muscles around the airways are relaxed, letting air move easily and quietly.
But during an asthma attack, three things can happen -

- *<u>Inflammation</u>*: Lining of airways becomes swollen.
- *<u>Broncho-spasm</u>*: Muscles around the airways constrict, or tighten.
- *<u>Increased mucus production</u>*: Which clogs airways.

When the airways narrows, due to these reasons, air flow becomes restricted, causing difficulty in breathing, and a sound called wheezing occurs, usually while breathing out.

Asthma attacks have multiple triggering factors such as allergens (like dust, pollen, pet hair), stress, exercise, smoke, strong chemicals or smells, illness and variations in seasons or climate, to name a few.

Genetics, even though a causative factor, does not play a major role as much as the other causes do, in the case of asthma. Respiratory as well as gut infections, which causes a hyper-active immune system, is the actual issue that needs to be dealt with.

Common symptoms of asthma resemble other respiratory infections, such as chest tightness, with pain or pressure, coughing (especially at night), breathlessness and wheezing.

It is common to have other diseases of an elevated scrum IgE, along with asthma, such as eczema or urticaria, and letting the physician know of these details, is important to diagnose and treat asthma.

Spirometry, chest X-ray, and blood tests are the common tests done to diagnose the issue.

Commonly prescribed medications to suppress the symptoms include –

- *__Bronchodilators__*: Relax muscles around the airways, allowing free flow of air.
- *__Anti-inflammatory__*: Reduces swelling and mucus production in the airways.

During a severe asthma attack, immediate medical care is required especially when regular maintenance inhalers are not effective.
In this case, a ***rescue inhaler*** must be used, which contains fast-acting medicines to open up the airways.

And when the rescue inhalers, are not being effective, the individual must be taken to the nearest emergency department, especially if they show signs of anxiety or panic attack, coughing that won't stop, rapid breathing, severe wheezing, difficulty to talk, or have bluish or grey fingernails or lips, whitish lips or gums, or a pale, sweaty face.

Keeping away from known irritants and triggering factors, and taking cold or warm showers (depends on each individual), are various steps to manage mild asthma at home, while ongoing treatments for the underlying condition.

And as the root cause of the issue lies in gut flora infection and a leaky gut, explained in Chapter-13, the treatment should coincide with a dietary habit that supports friendly gut flora and prevents indigestion or gastritis. The changes that need to be included, in the diet, to treat and manage **Bronchial Asthma**, is explained in the sample diet charts, in Chapter- 25.

- ## 24.48 – <u>Urticaria (Hives)</u>

Urticaria is a type of allergic reaction that creates itchy bumps on the skin, which appear as red bumps (welts) or splotches on the skin, and are often very itchy, but is usually felt as a burn or sting.

These bumps can either be very small, or join together to form larger areas called plaques.

Urticaria also appears as painful swelling under the skin causing puffiness (angioedema), especially on the lips, face, eyes and inside the throat. It tends to fade within 24 hours, but may be noticeable for several days or longer.

Anyone with a hyper-reactive immune system can get urticaria attacks especially when triggered by allergens specific to each case.

People suffering from prolonged periods of stress and allergic issues such as asthma, allergic rhinitis and atopic dermatitis, especially children, have an increased chance to have an urticaria attack.

There is also a condition called physical urticaria, which is triggered by exposure to cold, heat, vibrations or pressure, exercising or sweating etc. Physical urticaria usually appear within an hour after exposure.

The skin has immune cells called mast cells. When these cells go into action, they release chemicals, including one called *histamine*.

Histamine is the reason that urticaria form. Histamine can form from certain foods, but in normal circumstances get metabolised.

But this this normal breakdown and excretion can be impaired during the presence of elevated IgE in the body, and can also form unnecessarily during the same.

Vitamin-B$_9$ (folate) is essential for the proper breakdown and excretion of histamine. Folate deficiency, as well as genetic mutations in the enzyme that converts folate to its active form, can contribute to histamine related issues like urticaria, asthma and rhinitis.

MTHFR (*methylene-tetrahydro-folate reductase*) is the enzyme responsible for the conversion of folate, and genetic mutations in the MTHFR gene are quite common.

About **15%** of the world population have a significantly reduced MTHFR activity, while around **40%** experience partial reduction. The prevalence of these mutations varies by ethnicity, with higher rates in South American, Mediterranean, and Asian populations.

Fatty liver and other liver dysfunctions can impair histamine metabolism as well, due to the reduced production of HNMT (*histamine N-methyl-transferase*), an enzyme involved in histamine inactivation. HNMT is also produced in tissues like the kidneys, lungs, and brain, but in the liver, it plays a key role in detoxifying histamine from the bloodstream.

Allergies can also often be mistaken for *'food intolerances'* which are not immune responses but digestive issues. Food intolerances, such as *histamine intolerance*, occur when the body struggles to break down certain foods, leading to symptoms like bloating or skin rashes. Unlike true allergies, food intolerances are typically caused by digestive dysfunction (hypo-acidity) rather than an immune system reaction.

Histamine rich foods, such as fermented products, aged cheeses, cured meats, and alcoholic beverages, either contain high levels of histamine, or trigger its release. For individuals with histamine intolerance, avoiding these foods may help alleviate symptoms. DAO (*diamine oxidase*) supplements have also been often found to be helpful in managing histamine intolerance due to indigestion issues.

Gluten intolerance is one of the most commonly seen issues that triggers allergic reactions. Gluten is (in normal and healthy conditions), partially digested by salivary enzymes produced by gut bacteria in the mouth before reaching the gut.

In a healthy body, the gliadin peptide in gluten is further broken down into amino acids by the transglutaminase enzyme.

However, in cases of indigestion issues, or gut bacterial dysbiosis conditions, gluten is not adequately digested by the salivary enzymes, leading it to pass undigested into the gut.

This undigested gluten then triggers an immune response, binding to HLA-DQ2 molecules, activating TH1 cells that can cause diseases that initiate an inflammatory response in the gut lining, and that which can show up on the skin of the individual as well.

Unlike acute urticaria, chronic urticaria aren't caused by allergies, but due to presence of other auto-immune factors such as ANA, lupus etc.

To diagnose urticaria, a detailed evaluation starting with questioning, lab investigations and tests that include allergy tests, blood tests to reveal vitamin and mineral deficiencies, or other issues with the internal organs, imaging tests such as X-ray or MRIs, etc.

Skin biopsies might be required in certain cases.

Most of the time, urticaria go away without treatment, but anti-histamine and steroid medications, in various forms are administered depending on the severity and persistence of the attack.

Epinephrine shots are given during life-threatening emergencies where throat and breath ways are severely swollen.

Keeping away from known irritants and triggering factors, and taking cold or warm showers (depends on each individual) are various steps to manage mild urticaria at home while ongoing treatments for the underlying condition.

And as the root cause of the issue lies in gut flora infection and a leaky gut, (explained in Chapter- 13), or liver infections, the treatment should coincide with a dietary habit that supports the liver, growth of friendly gut flora and prevent indigestion or gastritis.

The changes that need to be included, in the diet, to treat and manage **Urticaria**, is explained in the sample diet charts, in Chapter- 25.

> *Let us next discuss about a few common disorders caused due to an imbalance in bowel movements, regardless of its causative origin being of Functional or* **Auto-Immune** *reasons.*

24.49 – Fissures, Fistula & Haemorrhoids

Haemorrhoids / Piles	Fissures	Fistula
Veins in the rectum swell causing an internal or external haemorrhoid.	Skin crack or tear, that occurs in and around the anus.	Tunnel which connects an infected gland, inside the rectal walls, to another area or organ.
Causes		
Chronic constipation. Straining to pass stool.	IBD, frequent diarrhoea or laxative abuse, tight anal sphincter.	Anal glands infections, ulcers, UTI, rectal cancer, Crohn's.
Symptoms		
Often painless rectal bleeding and pus discharge is seen from the anal opening. There is a constant discomfort in rectum, even when empty. A constant itching is felt in and around the opening of the anus causing it to be red and sore.	• Blood is released from the anal opening during bowel movements. • Severe pain felt during and after passing stool. • A crack is easily noticed around the opening of the anus.	• Pus is released from the anus, and other openings. • A redness, soreness or itching sensation is felt around the anus and other openings. • Pain during bowel movement.
Home Remedies		
Use of laxatives, increase fluids and fiber, do not strain or force to excrete stool, avoid long hours of sitting.	Use of laxatives, increase fluids and fiber, apply moisturizers, sitz bath with epsom salt to the rectum, avoid straining.	Topical anaesthetics, use of laxatives, increase fluids and fiber, avoid straining during excretion, maintain hygiene.

Treatments		
Haemorrhoids / Piles	*Fissures*	*Fistula*
• Laser Haemorrhoido-plasty, where a laser is used to heat the haemorrhoid in order to destroy it. • Sclerotherapy where piles is injected with a mild chemical which shrinks the piles. • Rubber band ligation, where the haemorrhoid is tightly bound at the base, thus cutting off blood supply, causing it to wither and fall off.	• Laser surgery for the fissure. • Topical anaesthetics to promote recovery. • Applying nitro-glycerine on the fissure so as to promote healing.	• Laser surgery where the tip of the laser is inserted into the fistula and pulled bac effectively closing it. • Seton placement, do for deep fistulas, whe the seton drains the tract and is expected heal in around 6 wee • Fistulotomy, an incis made into the fistula tract to drain the pus out.

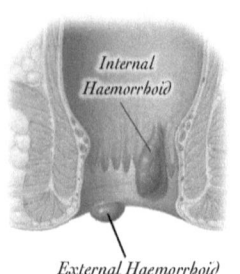
External Haemorrhoid / *Internal Haemorrhoid*

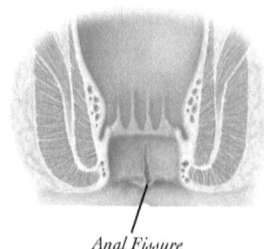
Anal Fissure

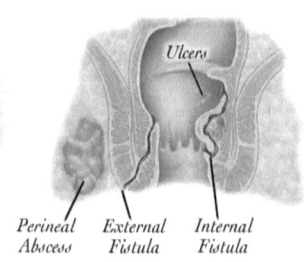
Perineal Abscess / *External Fistula* / *Internal Fistula* / *Ulcers*

Lay open surgery, is the go to surgical procedure to treat anal fistulas, where the fistula tract is cut open, and the wound is left open to heal. It is usually effective for fistulas that do not pass through much of the sphincter muscle.

But prolonged hospitalization, anal incontinence and high rate of recurrence, is the major issue with this procedure.

Moreover, the initial recovery period, also causes much discomfort to the patient, and they will not be able to do any other activities for a few days.

A highly efficient, and cost effective alternative solution for this issue, is the traditional Indian medical minor surgical procedure called - '*Ksharasutra.*'

Ksharasutra is the application of a sterilized, medicated cotton or linen thread, coated with herbal medicines, through the fistula, and replaced every 3 to 5 days, until the fistula completely heals.

The application and follow-up of Ksharasutra is quite easy, have little to no pain, and have an extremely low rate of complications, and have been subject of multiple scientific researches due to its high success rate.

Similarly, laxatives (substances that promote bowel movements), come in several types, each functioning in different ways, with their own set of side effects such as, nausea, flatulence, bloating, cramping, dehydration, electrolyte imbalance, diarrhoea, interference with the absorption of fat-soluble vitamins, and even dependence with prolonged use.

Bulk-forming laxatives, stimulant laxatives, osmotic laxatives, saline laxatives, emollient laxatives (stool softeners), lubricant laxatives, chloride channel activators etc. are some of the different varieties that are used for constipation.

Each type of laxative has its own indications, and the choice of which to use, depends on factors such as the severity of constipation, presence of underlying medical conditions, and the patient's tolerance to side effects.

Always consult your Physician before using laxatives regularly, to avoid dependence or any other complications.

Even though various surgeries and medication are helpful for treating haemorrhoids, fissures, and fistula, unless the underlying issue is resolved, these problems will arise after a few weeks or months' time.

Keep in mind to maintain a healthy balanced diet along with all other treatments, that which supports a friendly gut flora and prevents indigestion or gastritis and other diseases of the gut or bowels.

The changes that need to be included, in the diet, to treat and manage **Fissures, Fistula & Haemorrhoids**, is explained in the sample diet charts, in Chapter- 25.

Let us next discuss a few issues related to Redox Health, or ones that are caused majorly due to the harmful effects of **Oxidative Stress** *explained in* **Chapter- 5** *and* **Chapter- 20.**

24.50 – **Pigmentation**

Pigmentation is when the colour of our skin becomes different from our normal or usual complexion. Skin discoloration looks different on everyone, depending on the skin tone and reason for discoloration.

Melanin is that which gives the skin, hair and eyes its colour.

When the damaged melanin cells produce too much melanin, it causes darker tones, and causes lighter skin tones in cases of scarcely produced melanin. Some skin conditions cause the skin to become dry, scaly and itchy, while others only affect the skin's colour.

Some causes of skin discoloration (like birthmarks or due to genetic issues) are beyond our control. Major causes of pigmentation due to epigenetics are classified as either **'extrinsic'** (pollution, cosmetics, UV radiation etc.) or **'intrinsic'** (insulin resistance, heavy metal poisoning, adrenal fatigue, hormonal imbalance etc.)

Heavy metal poisoning (such as mercury, cadmium, lead, arsenic etc.) have been found to be one of the leading factors, causing pigmentation on the face and throughout the body.

Postural hypotension, symptoms of IBS, red eyes etc. are also commonly associated in these cases of heavy metal poisoning. Too much cereals or grains in the diet, smoking, consuming contaminated food, and direct consumption of tap water, are the most common sources.

Diagnosing the cause of pigmentation, is through physical examination, biopsy and blood tests depending on other specific signs and symptoms shown by the body. You should consult a medical physician if you notice any spots on the skin that look different from others, or if it itches or bleed, or if you have moles or lesions that change shape, or doesn't heal.

Treating the pigmentation depends on the cause, and addressing the underlying issue can help fix the issue in the long run.
Most pigmentations heals by itself or with minor treatment.

Creams or lotions to lighten or fade dark spots or patches, laser treatments, oral or topical medication like antibiotics, antifungal medications or steroids etc. are the commonly used first line modes of treatment. If the pigmentation or moles are cancerous, radiation therapy, chemotherapy or even surgery might be required in rare cases.

At home treatments like sauna or steam baths are great at detoxifying heavy metals from the system, along with glutathione and other chelating medicines.

Sandalwood paste application in cases of melasma (primarily caused due to excess estrogen), is also found to be highly effective due to its anti-inflammatory and antioxidant properties as well as its ability to inhibit the enzyme tyrosinase, which plays a key role in melanin production.

Covering the skin with loose, comfortable and breathable clothing when outside, avoiding direct sunlight between 11:00 a.m and 3:00 p.m. (when ultraviolet, or UV, rays are strongest), and applying sunscreen when spending time outdoors (particularly for light-skinned individuals), are preventive steps that can help avoid damage to the skin.

Maintaining a healthy balanced diet, rich in antioxidants and which supports our body's own anti-oxidant production, along with the other treatments, is of utmost importance.

The changes that need to be included, in the diet, to treat and manage **Pigmentation**, due to epigenetic reasons, is explained in the sample diet charts, in Chapter- 25.

- **24.51 – <u>Acne</u>**

Acne is when the pores of the skin get clogged, leading to bumps on the skin, often times pus-filled, and painful, or causes black-heads, white-heads or other types of pimples, and commonly occurs on the face, chest, chest, shoulders, upper back (where oil glands exist the most).

Acne usually affects everyone at some point in their lifetime, but most commonly teenagers and women are affected, commonly due to the excess production, or imbalance in hormones.

Usually acne are formed as pimples or *pustules* (pus-filled bumps), *papules* (small, discoloured bumps, often darker than natural skin tone), *cyst* (painful, fluid or pus filled lumps, with a high chance of scarring), *nodules* (large, painful lumps under skin), black-heads and white-heads.

Acne is caused due to the overgrowth of micro-organisms, in clogged skin pores or hair follicles due to excess secretion and presence of sebum, which is our body's natural oil.

Fungal infections, leaky gut, hormonal imbalances, over stimulation of mTOR pathway, insulin resistance, PCOD and high cortisol, are all common reasons for the excess secretion of sebum.

This suitable environment causes the over growth of bacteria (particularly *Propionibacterium acnes*), which release several chemicals, that activate TLR2 causing our body to respond through creating inflammation, which results in various acne formation.

Isotretinoin, a common treatment for severe acne, is a TLR2 blocker. While effective in treating acne, isotretinoin has been known to cause mood and behavioural side effects, including depression, anxiety, and even schizoid-like disorders during long-term use.

In contrast, sulfur found in cruciferous vegetables (like broccoli, cabbage etc), garlic, and onions, acts as a natural TLR2 blocker, without the adverse side effects linked to synthetic drugs like isotretinoin. Curcumin (turmeric) and zinc are also potent TLR2 blockers.

When it comes to hormones, androgens and testosterone are primary contributors to acne, as they increase the size and activity of sebaceous glands, leading to excess oil production.

DHT (*dihydrotestosterone*) is a testosterone derivative, and has an even stronger effect on the sebaceous glands, playing a critical role in exacerbating acne. **5AR** (*5-alpha reductase*) is the enzyme responsible for converting testosterone into DHT.

Cinnamon and nettle leaf extracts, are mild *5-alpha reductase* inhibitors, offering a safe and natural home remedy, to manage acne.

Additionally, estrogen influences acne by increasing the **SHBG (sex hormone-binding globulin)**, which binds to free flowing testosterone in the body, and making it inactive.

When estrogen levels drop, SHBG decreases, allowing more free testosterone to circulate, contributing to acne development and male pattern facial and body hair growth in females called *hirsutism*.

The compounds ***Resveratrol*** (found commonly in grapes and berries), and ***oleic acid*** (found commonly in olive oil) has been shown to influence the liver and increase the production of SHBG, which reduces amount of free testosterone circulating in the body, which then balances the hormone levels, and minimises the risk of acne formation.

Fungal acne is primarily caused by *Malassezia folliculitis*, a yeast species that naturally resides on our skin, along with other fungal species like Candida. These fungi can proliferate or cause infections in favourable conditions, such as humidity, excessive sweating, skin occlusion, antibiotic abuse, or weakened immunity.

Areas prone to fungal acne include skin folds like the armpits, nape of the neck, and groin. Dandruff, a thick white-coated tongue, seborrheic dermatitis, and psoriasis etc. often occur alongside fungal acne due to the same underlying factors that promote fungal overgrowth.

	Fungal Acne (*Malassezia folliculitis*)	*Regular Acne* (*Acne vulgaris*)
Appearance	Lots of tiny, identical white-heads or red bumps.	Inflammatory pimples in a range of sizes, plus white-heads and black-heads.
Location	Face (particularly T-zone), on the back and chest.	Anywhere on the face and less common on the back and chest.
Symptoms	Often itchy, rarely sore.	Sometimes sore, rarely itchy.
Triggers	Worsens in high humidity.	Not much affected by climate.
Response to treatment	Does not improve with antibiotics and other acne treatments (may worsen).	Often improves with antibiotics and other conventional acne treatments.

SBO probiotics (soil based organisms), in combination with Vitamin-D, zinc, and selenium, work collectively to improve the immune function, reduce inflammation, and support skin health, helping to manage fungal acne and associated flare-ups.

A more targeted approach, is to address the excess sebum being produced, and vitamin-B_5 does wonders in regulating sebum production, regardless of the underlying issue.

Diagnosing the cause of acne, is through physical examination, blood tests (such as testosterone, DHEAS, SHBG, LS-FSH ratio, prolactin, cortisol, CBC, lipid profile etc.) and other tests depending on the various specific signs and symptoms shown by the body.

Topical or oral medications including retinoids, hormone therapy and anti-biotics are commonly prescribed to treat acne. In extreme cases, steroids, laser therapies etc. are also suggested.

At-home skin care routines, and mild home-remedies are helpful, and advised for individuals suffering from acne, especially for teenagers, pregnant women, or women who are planning on becoming pregnant, feeding mothers etc. as these gentle approaches can help manage acne without the risks associated with stronger medications

And without a doubt, maintaining a healthy balanced diet, along with or without the other supportive treatments, is of utmost importance, as it can address the various factors leading to, and sustaining different types of acne. The changes that need to be included, in the diet, to treat and manage **Acne**, is explained in the sample diet charts, in Chapter- 25.

Let us next discuss about a few common disorders related to **bones**, **joints**, **muscles**, **tendons** *and* **ligament** *health.*

- **24.52 – <u>Osteo Arthritis (OA)</u>**

Osteoarthritis is the most common issue that affects the joints.
The ends of bones in the joints are capped by a layer of tough, smooth cartilage, that functions as a lubricant and shock absorber.

Osteoarthritis happens when the cartilage that lines the joints is worn down due to various causes, and eventually, the bones end up rubbing against each other, adding up to the existing issue.

Osteoarthritis can affect any joints, but most commonly develops in the weight bearing joints, which are the hips and knees.
It is also common in the shoulders, lower back and neck.

Osteoarthritis is quite common, and is estimated that more than **80%** of adults older than **55 years** of age have osteoarthritis, even if some of them never experience symptoms.

But lately, osteoarthritis have become common in the **30 to 40 years** age groups as well, due to increase in metabolic disorders.

Pain in the joint (especially when moving), stiffness, swelling on or around the joint, decreased range of motion, sounds from the joint while moving (crepitus), and joint deformity are the most common symptoms of osteo arthritis.

Even though osteoarthritis is attributed primarily to age and weight, it is nutrition that plays the actual pivotal role for formation of OA.

It is common knowledge, that each and every cell in our body dies off, and are replaced by new ones regularly. The rate of regeneration must be higher than, or at the least, almost equal to degeneration, in order to prevent issues like osteoarthritis.

Stage - I	Stage - II	Stage - III	Stage - IV
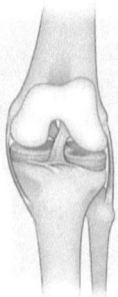	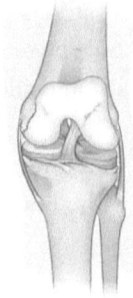	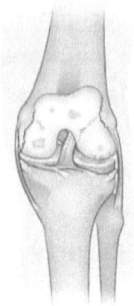	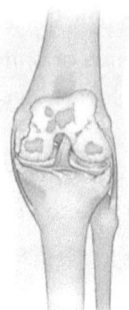
Minimum disruption. But there is already 10% loss of cartilage.	*Joint-space narrows. Cartilage begins breaking down. Occurrence of osteophytes.*	*Moderate joint-space reduction. Gaps in the cartilage expand until they reach the bone.*	*Joint space greatly reduced (more than 60%). Large osteophytes are also formed.*

But if a person is on a regular carbohydrate rich diet, this can increase the oxidation of cells, and in turn, increase the degenerative process.

It also does not give the individual enough space to consume nutrition dense foods, leading to the rate of regeneration, to become lower than degeneration.

Additionally, a carbohydrate rich diet also leads to weight gain.

So the actual major reasons for OA are –

- **Excess intake, or production of oxidants** such as sugars, ox-LDL, AGE, HCA, *omega*-6 etc.
- Not enough intake of **replenishers** (minerals, vitamins and proteins).
- Not enough intake or production of **anti-oxidants** such as glutathione, vitamin-C etc.
- **Overburden of joints** due to over-weight or excessive exercise without proper nutrition uptake.

In my clinical practice, I have quite often found hypo-chlorhydria (hypo-acidity) to be the root cause for osteoarthritis as well (particularly if found in young individuals), as the inefficiency in digestion, and absorption of valuable nutrients from ingested food during this condition, prevents the normal regeneration of joints.

X-rays, MRI and CT scans are helpful in diagnosing and evaluating the current stage of degeneration at a joint, and blood tests can help rule out any auto-immune factors.

Pain killers in various forms (as tablets, creams, ointments or patches), calcium supplements, PRP therapy, exercise, and application of hot or cold packs, are the usual method of treatment for OA, with joint replacement surgery being the last resort. But these are not aimed at resolving the issue efficiently, or at it its underlying cause.

As mentioned in Chapter- 14, concentrate on other vitamins and minerals that help the body to efficiently absorb calcium to the targeted area in the body, such as vitamin-D, vitamin-A, vitamin-K, vitamin-C and magnesium.

Ample amounts of collagen (makes up **40%** of bones), along with other trace minerals such as phosphorous, fluoride, manganese, boron, and zinc, along with a healthy diet, and resolving indigestion (if present), is the best treatment for early cases of osteo arthritis.

The changes that need to be included, in the diet, to treat and manage **Osteo Arthritis**, is explained in the sample diet charts, in Chapter- 25.

- **24.53 – <u>Osteopenia & Osteoporosis</u>**

Osteoporosis is a when the bones in the body reduces in density, becomes thin and weak, which causes it to break more easily (fracture). Most people don't know that they have this condition, until it causes them to break a bone. The most commonly affected bones are ones at the, hips, wrists and back bones.

It is estimated that over half of all females, and a quarter of all males world-wide, have osteoporosis.
Studies have found that 1 in 3 adults over 50 years of age, suffer from the starting stages of osteoporosis, known as *osteopenia*.

Osteoporosis is a silent disease, as it doesn't have any symptoms like other diseases. Osteoporosis happens naturally, as we get older and the bones lose their ability to regrow, and reform themselves.
Bones are living tissue like any other part of the body, and constantly replaces their own cells and tissue. Up until around 30 years of age, the body naturally builds more bone than the degradation process.

After 35 years of age, bone breakdown happens faster than the body can replace it, and the process is even faster, especially if the individual does not regularly exercise, or if they consume alcohol regularly, or suffers from indigestion, or gastro intestinal diseases, or endocrine diseases like thyroiditis, metabolic diseases like PCOD, diabetes or other hormonal imbalances.

Nutritional deficiencies due to unhealthy eating habits, have also become a leading cause for cases of osteoporosis, in individuals under 30 years of age. The over consumption of soda, or carbonated drinks, which contain large amounts of phosphoric acids, high fructose corn syrup and other artificial sweeteners, have also been found to be a leading cause for osteoporosis.

Some medications or surgical procedures can increase the risk of osteoporosis, such as diuretics, corticosteroids, sema-glutide (weight loss drug, most commonly known by its brand name *Ozempic*), bariatric (weight loss) surgery, hormone therapies, anti-coagulants, and proton pump inhibitors (used to treat acidity, which can affect the calcium absorption).

You must go to the hospital, if you think you have a broken bone, or if you experience intense pain, can't move a part of your body, and can notice swelling in the area.

A bone density test, which uses X-rays to measure the strength of the bones, are most commonly done to identify osteoporosis.

The treatment plan for osteoporosis, must include a well and balanced diet, regular exercise (to strengthen the bones and all the tissue connected to them, such as the muscles, ligaments and tendons), nutritional supplements (similar to that of osteo arthritis), and medications for underlying diseases that could be accelerating the degradation of bones.

The changes that need to be included, in the diet, to treat and manage **Osteopenia & Osteoporosis**, is explained in the sample diet charts, in Chapter- 25.

- ## 24.54 – <u>Carpal Tunnel Syndrome (CTS)</u>

The carpal tunnel is a space in the wrist bones, that forms a passage to let tendon, ligaments, nerves and blood vessels to reach the hand.

Carpal tunnel syndrome is a condition that causes symptoms like pain, numbness, tingling and weakness in the wrist, hand or fingers, and causes inability or trouble, to use the hands to hold, or control objects.

Carpal tunnel syndrome happens when any of the structures passing through the tunnel, is damaged, especially the median nerve.
CTS usually develops slowly, and responds well to treatment, but it can permanently damage the median nerve, if not treated soon enough.

Commonly the symptoms are first noticed at night, with a feeling of pain or tingling while waking up. Over time though, the symptoms starts being noticeable during the day, especially for those who do repetitive works at their job like typing, writing or using tools.

Extra pressure on the wrist, repetitive strain injuries, arthritis, sprains, wrist fractures, are the various common causes for *carpal tunnel syndrome*.

Individuals with inflammatory and degenerative diseases such as auto-immune conditions, gastro-intestinal disorders, hyper-uricemia, thyroiditis, diabetes etc. have an increased risk of developing CTS.

Nutritional deficiencies, especially of vitamin-B_1, vitamin-B_{12}, vitamin-D, collagen, and other proteins, increased intake of oxalate rich food like spinach, almond, parsley, chocolate, peanuts etc. also cause the tightening of fascia and ligaments, leading to pain and formation of CTS.

A combination of physical and imaging tests, are used to diagnose *carpal tunnel syndrome*, including *Tinel's* sign, *Phalen's* sign, X-rays, and ultra sound and MRI scans.

Carpal tunnel syndrome is treated with nonsurgical treatments initially, which include modifying the daily routine, supporting and strengthening the wrist, by wearing a splint, or doing specific sets of exercise (physiotherapy), changing the posture or working environment, and taking anti-inflammatory medications.

When having to work repetitive jobs, the risk for *carpal tunnel syndrome* can be reduced by –

- Wear proper protective equipment, for all work and activities.
- Take frequent rest breaks, when working with the hands.
- Stretching the wrists and hands, before and after intense physical activities.
- Use proper technique, and maintain good posture, when working with tools, or typing on a keyboard.

Carpal tunnel surgery may be required in extreme cases, where the surgeon performs a carpal tunnel release, to create more space inside the wrist, by making an incision (cut) in the ligament that connects the wrist to the palm (transverse carpal ligament), which reduces tension on the carpal tunnel, and gives the tendons and nerves more space.

But this procedure is ineffective, in cases where the *carpal tunnel syndrome* is due to degeneration of the nerves, or inflammation of the ligaments and tendons, due to underlying diseases, or nutritional deficiencies, for which the appropriate medications and diet, is the most effective route.

The changes that need to be included, in the diet, to treat and manage **Carpal Tunnel Syndrome**, due to inflammatory and degenerative diseases, or nutritional deficiencies, is explained in the sample diet charts, in Chapter- 25.

- **24.55 – <u>Plantar Fasciitis (PF)</u>**

The plantar fascia is a strong, fibrous attachment (similar to a ligament) that runs from the heel, to the ball of the foot and toes. It is stretchy like a thick rubber band. It connects the bones in the foot together and forms the arch on the bottom of the foot.

Plantar fasciitis is when inflammation occurs in this fascia, due to various causes, which makes it painful to walk or use the foot.
Most people experience plantar fasciitis in one foot at a time, but it is possible for it to affect both the feet at once.

The most common symptoms of plantar fasciitis include, a dull aching pain in the arch of the foot and heel, stiffness and swelling around the heel, and also difficulty, pain, or the inability to squat.

The pain can change, depending on the type of movement, or the time of day, such as pain while standing up, after sleeping, or sitting down (pain usually fades after walking for a few minutes), and a sharp or stabbing pain, when pressure is applied on the affected foot or heel.

Exercising or moving, might temporarily relieve the pain, but the issue usually gets worse to the point, where exercise does not prove fruitful, unless the underlying issue is addressed.

Inflammatory and degenerative diseases such as auto-immune conditions, gastro-intestinal disorders, hyper-uricemia, thyroiditis, diabetes etc. have an increased risk of causing plantar fasciitis, and so does nutritional deficiencies, especially of vitamin-B_{12}, vitamin-D, collagen, and other proteins, which are necessary, for the healthy upkeep of ligaments and fascia.

Increased intake of oxalate rich food like spinach, almond, parsley, chocolate, peanuts etc. also cause the tightening of fascia and ligaments, leading to pain.

Along with these underlying issues, anything that irritates or damages the fascia, can fasten the process of developing fasciitis such as, being on the feet all day for work, playing sports, exercise or working on a hard surface, exercise without stretching or warming up, wearing flat shoes or slippers that do not support the arch of the feet well enough, etc.

A physical exam, along with X-rays, ultrasound and MRI scans, can help diagnose plantar fasciitis, but a blood work and further tests related to signs and symptoms of other underlying issues, will help with identifying, and treating the root cause.

Painkillers, anti-inflammatory drugs, arch support shoe inserts, immobilization with walking boot or walking cast, PRP (platelet rich plasma) therapy, percutaneous needle tenotomy, electrotherapy, physiotherapy and surgery are the various methods employed conventionally, to help relieve the symptoms of plantar fasciitis.

Icing the foot for 15 minutes, twice a day, with cold packs (or ice cubes covered with thin cloth) rolled along the bottom of the foot with a gentle massage, helps reduce the inflammation.

Despite the usual *'gut feeling'* to stretch the foot upward, it actually gives better symptomatic relief when the foot is repetitively stretched downward (around 20 times) twice or thrice a day, while taking necessary steps to internally treat the issue, through proper medicines, supplementations and a balanced diet.

The changes that need to be included, in the diet, to treat and manage **Plantar Fasciitis,** due to inflammatory and degenerative diseases, or nutritional deficiencies, is explained in the sample diet charts, in Chapter- 25.

- ## 24.56 – <u>Frozen Shoulder (Adhesive Capsulitis)</u>

Frozen shoulder occurs when the strong connective tissue surrounding the shoulder joint becomes thick, stiff and inflamed, limiting the shoulder movement and causing pain.

The condition is called *'frozen'* shoulder because the more pain one feels, the less likely they will use the shoulder. Lack of use, causes the joint to become even more tight, and difficult to move, leading to the shoulder being "frozen" in its position.

Even though various risk factors such as age, injury, and chronic diseases (such as thyroiditis or *Parkinson's*), increases the chance for developing frozen shoulders, the most common reason is the combination of nutritional deficiencies along with diabetes.
Around **20%** of those suffering from diabetes mellitus, have been found to develop frozen shoulder.

AGE (*advanced glycated end products*) are harmful compounds formed when excess blood sugar (glucose) binds to proteins, lipids, or nucleic acids in the body, and this binding process is called ***glycation***.
This occurs particularly in individuals with chronic high blood sugar, such as those with uncontrolled diabetes.

Accumulated AGEs bind to RAGE (*receptor for advanced glycation end-products*) present on various cells, which activates TLR4 and triggers an inflammatory response. This inflammation then produces *reactive oxygen species* (ROS) or free radicals, which damage cells and tissues leading to fibrosis and scarring of tissues around the shoulder joint.

Deficiency of vitamin-B_1, vitamin-D, and heavy metal toxicity are also found to be potent catalyst in the development of frozen shoulder. Managing blood sugar levels, reducing oxidative stress, and boosting antioxidants are required steps to downregulate this issue.

Frozen shoulder symptoms are categorized into three stages -

- The "**Freezing**" stage, is when the shoulder becomes stiff and is painful to move. The pain slowly increases. It may worsen at night. Inability to move the shoulder joint increases.
  This stage lasts from 2 to 9 months.
- The "**Frozen**" stage shows noticeable reduction in pain, but the shoulder remains stiff. This makes it more difficult to complete daily tasks and activities.
  This stage can last for 2 to 6 months.
- The "**Thawing**" (recovery) stage has even more reduction in pain, and the ability to move the shoulder slowly improves, as a result of treatment. Full or near full recovery occurs as typical strength and motion return. The stage lasts from 6 months to 2 years.

To diagnose frozen shoulder, a physical examination, X-rays, ultrasound scans, MRI and CT scans are commonly done, along with other tests for underlying issues, depending on the various specific signs and symptoms shown by the body.

Conventional methods to manage frozen shoulder includes the use of topical, oral and injectable medications, physiotherapy and electrotherapy. Surgery is preferred in severe cases.

The changes that need to be included, in the diet, to treat and manage **Frozen Shoulder (Adhesive Capsulitis),** due to inflammatory and degenerative diseases, or nutritional deficiencies, is explained in the sample diet charts, in Chapter- 25.

- ## 24.57 – Sciatica

Sciatica is a condition, where mild to severe pain is experienced, in any area with nerves that connect to the sciatic nerve, such as the lower back, hips, buttocks or the legs.

Tingling or numbness, with a characteristic radiating pain to the thighs, muscle weakness, and urinary or faecal incontinence, can also be involved with or without the pain, and it occurs due to an injury, or irritation to the sciatic nerve, because of various reasons.

The sciatic nerves are the largest nerves in our body, which runs through the hip and buttock on each side. They each go down the leg until just below the knee, from where, they split into other nerves that connect to parts farther down, including the lower leg, foot and toes.

Conditions that can cause sciatica include –

- **IVDP** (*inter vertebral disk prolapse*) due to overweight or obesity, bad posture, injury due to accidents, weakness of 'core muscles' and supporting muscles of the lower back, as a consequence of, an inactive or sedentary lifestyle.
- **PID** (*pelvic inflammatory disease*), due to PCOD, UTI, fungal infections, worm infestation, IBS, IBD etc.
- *Nutritional deficiencies*, especially of those which are needed for the upkeep of nerves, such as vitamin-B_1, vitamin-B_{12}, choline, and healthy fats.
- *Tightness of piriformis muscles*, situated in the buttocks, which can tighten due to an inactive or sedentary lifestyle, or due to nutritional deficiencies (especially magnesium), and cause sciatica, by pressing against the sciatic nerve.
- *Degenerative diseases*, including osteo arthritis, diabetes, etc.
- *Tumours*, *cysts* or other growths are uncommon causative factors.

The easiest test to help diagnose sciatica, from other causes of back pain, is the straight-leg raising test, which involves having the person lie on an examination table with legs straight out. The examiner slowly raises one leg at a time, upwards. A person suffering from sciatica, will not be able to raise the leg completely, and will feel an intense pain, in the back and inner part of their thighs, as well as the lower back.

Other common tests include, but aren't limited to X-rays, MRI and CT scans, myelogram, electromyography, nerve conduction velocity studies, as well as blood work, and further tests related to signs and symptoms of other underlying issues, which will help with identifying, and treating the underlying cause.

Treating sciatica involves trying to decrease pain, and increase mobility, while addressing the underlying causes as well. It is to be noted that moderate to severe pain, with numbness and tingling, or muscle weakness, may require professional medical care.
Do not try to self-treat.

In milder cases, self-treatments can include cold pack (preferred), or heat pad applications, and various types of backward arching stretches while lying down.

NSAIDs, painkillers, muscle relaxants, anti-seizure medications, corticosteroid or local anaesthesia spinal injections, and surgeries are the conventional options for treatment. Most causes of sciatica (around **90%**) are preventable, but others that happen unpredictably or due to accidents might require emergency surgery, which could be unavoidable.

The changes that need to be included, in the diet, to treat and manage **Sciatica,** due to inflammatory and degenerative diseases, or nutritional deficiencies, is explained in the sample diet charts, in Chapter- 25.

- **24.58 – Inter-Vertebral Disc Prolapse (IVDP)**

Vertebrae are the series of bones on the back, from the base of the skull to the tailbone. Between each vertebrae, are round cushions with a gel-like center, and a firmer outer layer, called disks.

These disks act as buffers between the bones, allowing us to bend and move with ease. Due to various causes, the disks become less effective, and may become displaced, which is called as a herniated / bulging / slipped / ruptured / protruding disk.

A herniated disk occurs, when one of the disks in the backbone tears, leaks, or is compressed excessively due to an injury, or wear and tear. This puts pressure on the spinal cord, and irritates the spinal nerves, leading to pain, numbness and weakness, at the site of herniation, and in the corresponding parts, that the nerve supplies to, such as the hands, thighs etc.

IVDP, is classified based on the affected vertebral region, with specific terminology corresponding to each spinal section, such as – ***Cervical** spondylosis*, ***Lumbar** spondylosis* and ***Thoracic** spondylosis*.

'***Radiculopathy***' is a broad term that describes the symptoms caused by a pinched nerve in the spine.
Sciatica, is the most common type of radiculopathy.

Overweight or obesity, bad posture, weakness of 'core muscles' and supporting muscles of the lower back, as a consequence of an inactive or sedentary lifestyle are easily the most common factors that cause IVDP. Traumatic injuries, like falls, improper lifting of heavy objects, degeneration due to natural ageing, and due to diseases, such as osteo arthritis, diabetes, nutritional deficiencies, especially of those which are needed for the upkeep of bones and intervertebral disk tissue, such as those mentioned in *osteo arthritis*, are the various causative factors as well.

A physical and neurological examination, X-rays, MRI and CT scans, electromyography, myelogram, nerve conduction velocity studies, as well as blood work and further tests related to signs and symptoms of other underlying issues, are the various diagnostic procedures that help with identifying, and treating the cause of IVDP.

Treating IVDP, involves trying to decrease pain, and increase mobility, while addressing the underlying causes. It is to be noted, that moderate to severe pain, with numbness and tingling, or muscle weakness, may require professional medical care. Do not try to self-treat.

In milder cases, self-treatments can include cold pack (preferred), or heat pad applications, traction, and backward stretches while lying down (forward stretches must not be done).

NSAIDs, painkillers, muscle relaxants, anti-seizure medications, corticosteroid or local anaesthesia spinal injections, and surgeries, are the conventional options for treatment. There are multiple surgical techniques for relieving pressure on the spinal cord and nerves.

In rare cases, a large ruptured disk might injure nerves to your bladder, or bowel which may require emergency surgery. For non-emergency cases, herniated disk surgery is an option, when other treatments don't work. *Microdiscectomy, diskectomy, laminotomy, laminectomy,* artificial disk surgery, spinal fusion etc. are various surgical procedures for IVDP.

The changes that need to be included, in the diet, to treat and manage **Inter-Vertebral Disk Prolapse,** due to inflammatory and degenerative diseases, or nutritional deficiencies, is explained in the sample diet charts, in Chapter- 25.

- **24.59 – Urinary Incontinence**

Urinary incontinence, is a condition where one experiences bladder control issues and involuntarily leaks urine.

The urinary bladder is like a storage tank, once full, the brain sends a signal, that it's time to urinate, and normally, our decision to release it, allows the urine to flow freely out of the body through the urethra. This is affected by various causes.

The different types of incontinence include -

- *Urge incontinence-*
  Characterized by an intense need to urinate right away, caused by weak pelvic muscles, nerve damage, infections, low estrogen levels, body overweight, certain medications, and abuse of beverages like alcohol and caffeine.

- *Stress incontinence-*
  When actions like a laugh, cough, sneeze, running, jumping or lifting heavy objects, are done, it increases the pressure inside the abdomen, putting a stress or pressure on the bladder. Without the support of strong pelvic muscles, this could cause urine to leak.

- *Overflow incontinence-*
  If your bladder is not emptied completely during each urination, it can result in overflow incontinence. Usually, this results in small amounts of urine dripping out over time instead of one big gush of urine. Common in people with chronic conditions like multiple sclerosis, stroke, diabetes, or prostatitis.

- *Mixed incontinence-*
  This type of incontinence, is a combination of several problems, that all lead to leakage issues. Identifying the triggers, and underlying issues of the mixed incontinence, is usually the best way to manage it.

Urinary tract infections (UTIs), constipation, pelvic floor disorders, stroke, diabetes and other metabolic issues, auto-immune disorders, prostatitis, pregnancy, menopause, certain medications and beverages, prolonged habit of holding in urine, and nutritional deficiencies are the various common, *'temporary'* and *'long-term'* causes for urinary incontinence.

Physical examinations, urinalysis, ultrasound scans, cystoscopy, urodynamic testing are the various diagnostic methods to find the root cause of the issue. Depending on the underlying cause, appropriate medications and treatments are prescribed.

Emptying your bladder when full or when the urge presents, practicing Kegel exercises to strengthen pelvic floor muscles, avoiding alcohol or caffeine or sugar abuse, maintaining a healthy body weight, and consuming a balanced, nutritious diet, is helpful to reverse most of the underlying issues, of a urinary incontinence.

The changes that need to be included, in the diet, to maintain and manage **Urinary Incontinence**, is explained in the sample diet charts, in Chapter- 25.

- ## 24.60 – Dental Health

Teeth and bones share some similarities, but are quite different. Bones can heal themselves when broken, thanks to living cells that regenerate, however, teeth do not regenerate like how a bone does.

When a tooth suffers damage, it loses something called dentin, a hard, bony tissue underneath the enamel, that forms the bulk of the tooth.

Each tooth's stem cells produce new dentin, in an attempt to repair the damage. However, this innate repair mechanism has its limits, and can only manufacture small amounts of tissue, while combating a cavity, injury, or infection. This is why, under normal circumstances, teeth cannot heal themselves, as well as other bones do.

According to a recent study from the journal '*Scientific Reports*' researchers may be able to stimulate stem cells in the teeth, to naturally repair defects including cavities, cracks, chips, and more.

Though no clinical studies have been conducted on humans as of yet, experts are hopeful that the findings will dramatically impact the future of dental care.

So far, tests on mice have produced successful results. After drilling holes into the molars, scientists stimulated the teeth's stem cells. Within six weeks, the mice regenerated much of the dentin lost in their teeth.

The ultimate goal, according to researcher Paul Sharpe, is to stimulate stem cells enough to 'regenerate a whole tooth.' If possible, stem cell treatments could eventually replace traditional dental procedures.

When looking through a preventive aspect, there are a few changes that can be done in the lifestyle and food habits of an individual, to take precautions for, in the case of teeth health.

Before humans 'settled down' and the emergence of agriculture began around 12,000 years ago, hunter-gatherers had much denser teeth and stronger jaw structures. Their diet, rich in proteins and fats, like meat and bone marrow, unprocessed foods, including fruits, and fibrous plants, naturally promoted the development of more robust teeth.

These remains, are still observable in archaeological findings, which show strong and well-formed teeth and skulls.

However, with the rise of agriculture and the increased reliance on grains, particularly over the last several hundred years, dietary changes led to a decline in tooth density and overall dental health.

The shift to softer, processed foods such as grains that require less chewing resulted in a decrease in jaw and tooth strength.
Additionally, grains can be acidic and require more effort from the body to maintain oral health, potentially contributing to tooth decay and other dental issues over time.
This dietary shift marks a clear transition in human evolution, where teeth and jawbones became less dense, showing the long-term impact of our current food practices on the overall human physique, beyond that of metabolic diseases.

The common dental disorders due to nutritional deficiencies and unhealthy food habits are, **bruxism** (habit of teeth grinding or jaw clenching), scurvy, tooth decay and gum disease or periodontal disease, that leads to tooth sensitivity and erosion.

This is caused by the breakdown of tooth enamel, due to acid producing bacteria in the mouth, and plaque buildup along the gumline that lead to inflammation, or gingivitis, and even cancers, often from extra sugar or carbohydrate consumption.

Bacteria does all of this so effectively, as they tend to grow in large, stable collectives called **biofilms**, which are an indestructible fortress, and the plaque formations on the teeth are biofilm.

One powerful nutrient that can address the combination of these issues, is **ascorbic acid**, which is part of the vitamin-C complex, and is one of the most essential nutrients for teeth health. It prevents and cures scurvy (bleeding, loose gums), by helping in the absorption and synthesis of collagen which is vital for the skin, bones, teeth, ligaments, cartilage, discs, gums of teeth, and the integrity of blood vessels.

Vitamin-C, also boosts the immunity, which prevents the overgrowth of mouth bacteria, and can help prevent and control bad breath and gingivitis. Vitamin-C, not only directly prevents and disrupts the formation of biofilm, but also indirectly disrupts biofilms and plaques, by producing low levels of hydrogen peroxide in the body.
Lemon, guava, other citrus fruits, sauerkraut, and green vegetables are good sources of the vitamin-C complex.

Bruxism or involuntary teeth grinding, has been found to be commonly caused due to the lack of serotonin (happy hormone) and dopamine, due to increased stress, and nutritional deficiencies such as vitamin-B_1 which is a precursor, and vitamin-D which is an activator of the serotonin hormone.

Oral infections, and other dental issues, can also lead to more serious issues like auto-immune conditions, and are even attributed to increasing the risk of heart attacks.

Bacteria from cavities and gum disease, can enter the bloodstream and contribute to plaque buildup in the arteries, which can lead to atherosclerosis, causing inflammation and increasing the risk of heart attack. Bacteria from the mouth can spread to the heart and cause infections of the heart lining, called endocarditis as well.

Porphyromonas gingivalis (P. gingivalis) is a bacterium that can increase the risk of developing rheumatoid arthritis (RA), in a number of ways, including molecular mimicry.

Molecular mimicry is where the bacteria produces enzymes, that influence immune system responses, and causes an auto-immune response by the body. This happens because the enzymes produced by the bacteria has a molecular structure similar to that of another enzyme, naturally present in our body, confusing our body into attacking itself. The bacteria also causes harm, by affecting our gut barrier permeability.

Other examples include -

Disease	*Associated Oral Bacterial Species*
IBS (*irritable bowel syndrome*).	• Streptococcus (genus). • Streptococcus thermophilus. • Veillonella (genus).
IBD (*inflammatory bowel disease*).	• Veillonellaceae (family). • Pasteurellaceae (family). • Neisseriaceae (family).
Colorectal cancer.	• Porphyromonas gingivalis. • Fusobacterium.

Mouth washes do help in controlling the infections in the mouth, but the regular use of mouth washes have been linked to an increased risk of colorectal cancer due to its potential to disrupt the natural balance of oral bacteria.

Certain mouthwashes, particularly those containing strong antibacterial agents, causes the elimination of both harmful as well as beneficial bacteria in the mouth. This disruption allows harmful bacteria with a better antibiotic-resistance, such as *Fusobacterium*, to thrive.

Research suggests that the overgrowth of these bacteria potentially increases inflammation and the development of cancerous cells.

Cancer can occur particularly in the digestive system, due to its various metabolic end-products, and as a result, a leading mouthwash brand is currently facing a lawsuit, for not adequately warning about these risks to the customers.

Using mouth washes must be limited to the time of need (as in times of infections), and should not be used for the day-to-day requirements of maintaining dental hygiene.

The same can be said about the *fluoride* content in toothpaste. Even though it has an ability to prevent decay, when it is over-used, in high concentrations, it leads to the discoloration and weakening of teeth, due to damage of the enamel, especially in children.

As an alternative, *hydroxyapatite* is a compound that is being used as the major ingredient in toothpastes, in countries like Japan, South Korea and Germany, and has been gaining attention in other regions for its tooth remineralizing properties.

Hydroxyapatite is a naturally occurring mineral form of calcium apatite, which makes up around **97%** of our tooth enamel.

Research suggests *nano-hydroxyapatite* works by directly restoring lost minerals to the enamel, which helps to strengthen and repair it without the potential risks associated with fluoride.

It forms a protective layer on the teeth, providing a barrier against decay, lowers sensitivity, reduces plaque buildup, and improves the overall tooth appearance.

And since *hydroxyapatite* is biocompatible and safe when ingested in small amounts, it is seen as a gentle and effective solution for children as well.

Advanced stages of tooth infections, cavities and plaque or tartar buildup require the intervention from expert dental specialists, but a healthy diet can go a long way in the prevention of oral and dental health issues, and is a powerful supportive treatment to integrate during other procedures as well.

The changes that need to be included, in the diet, to maintain and manage **Dental Health**, is explained in the sample diet charts in Chapter- 25.

Let us next discuss about the infamous disease feared by all, **Cancer**.

- **24.61 – <u>Cancer</u>**

One thing most of us don't realize about cancer, is that each and every person in the world, including you and me, we all have cancers in our body right now.

When there is an uncontrolled, abnormal growth, and spread of cells in the body, it is known as cancer.
This happens in each and every one of our bodies, on a daily basis.

But what differentiates those who are suffering from cancer as a disease, is that their bodies, are not strong enough to suppress, and dispose these cancerous cells, as a healthy body would.

Decades of detailed genetic analysis have revealed, that there are nearly **1000 known cancer associated genes in humans**, of which, roughly –

- **250 are oncogenes** (that which **causes** cancer).
- **700 are tumor suppressors** (genes that regulate cell growth and division, and **prevent** the development of cancer).

Cells typically need two or more mutations in the cancer associated genes, to become carcinogenic, which means that there are more than 1 million different cancer genotypes.

How can anyone hope to treat a million different types of cancer?

When put in simple terms, using genetic fingerprinting of tumors in order to design custom, tumor-specific drugs, is a formidable challenge. But a breakthrough can be achieved, if we follow the lead, that is, the detailed analysis of these cancer associated genes, suggest that they play a key role in cellular metabolism.

So, the central question is, whether cancer should be considered a **metabolic disease** or a **genetic disease**.

Interestingly, prior to 1970, most cancer researchers believed cancer to be a metabolic disorder, and not to be a genetic one.

In 1927, Dr. Otto Warburg noticed that cancer cells exhibited a distinct behavior, consuming up to 200 times more glucose than normal cells, which came to be known as the '**Warburg effect**'.

Based on Warburg's influence, most cancer drugs discovered in the 1950s and 1960s were called "*anti-metabolites*".

However, with Warburg's death in 1970 and the discovery of oncogenes in 1971, most cancer researchers shifted to viewing cancer, as a genetic disease rather than a metabolic disease.

The "**re-discovery**" of cancer as a metabolic disorder, largely occurred in the last five years, driven by advances in metabolomics, and the discovery, of '**oncometabolites**' (which are endogenous metabolites, whose accumulation can initiate or encourage tumour growth and the **metastasis**, or the spread of it).

Many of the seemingly infinite number of cancer mutations and cancer genes in humans, affect three major metabolic pathways,

        i.   **Aerobic glycolysis.**
       ii.   **Glutaminolysis.**
      iii.   **One-carbon metabolism.**

These pathways allow cancer cells to shift from being simple ATP (energy) producers, to ones that can generate large quantities of amino acids, nucleotides, fatty acids and other intermediates, needed for rapid cell growth and division.

Warburg had hypothesized that the shift from respiration, to aerobic glycolysis in cancer cells, was due to defective mitochondrial respiration (as mentioned in Chapter- 20), and that all the other characteristics of the disease, including the errors and damages in the DNA, arise either directly or indirectly, from defective respiration.

New evidence indicates, this to be true, and that cancer originates from damage to the mitochondria in the cytoplasm, rather than from damage to the DNA in the nucleus, which means that, the DNA or genomic damage in tumor cells, is not the causative factor, but is a result from the action of defective mitochondria.

Results from Prof. Seyfried's research indicate that DNA defects alone, cannot account for the origin of tumors, and that normally functioning mitochondria can suppress tumorigenesis (growth of tumors).

The conventional treatment of cancer is a targeted, disease focused approach that utilizes immunotherapy, hormone therapy, radiation therapy, chemotherapy, transplantations and surgery to fight against, and keep the cancerous growths in check.

In 2022, the projected number of new cancer cases in India was **1,461,427** which means that around **100 people, per 100,000** (1 lakh) individuals of the population, were affected.

- *Lung cancer* ranked highest among males.
- *Breast cancer* held the top spot for females.
- *Lymphoid leukaemia* emerged as the highest in childhood cancers (up to 14 years of age), with around **30%** in **boys**, and **25%** in **girls**.

As compared to 2020, an estimated **13%** increase in cancer cases is expected by 2025 (up to about 30 million cases),
and around 1 in 10 people in India, are expected to face a cancer diagnosis during their lifetime.

So unless, a treatment method that addresses the underlying issue that leads to cancer, is not integrated with the conventional treatment approach, the cases of cancer emergence, and the re-emergence in cases that had seen remission, are going to be the norm of tomorrow.

Increased cortisol, mitochondrial dysfunction, vitamin-C deficiency, tissue hypoxia, acidic tumour micro-environment, oxidative stress, increased action of mTOR, and dysfunctional autophagy are the major metabolic issues, faced by an individual with an unhealthy lifestyle, and a nutrient deficient food habit.

This in turn, causes an increase in vascular endothelial growth factor, aerobic glycolysis, glutaminolysis, uncontrolled angiogenesis, DNA mutation and aberrations, and aggravates the inflammatory response and much more, all leading to the uncontrollable growth, and spread of cancer cells in the body.

Current cancer diagnostic procedures, while advanced, have several limitations like late detection, invasiveness, high costs, and false results.

Continued innovation and investment in more accurate, accessible, and non-invasive diagnostic technologies are essential for improving the outcomes of patients suffering from cancer.

Live Blood Analysis and *Thermal Scans* are emerging diagnostic methods, that offer unique advantages when it comes to detecting and monitoring cancer. While both techniques are not yet mainstream or universally accepted in clinical practice, they offer promising insights that could complement traditional methods.

Some of the benefits of live blood analysis, is that it is non-invasive and quick, allows real-time insights on the cell behaviour, helps in early detection, can help track the progression of the cancer, which helps in making needful personalized adjustments for each patient, and most importantly, helps in identifying the underlying causes.

CEA (*carcinoembryonic antigen*), **CRP** (*C-reactive protein*), ***ionic calcium levels***, 25-OH **vitamin-D**, **IPTH** (*parathyroid hormone*), **CBC** (*complete blood count*), **LFT** (*liver function test*), **RFT** (*renal function test*), **ferritin** (a helpful marker for proliferation, angiogenesis, immunosuppression, and iron delivery which is increased to cancerous cells), **TSH** (*thyroid stimulating hormone*), **LDH** (*lactate dehydrogenase* indicate oncogenic signaling pathways, invasiveness and immunogenicity), and **D-dimer** (indicates abnormality in blood clotting process), are all, some of the important tests which help in this regard.

Thermal imaging, or thermography, is a technique that uses infrared cameras to detect heat patterns and blood flow in body tissues. Since cancerous tissues tend to have increased blood flow and metabolic activity, thermal scans can sometimes identify areas of concern where abnormal growth may be occurring.

This procedure is non-invasive, painless and doesn't require physical contact, helps in the early detection of tumours (by detecting the tumour inflammation), do not have radiation like other scans (mammogram, MRI or CT which increases the risk of growth, and spread of the disease), helps to monitor the progress of the treatment, which enhances the early detection, and significantly improves patient outcomes.

Molecular hydrogen therapy, hyperbaric ozone therapy, liposomal curcumin, coenzyme Q-10, high dose vitamin-C and vitamin-D supplementation, chelation therapy (to remove heavy metal toxicity), are some of the supportive treatments that can be integrated with the conventional approach, along with a time-restricted, calorie-deficit, nutrition-dense diet, and intermittent fasting, which addresses the root cause, as well as help in the suppression of the cancer cells.

A quite interesting way to ***fight cancer with fat cells*** was discovered recently. Cancer cells constantly need a lot of glucose to grow. Our body has different types of fat cells, as explained in Chapter- 20.

When the *beige* or *brown* type of fat is active, it uses up the glucose quickly, causing various types of cancer cells to get less glucose, essentially starving it and causing it to stop growing and shrink in size. When the body is exposed to cool temperatures, around 4°C to 10°C, beige and brown fat become more active. They burn more glucose to produce heat. Scientists created beige fat in the lab and placed it next to cancer cells. The result was surprising, the cancer cells were not efficient enough to compete for glucose, and the majority died or got shrunken. Instead of attacking cancer cells directly, we can activate fat cells to take away their food (glucose). This method, though in need of more research, is better and less harmful than some current treatments, and is a promising step forward.

It is important to note that in advanced stages of cancer, particularly when the disease metastasizes, *autophagy* plays a critical role in the cancer cells' survival, respiration, division, and expansion.

Autophagy actually allows the cancerous cells to maintain their energy balance and continue growing, even under the stress. In this context, intermittent fasting can serve as a dangerous approach to treat cancer.

However, when autophagy is combined with chemotherapy, research shows it can enhance the effectiveness of the treatment, potentially making it more successful in targeting and killing cancer cells.

Despite these potential benefits, cancer treatment should never be self-administered or approached without medical guidance. Always seek advice from a qualified healthcare provider to ensure the safest and most effective treatment strategy.

The changes that need to be included, in the diet, to treat and manage **Cancer**, is explained in the Sample Diet Chart, in Chapter- 25, but the patient must be under the guidance of a licenced Medical Doctor or Physician while doing so.

Chapter XXV – Sample Diet Charts.

General Instructions:-

- Avoid all bakery products (like bread, biscuits, cakes, muffins), fast food, chocolates, and any kind of sugars, completely.

- Avoid any, and all kinds of grains and millets such as rice, wheat, maize, ragi, oats etc. (50_g can be included, better if fermented, when on a maintenance diet).

- Avoid all refined oils. Include only good fats, like that from whole milk, yoghurt, ghee, butter, cheese, paneer, olive oil, coconut oil and other nuts, and fish and meat fats.

- Avoid any alcohol consumption, including beer and wine (for those who believe that it only contains negligible amounts of alcohol).

- Replace common iodised salt, with sea salt. For patients suffering from high blood pressure, reduce intake of salt to 1 tsp. per day, use pepper and lime for enhancing taste.

- Intermittent Fasting- by finishing dinner before 7 p.m, and having breakfast by 10 a.m, the next morning. It should be a complete dry fast, without water as well.

- For friendly gut bacteria, consume yoghurt or curd, after allowing it to ferment, so that good bacteria overgrowth is present. If it is too sour for the individuals palate, mix it with fresh yoghurt and consume daily. Home-made *'Kimchi'* is also preferable.

- All types and varieties of vegetables can be consumed, except *tapioca* and *potato*, or such high starch (sugar) vegetables.

- Cooked vegetables must be consumed during 3 meals a day. (Lentils, pulses, sprouts must also be included but limited to 30%, and the rest 70% must be vegetables). These can be cooked as Gravies or Sautéed or Soups. Cooked vegetables are preferred than raw.

- For those with access to plenty of coconut, it is preferable to include at least a quarter of it a day, preferably grated and included without cooking, during mealtime with other foods.

- All meats and fish must be steamed, or cooked as gravies, or grilled (occasionally) and not be consumed as deep-fried dishes.

- It is preferred to include collagen rich 'Bone Soups' at least thrice a weak for a healthy gut bacterial flora and gut wall integrity, skin, bones and ligament health.

- Fatty liver, PCOD, Type-2 Diabetes (those who has not started injecting insulin), Obesity, Functional Thyroiditis patients, who do not have any other complications or allergies can follow the charts as it is, without the need for major changes.

- Auto-immune Thyroiditis patients must avoid milk, soy products and all grains, strictly for at least 2 months or until the doctor's advice.

- Gastritis patients must include more curd and fruits (especially ones high in vitamin-C like orange, amla / gooseberries, guava), and can include overnight fermented grains with curd (a potent probiotic combination that helps battle H. Pylori infections).

- Gastritis patients need to carry out the *'Baking Soda Test'* and consume ACV if necessary. In cases of severe indigestion, it is best to consume soups for meals, and buttermilk during snack times.

- Patients with extreme auto-immune conditions such as IBS, Rheumatoid arthritis, Ulcerative colitis, Crohn's disease etc. must exclude fruits as well, from the diet and must be under the doctor's consultation and guidance.

- Patients with kidney diseases, allergy or skin disorders such as psoriasis, eczema etc. (IgE elevated cases), must avoid all proteins that they are specifically allergic to, or that may aggravate their condition, for the time being, or may consume it along with **ACV** (apple cider vinegar) and digestive enzyme supplements, if it proves to not trigger their symptoms.

- Patients suffering from hyper-uricemia or high uric acid levels, need not worry about low purine protein foods (such as eggs and dairy), and can enjoy them in plenty.

  Moderate and high purine protein foods, need only be avoided in case the patient experiences pain or joint aches, immediately or after a while after its consumption.

  In those cases, stick to the *Insulin Resistance Diet Chart*, by avoiding moderate and high purine foods, or those foods that specifically trigger their gout attack, until the root cause is resolved, and then they can resume consuming the moderate and high purine foods, according to their liking.

Total Purine Content per 100$_g$ of Protein –

	Purine Content	*Food Groups*
Safe to Consume	Less than 50$_{mg}$	Eggs, Almonds & Dairy Products.
Potential to trigger Gout	Moderate (50 - 140$_{mg}$) & High (more than 150$_{mg}$)	Poultry, Red Meats & Organ Meats Fish & other seafood Wholegrains, Nuts, Pulses & Lentils Cruciferous vegetables & Mushrooms

Even though the following are completely healthy sample diet patterns, it has not been customized to patient's individual needs, and it also does not mean, that these are the only steps needed, to completely treat the disease for all cases. If you are under medications or in a serious health risk, please do not try to treat yourself without the consultation, diagnosis or professional guidance from a competent, registered Medical Doctor or Physician

- **Traditional Indian Diet -**

    The traditional Indian diet is largely carbohydrate-centric, with staples like rice, wheat, millets, and lentils making up over **80%** of daily food intake.

    This heavy reliance on carbohydrates provides ample energy, but for individuals genetically predisposed to metabolic disorders, this dietary pattern can be problematic.

    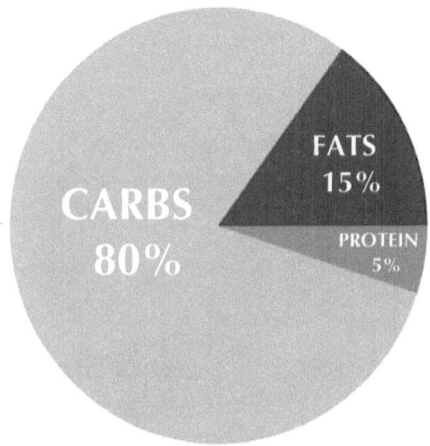

    Although fats contribute around **15%** to the diet, they are often of lower quality, with reliance on cooking oils that are high in *omega*-6 fatty acids. Proteins, essential for muscle repair, immune health, and metabolic function, tend to be under-represented in traditional diet.

    This imbalance can aggravate the metabolic dysfunction, making it critical for those at risk of conditions like diabetes, obesity, and cardiovascular diseases to reassess their nutritional intake.

- **Reversal Diet Plan -**

    The disease reversal diet plan should prioritize a shift in macronutrient distribution, focusing **75%** on healthy fats to encourage fat adaptation and to combat insulin resistance.

    This fat-rich approach allows the body to rely on fat for energy, improving metabolic efficiency and supporting the reduction of blood sugar levels. Protein should comprise around **20%** of the diet, playing a vital role in muscle repair, immune function, and overall tissue maintenance.

    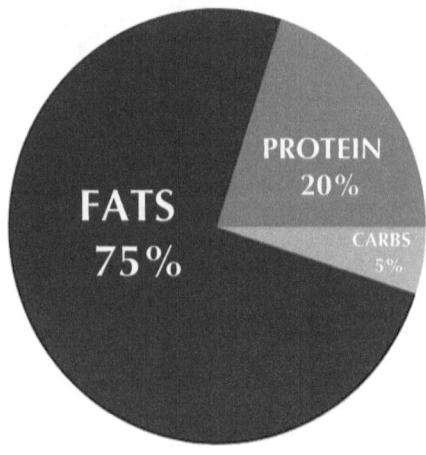

    By significantly reducing carbohydrate intake, especially that of refined sugars and grains, this plan helps to stabilize blood glucose, lower inflammation, and improve fat metabolism.

    The reduction in carbohydrates also regulate hormones, supports weight loss and aids for better cardiovascular health.
    This macronutrient strategy not only optimizes metabolic function but can also aid in the reversal of various chronic metabolic as well as auto-immune diseases.

- **Maintenance Diet Plan** –

    A maintenance diet should strike a balanced approach, with **40%** of the total daily calories coming from both healthy fats and complex carbohydrates.

    This equilibrium helps maintain energy levels and supports metabolic functions without excessive blood sugar spikes or crashes.

    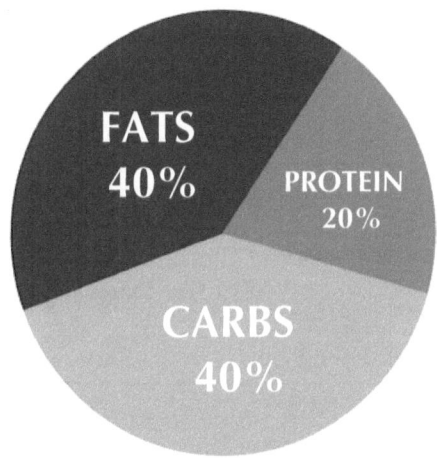

    Healthy fats from sources like avocados, nuts, coconut oil, olive oil, animal fats and dairy, help regulate hormone production and inflammation. Carbohydrates from whole grains, vegetables, and whole fruits provide essential fiber and micronutrients.

    The remaining **20%** of the diet should consist of protein, which is vital for muscle and organ repair, hormone and enzyme production, immune function, and overall body maintenance.
    This balanced macro-nutrient ratio supports long-term health.

Sample _Insulin Resistance (Pancreatic Body Type)_ Diet Chart –

TIME	MEALS
Breakfast 9:00 a.m	_**Spanish Omelette**_ (3 Eggs + equal amounts of all varieties of Vegetables + 2 tsp. Ghee) + 1 glass Milk **(OR)** Orange / Pomegranate / Pineapple / Guava juice.
Snack 11:00 a.m	Milk Coffee / Tea without sugar. Half teaspoon Ghee or Butter can be added. + 20 Nuts (unsalted) or 50g Coconut pieces.
Lunch 1:00 p.m	1 bowl steamed Vegetables + Pulses + Legumes + Sprouts. + 100g steamed Chicken / Fish / Meat / Paneer **(Do Not Deep-Fry)** + 1 small cup Curd or Buttermilk (70 ml)
Snack 4:00 p.m	Milk Coffee / Tea without sugar. Half teaspoon Ghee or Butter can be added. + 10 Nuts (unsalted) or 50g Coconut pieces + 4 Dates
Dinner 7:00 p.m	1 bowl steamed Vegetables + Pulses + Legumes + Sprouts. + 100g steamed Chicken / Fish / Meat / Paneer **(Do Not Deep-Fry)** + 1 small cup Curd or Buttermilk (70 ml)

Total Average Caloric Count of Diet Plan – **1700 kcal.**

Pancreatic Body Type

Sample _Ovarian Body Type_ Diet Chart –

TIME	MEALS
Breakfast 9:00 a.m	*Mushroom Scrambles* (3 Eggs scrambled in 2 tsp. Ghee or Olive-oil with sautéed Mushrooms, Onions and Tomatoes) + 1 cup Green Tea **(OR)** Cinnamon-infused Tea (without sugar).
Snack 11:00 a.m	12 raw Peanuts / Almonds / Walnuts (unsalted) + 1 small orange.
Lunch 1:00 p.m	Plantain-leaf wrapped grilled Fish (150g) or grilled Chicken (100g). + Large bowl raw salad with mixed greens – Cabbage, Spinach, Lettuce, Cucumber, Tomato, Avocado, with Olive-oil, and *Apple Cider Vinegar* dressing.
Snack 4:00 p.m	1 Avocado / 2 boiled Eggs for additional healthy fats
Dinner 7:00 p.m	1 bowl Chia-seed and Yoghurt mix with Pomegranate garnish. + Grilled Fish / Chicken / Mutton or Beef (50g) in Olive-oil or Coconut-oil.

Total Average Caloric Count of Diet Plan – 1600 kcal.

Ovarian Body Type

Sample *Thyroid Body Type* Diet Chart –

TIME	MEALS
Snack 8:00 a.m	1 small handful (10 to 12) of raw Cashews / Almonds / Walnuts (unsalted) + 1 glass Goose-berry juice (3 large Goose-berries deseeded, and combined in a blender with enough water. Add 1 tbsp. soaked Chia-seeds and 2 tsp. Honey).
Breakfast 10:00 a.m	*Cheesy Fresco* (3 Eggs cooked in 1 tsp. Ghee or Coconut oil with sautéed Spinach, Onions, and Tomatoes, topped with 3 slices of Cheese) + 1 cup Green Tea **(OR)** Cinnamon-infused Tea (unsweetened).
Snack 1:00 p.m	1 boiled Egg with 1 Carrot
Snack 2:30 p.m	1 small cup of Greek Yoghurt (unsweetened) with a tablespoon of Chia-seeds or powdered Flax-seeds + 1 small orange.
Snack 4:30 p.m	1 small bowl of steamed Chick-peas with sautéed Vegetables.
Dinner 07:00 p.m	1 small bowl of steamed Vegetables + Plantain-leaf wrapped grilled Fish or grilled Mutton or grilled Chicken (100g) with sautéed Brinjal or Ladies-finger in Olive-oil or Coconut-oil. **(OR)** Fish / Beef / Mutton / Chicken (100g) gravy with Brinjal or Cauliflower in Olive-oil or Coconut-oil.

Total Average Caloric Count of Diet Plan – 1800 kcal.

Sample *Adrenal Body Type* Diet Chart –

TIME	MEALS
Breakfast 9:00 a.m	*Nira Omelette* (3 Eggs + sautéed Spinach, Onions, Brinjal, Tomato and Capsicum in 2 tsp. Ghee or Coconut-oil) + 1/4 Avocado for healthy fats. + 1 cup Herbal Tea (with Cinnamon and Tulsi leaves with no sugar)
Snack 11:00 a.m	1 small handful of unsalted mixed Nuts (Almonds, Pistachios, Cashews, Peanuts, Walnuts). + Green Tea **(OR)** 1 cup of unsweetened *Tender Coconut Water*
Lunch 1:00 p.m	Sautéed Brinjal or Cauliflower gravy in Olive-oil or Coconut-oil. + 1 bowl Chia-seed and Yoghurt mix with Pomegranate garnish
Snack 4:00 p.m	1 glass *Lemon Honey Water* (1 small Lemon + 2 teaspoon Honey) **(OR)** 1 glass Pineapple juice (unsweetened)
Dinner 7:00 p.m	Plantain-leaf wrapped grilled Fish (150g) or grilled Chicken (100g). + Large bowl raw salad with mixed greens – Cabbage, Spinach, Lettuce, Cucumber, Tomato, Avocado, with Olive-oil, and *Apple Cider Vinegar* dressing.

Total Average Caloric Count of Diet Plan – **1500 kcal.**

Sample _Liver Body Type_ Diet Chart –

TIME	MEALS
Breakfast 9:00 a.m	*Turkish One-sides* (3 Eggs poached in soupy mix of cooked Onions and Tomatoes in 2 tsp. Ghee or Olive-oil, with sautéed Spinach). + 1 cup Green Tea **(OR)** Cinnamon-infused Tea (no sugar)
Snack 11:00 a.m	10 Almonds or Walnuts (unsalted) + 1 Cucumber or Carrot.
Lunch 1:00 p.m	Plantain-leaf wrapped grilled Fish (150g) or grilled Chicken (100g). + Large bowl raw salad with mixed greens – Cabbage, Spinach, Lettuce, Cucumber, Tomato, Avocado, with Olive-oil, and *Apple Cider Vinegar* dressing.
Snack 4:00 p.m	1 small cup of Greek Yoghurt (unsweetened) with a tablespoon Chia-seeds or Flax-seeds. + 1 small Pomegranate.
Dinner 7:00 p.m	Fish or Beef or Mutton or Chicken (100g) grilled or gravy, with sautéed Vegetables in Olive-oil or Coconut-oil + 1 glass *Lemon Honey Water* (1 small Lemon + 2 teaspoon Honey)

Total Average Caloric Count of Diet Plan – 1600 kcal.

Liver Body Type

Chapter XXVI – Sample Healthy Recipes.

"Our Creativity is Only Limited By Our Imagination."

And in the case of cooking and recipes, no other statement stands more true. I say this because the majority of the population are under the impression that food must have specific recipes to taste perfect.

Personally I find this not true.

Recipes are only a guiding structure, for us to improvise and experiment with food.

This feeling of restriction, is one of the main reasons, why people are not willing to get into eating healthy. The most common question I face when I tell my patients to avoid all kinds of grains including millets -

"Then what else are we supposed to eat?"

It is distressing for people to avoid grains because it is the staple food world-wide. But if you are ready to look beyond grains for a moment, you will find that there are six other major food groups, and countless other foods in these groups, from which we can choose, to cook healthy and tasty food.

The same can be said for each recipe mentioned here, and the thousand others available in the world. Do not let yourself be limited by the ingredients, as they can all be substituted by any other healthy ingredient, belonging in the same food group.
For example, if the recipe calls for pumpkin and chickpeas, we can substitute pumpkin with zucchini or ash-gourd, and substitute chickpeas for any other kind of lentils or pulses.

Even the ratio for each ingredient are customizable, and as long as all the ingredients are ones which are mentioned as allowed, in the general instructions, from the previous chapter, you can feel free to explore and enjoy the world of cooking.

Even if the recipe is a vegetarian one, you can easily make it into a non-vegetarian recipe, simply by adding eggs, or any type of meat, that you prefer.

One other reason that eating healthy is a scary experience for some, is because of the false notion, that spices should be avoided as well.

As we all know, a food is given flavour and aroma through different spices and *masala*, without which, the food may seem bland to the taste buds. But spices **need not** be avoided.

Spices actually possess anti-inflammatory, anti-oxidant, anti-microbial properties, and helps in digestion as well, among many other health benefits.

Just as important as the other reasons, yet another main cause for people being reluctant to get into healthy eating, is because of the familiarity with how a dish is perceived.

For example, Indians, love a good '*sambar*.'
And in our subconscious minds, we can only use sambar as an accessory to either rice, idli, dosa, or with any other staple.

But if you are ready to look at this dish through a different perspective, sambar can be the main dish. It can be poured into a bowl, and be consumed with a spoon just like we would, for a bowl of soup.

So getting out of your comfort zone, and letting go of a few familiarities, may be needed to bring about healthy changes in our diet.

Let's explore a few simple, healthy recipes that can kick-start your journey toward mindful eating, whether you're someone who's facing health challenges or not.

Natural Health Drinks

- *Hot Beverages*
  1. Apple Tea.. 389
  2. Herbal Blend... 390
  3. Orange Peel Tea.. 391
  4. Lemon Grass Tea... 392
  5. Sweet Ginger Cup.. 393

- *Milkshakes*
  1. Smoothie Bowl.. 394
  2. Raw Coconut Milkshake....................................... 395
  3. Peanut Butter Banana Milkshake........................... 396

- *Mix Juices*
  1. ABC Juice.. 397
  2. Celery, Apple, Ginger Juice................................... 398
  3. Carrot, Celery and Tomato Juice............................ 399

Healthy Chutneys / Dips

1. Lemon Chutney... 400
2. Peanut Chutney... 401
3. Beetroot Chutney.. 402
4. Healthy Mayonnaise... 403
5. Mint-Coconut Chutney... 404
6. Sesame Chickpea Humus....................................... 405

Healthy Salad Meals

1. Egg Salad... 406
2. Paneer Salad... 407
3. Sprouts Salad... 408
4. Sautéed Vegetable Salad.. 409
5. Chickpea-Avocado Salad....................................... 410

Healthy Soupy Meals

1. Carrot Butter Cashew Soup.................................... 411
2. Spinach Mushroom Soup....................................... 412
3. Traditional Herbal Rasam...................................... 413
4. Instant Bone Broth... 414
5. Steamed Vegetables in Coconut Milk....................... 415

Healthy Sandwiches

1. Grilled Cheese Sandwich....................................... 416
2. Cuban Roast Sandwich... 417
3. Lettuce Wrap Sandwich.. 418
4. Pro-Steak Sandwich... 419
5. Layered Top Sandwich... 420

Healthy Fillers

1. Sprouts Dosa.. 421
2. Millet Upma... 422
3. Meat Loaf.. 423
4. Millet Idli & Dosa.. 425
5. Keto Curd Rice... 427

Natural Health Drinks

Hot Beverages

1. *Apple Tea.*

Total Average Calories: 75 kcal per serving.
Preparation Time: 5 minutes.
Cooking Time: 10 minutes.
Servings: 4 persons.

Ingredients-

- 3 tbsp honey.
- 2 mint leaves.
- 1 tsp cinnamon.
- 2 green tea bags.
- $1/2$ tbsp lemon juice.
- 1 cup grated apples.

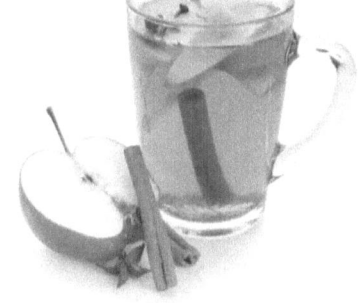

Preparation-

- Heat 4 cups of water in a pan, bring up to boil.
- Add the apples, cinnamon powder and lemon juice.
- Mix well and cook on a medium flame for 2 minutes.
- Keep stirring occasionally.
- Add green tea and mint leaves.
- Allow it to rest for 15 minutes.
- Strain the apple tea and serve immediately with honey.

2. *Herbal Blend*.

Total Average Calories: 200 kcal.
Preparation Time: 5 minutes.
Cooking Time: 10 minutes.
Servings: 1 person.

Ingredients for the powder-

- 1 cup coriander seeds.
- ½ cup cumin seeds.
- ¼ cup fennel seeds.
- ¼ cup fenugreek seeds.
- ¼ cup dry ginger powder.
- 1 tbsp black pepper (can be used when you have cough, cold or sore throat).

Dry roast all the ingredients in low flame till fragrant. Let it cool completely and grind into a powder. Store in an airtight container.

Ingredients for the blend-

- 2 to 4 tbsp coconut milk (optional).
- 1 tbsp jaggery.
- 1 tsp Herbal powder.

Preparation-

- Boil 1 cup water with 1 tsp herbal powder and 1 tbsp jaggery for 2 mins. Allow it to cool a bit and add 2 to 4 tbsp coconut milk and turn off the heat. Strain and enjoy the drink hot.

3. *Orange Peel Tea*.

Total Average Calories: 45 kcal per serving.
Preparation Time: 30 minutes.
Cooking Time: 30 minutes.
Servings: 2 persons.

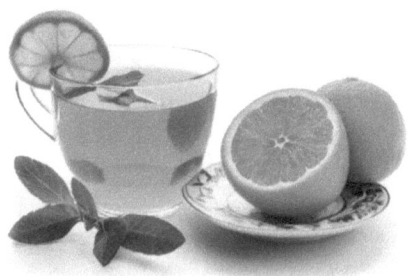

Ingredients-

- 2 dry citrus peel.
- Remove peel from the fruit.
- Cut the peel into small pieces and spread it on a cookie sheet.
- Place it in the oven on the lowest setting until the peels dry, but be careful not to let them burn.
- Store dry peels in a jar with a lid and use in teas.

Preparation-

- Add 2 cup water and peel from one orange to a pot.
- Put the lid on, bring water to a boil and turn off the heat.
- Let it steep for 30 minutes.
- Strain out the peel, re-heat and enjoy with 3 tsp honey

4. *Lemon Grass Tea.*

Total Average Calories: 25 kcal per serving.
Preparation Time: 5 minutes.
Cooking Time: 15 minutes.
Servings: 3 persons.

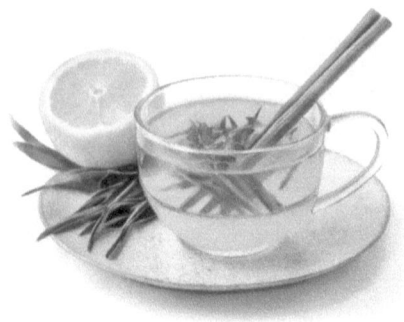

Ingredients-

- ½ cup lemon grass, finely chopped.
- ½ cup mint leaves (pudina), finely chopped.
- 1 tsp tea leaves (optional).
- Honey to taste.

Preparation-

- Combine lemon grass & mint leaves with 5 cups of water in a pan and bring it to a boil.
- Lower the flame and simmer till it reduces to about 3 cups.
- Remove from the flame, add the tea leaves, cover and allow it to infuse for a few minutes.
- Strain and serve hot, with 3 tsp. honey.

5. *Sweet Ginger Cup*.

Total Average Calories: 120 kcal.
Preparation Time: 5 minutes.
Cooking Time: 15 minutes.
Servings: 1 person.

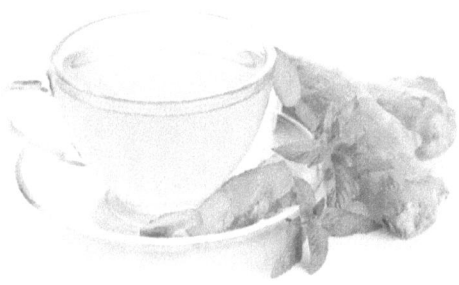

Ingredients-

- ½ cup tulsi (Indian basil) leaves.
- ¼ cup mint leaves (pudina).
- 1 tbsp roughly chopped ginger.
- 2 tbsp honey / jaggery.

Preparation-

- Combine the tulsi, mint and ginger and blend in a mixer to a coarse paste using very little water.
- Transfer the paste into a non-stick saucepan, add 1½ cups of water and mix well and boil for 5 to 7 minutes,
- Keep stirring occasionally.
- Strain the mixture using a strainer, add the honey and mix well. Serve immediately.

Milkshakes

1. *Smoothie Bowl*.

   Total Average Calories: 600 kcal.
   Preparation Time: 30 minutes.
   Cooking Time: 7 minutes.
   Servings: 1 person.

   Ingredients-

   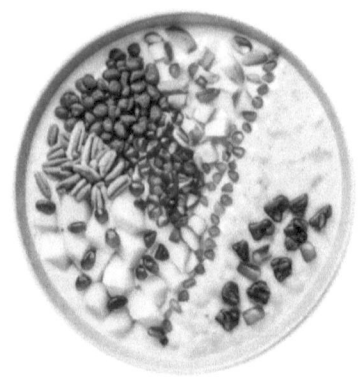

   - 2 tbsp basil seeds.
   - 1 cup coconut milk.
   - ½ of an apple.
   - 1 banana.
   - ½ cup pomegranate.
   - 5 cashew nuts.
   - 5 almonds.
   - 10 raisins.
   - 5 dried or fresh fig.
   - 5 dried or fresh apricots.

   Preparation-

   - Soak basil seeds for half an hour.
   - Chop up all the other ingredients, into small cubes.
   - In a mixing bowl, add coconut milk, other chopped ingredients with pomegranate and mix well.
   - Add 3 tbsp honey for taste.

2. _Raw Coconut Milk-shake._

Total Average Calories: 500 kcal.
Preparation Time: 5 minutes.
Cooking Time: 5 minutes.
Servings: 1 person.

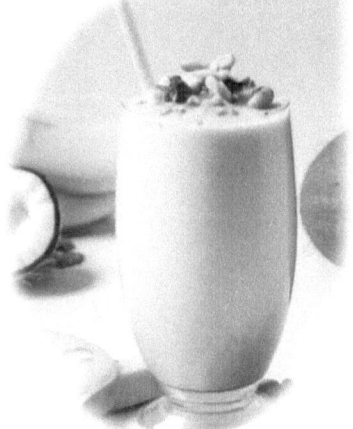

Ingredients-

- 1 glass coconut milk.
- 1 banana.
- ½ tsp cardamom powder.
- 5 chopped cashew nuts.
- 5 chopped almonds.
- 5 raisins.
- 15 gm ghee.

Preparation-

- Blend coconut milk, banana and cardamom powder.
- Heat ghee and sauté cashew nuts, almonds and raisins and add to the blended coconut milk.

3. *Peanut Butter Banana Milk-shake.*

Total Average Calories: 400 kcal.
Preparation Time: 5 minutes.
Cooking Time: 5 minutes.
Servings: 1 person.

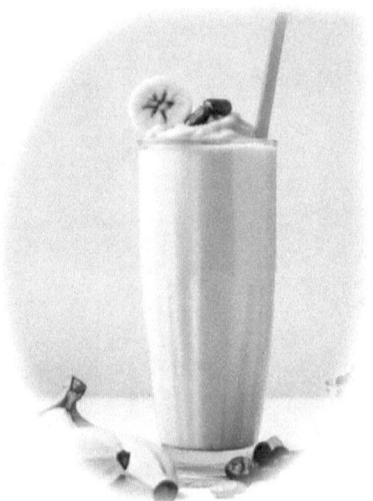

Ingredients-

- ½ glass milk.
- Two medium size banana.
- 2 tsp peanut butter.
- 5 chopped cashew nuts.
- 5 chopped almonds.

Preparation-

- Blend peanut butter, banana and milk.
- Garnish with cashew nuts and almonds.

Mix Juices

1. *Amla, Beetroot, Coconut-* ABC *Juice*.

Total Average Calories: 125 kcal per serving.
Preparation Time: 15 minutes.
Cooking Time: 5 minutes.
Servings: 2 persons.

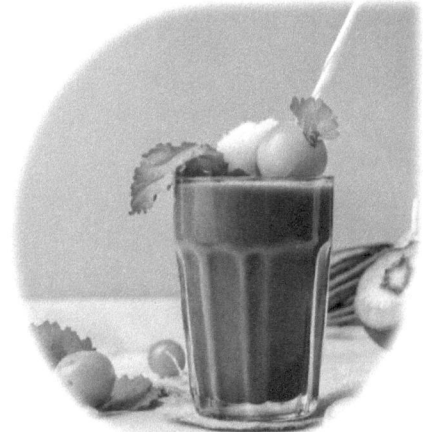

Ingredients-

- 1 large beetroot.
- 4 gooseberries (amla).
- 1 whole coconut and its water.

Preparation-

- Remove the seed from the gooseberries.
- Peel and dice the beetroot.
- Break the coconut and set and aside its water.
- Grate or cut the pieces from the coconut shell.
- Blend the ingredients along with the coconut water.
- Strain and separate the solids (optional).
- Transfer to a large jug and stir to combine.
- Serve with ice and honey.

2. *Celery, Apple, Ginger Juice*.

Total Average Calories: 50 kcal per serving.
Preparation Time: 5 minutes.
Cooking Time: 5 minutes.
Servings: 4 persons.

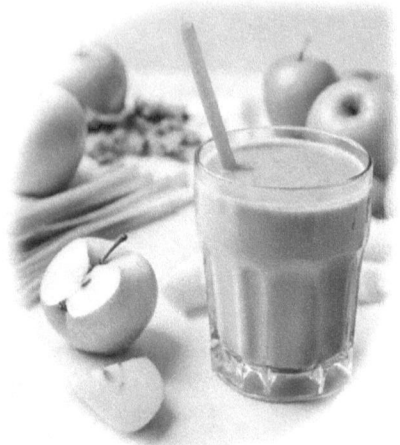

Ingredients-

- 6 sticks celery trimmed.
- 6 green apples.
- 5 cm piece fresh ginger.

Preparation-

- Trim the celery sticks.
- Cut each apple into 8 wedges.
- Peel and slice or crush the piece of ginger.
- Blend the celery, apples and ginger.
- Strain and separate the solids.
- Transfer to a large jug and stir to combine.
- Serve immediately, with ice and honey.

3. *Carrot, Celery and Tomato Juice.*

Total Average Calories: 37 kcal per serving.
Preparation Time: 5 minutes.
Cooking Time: 5 minutes.
Servings: 4 persons.

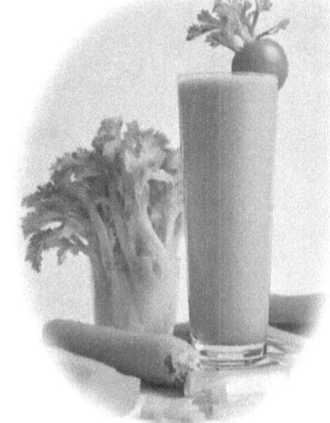

Ingredients-

- 1 cucumber.
- 5 stalks celery.
- 2 tomatoes.
- 3 medium sized carrots
- ½ the lemon peeled.
- Handful of parsley.

Preparation-

- Peel and dice the carrots.
- Dice the cucumber.
- Trim the celery sticks.
- Dice the tomatoes.
- Blend the ingredients.
- Strain and separate the solids (optional).
- Transfer to a large jug and stir to combine.
- Serve immediately, with ice and lemon squeezed.

Healthy Chutneys & Sauces

1. *Lemon Chutney.*

Total Average Calories: 150 kcal.
Preparation Time: 10 minutes.
Cooking Time: 7 minutes.
Servings: 1 person.

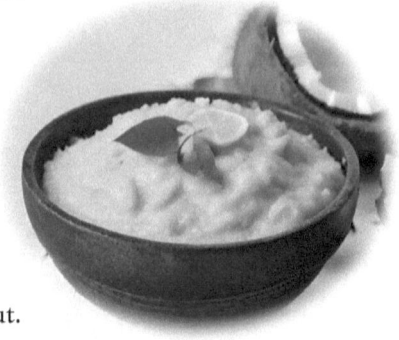

Ingredients-

- ½ cup grated coconut.
- 2 tbsp coriander leaves.
- Finger length piece of ginger.
- 1 pod of garlic.
- Juice of 1 lemon.
- Zest of 1 lemon.
- Salt as per taste.

Preparation-

- Heat oil in a small pan and sauté the garlic and ginger, with pinch of mustard seeds, cumin, and zest of one lemon.
- Remove this mixture from the pan and add it to a chutney grinder or blender, along with the rest of the ingredients.
- Add about ¼ or ½ cup water and grind to a smooth paste.
- Squeeze the lime juice in the blend.
- Add salt to taste, stir well and serve.

2. *Peanut-Tomato Chutney*.

Total Average Calories: 150 kcal per serving.
Preparation Time: 5 minutes.
Cooking Time: 15 minutes.
Servings: 2 persons.

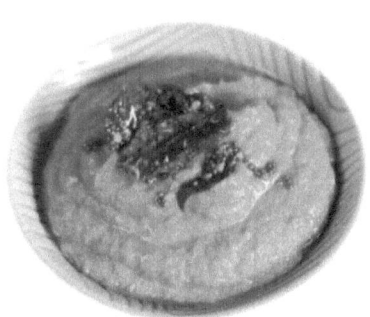

Ingredients-

- ¼ cup peanuts.
- 2 small onions.
- 1 green chili.
- ¼ inch ginger.
- 12 to 15 curry leaves.
- 2 tomatoes.
- ¼ cup roasted split chickpeas (channa dal).
- Half of a handful coriander leaves.
- Salt as required.

Preparation-

- Roast the peanuts on a medium flame for 5 minutes.
- Add the roasted channa dal, asafoetida and fry for 3 minutes on a low flame.
- Roast the tomatoes on a high flame for 5 minutes and stir
- Add in all the ingredients, in a chutney grinder or a small blender.
- Pour some water and grind the chutney to a smooth consistency.
- You can make the chutney thick or of medium consistency.
- Check the salt and add more if required.

3. *Beetroot Chutney*.

Total Average Calories: 150 kcal.
Preparation Time: 5 minutes.
Cooking Time: 10 minutes.
Servings: 1 person.

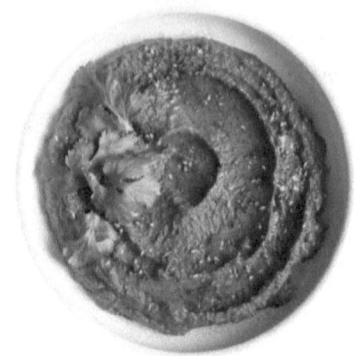

Ingredients-

- ½ cup beetroot gratings.
- ¾ cup of coconut gratings.
- One small chilli, finely chopped.
- 2 shallots.
- 1 tsp lemon juice.
- Curry leaves, one string.
- 2 tsp coriander leaves.
- Pinch of salt.

Preparation-

- Sauté the chili, shallots and curry leaves on a medium flame for 5 minutes.
- Add all the ingredients in a chutney grinder or a small blender.
- Pour some water and grind the chutney to a smooth consistency.
- You can make the beetroot chutney thick or of medium consistency.
- Check the salt and add more if required.

4. *Healthy Mayonnaise*.

Total Average Calories: 150 kcal per serving.
Preparation Time: 5 minutes.
Cooking Time: 10 minutes.
Servings: 2 persons.

Ingredients-

- 2 large boiled eggs.
- 3 cloves of garlic.
- Chilli flakes.
- 1 tbsp lemon juice or white vinegar.
- 1 tbsp olive oil or coconut oil.
- Salt and pepper to taste.

Preparation-

- In a blender, combine eggs, garlic, lemon juice or vinegar.
- Blend on medium speed for few seconds until well mixed.
- With the blender running on low speed, add the oil and chilli flakes.
- Keep blending until mayonnaise thicken and become smooth.
- If the mayonnaise is too thick, add a teaspoon of water to adjust the consistency.
- Taste and add salt and pepper as needed. You can also add a little more lemon juice or vinegar to adjust the tanginess.
- The healthy mayonnaise is ready to serve.

5. *Mint-Coconut Chutney*.

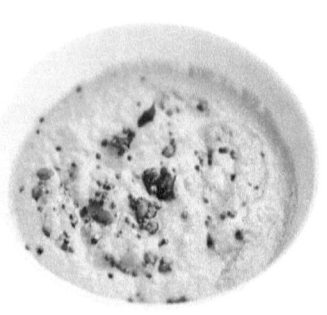

Total Average Calories: 200 kcal.
Preparation Time: 5 minutes.
Cooking Time: 10 minutes.
Servings: 1 person.

Ingredients-

- ¼ cup mint leaves.
- ½ cup grated coconut, fresh or frozen.
- 1 tbsp roasted channa / bengal gram.
- ½ inch ginger, roughly chopped.
- 10 curry leaves.
- 1 or 2 green chilies, chopped.
- 1 tbsp oil.

For tempering-

- ½ or ¾ tsp mustard seeds.
- 10 curry leaves.
- a pinch of asafoetida.

Preparation-

- Heat oil in a small pan .Fry the mint leaves, curry leaves and ginger till the mint and curry leaves become crisp.
- Remove this mixture from the pan and let it cool.
- In a chutney grinder or blender, add rest of the ingredients along with the fried mint leaves, curry leaves and ginger.
- Add about ¼ or ½ cup water and grind to a smooth paste.
- In the same pan, add oil if required.
- Stir well and serve.

6. *Sesame - Chickpea Humus*.

Total Average Calories: 250 kcal per serving.
Preparation Time: 5 minutes.
Cooking Time: 20 minutes.
Servings: 2 persons.

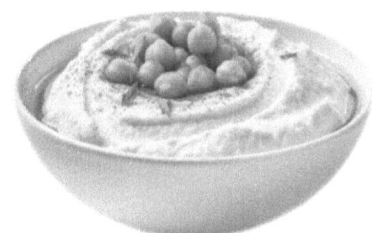

Ingredients-

- 5 tbsp sesame seeds.
- 1 bowl chickpeas, big chana.
- 2 tsp olive oil.
- 1 pod of garlic.
- 2 tsp lemon juice.
- Pinch of salt.

Preparation-

- Boil and drain chickpeas in a strainer, reserving the liquid.
- Dry roast sesame seeds for around 3 mins. constantly stirring.
- Blend sesame seeds, big chana, olive oil, garlic, lemon juice and pinch of salt and pepper.
- Blend until smooth past like consistency.
- Taste and adjust seasonings. Taste and add more of any of the ingredients to taste. If your hummus is thicker than you'd like, blend 2 to 3 tablespoons of the reserved chickpea liquid to thin it out and make the hummus creamier.
- Garnish with a few chickpeas and a generous drizzle of extra virgin olive oil.

Healthy Salad Meals

The following recipes are called "Salad Meals" because they have the potential in itself to be a one-time meal, without the hassle of having to cook more than one dish, in order to bring a complete meal to the table. But of-course other elements can be included, to enhance the experience and joy of consuming healthy meals.

1. *Egg Salad*.

    Total Average Calories: 350 kcal.
    Preparation Time: 20 minutes.
    Mixing Time: 5 minutes.
    Servings: 1 person.

    Ingredients-

    - 1 bunch spinach.
    - 3 boiled eggs.
    - 2 tomatoes.

    Dressings-

    - Tahini / sesame seed sauce.
    - Lemon juice.
    - Salt and pepper.

    Preparation-

    - Cut the boiled eggs and tomato into slices or dices
    - Add the spinach leaves and mix well.
    - Sprinkle salt and pepper.
    - Squeeze half of a lemons juice
    - Pour around 3-5 tbsp tahini sauce on top and serve.

2. *Paneer Salad*.

Total Average Calories: 225 kcal per serving.
Preparation Time: 15 minutes.
Mixing Time: 5 minutes.
Servings: 2 persons.

Ingredients-

- 100 gm cubed paneer.
- 25 gm butter.
- 2 tsp roasted watermelon seeds.
- 1 tsp lemon juice.
- 2 tsp virgin coconut oil / olive oil.
- One small size onion, finely chopped.
- ½ small size red bell pepper, finely chopped.
- ½ small size red kraut (cabbage), finely chopped.
- ½ medium size cucumber, finely chopped.
- Pinch of salt and pepper.

Preparation-

- Heat butter in a pan. Add paneer cubes and stir fry on high heat till it becomes brown, and keep it aside.
- In a mixing bowl, add chopped cucumber, red bell pepper, onion, red kraut and 2 tsp of virgin coconut oil / olive oil.
- Add the paneer and toss the salad.
- Squeeze 1 tsp lemon juice. Add pinch of salt and pepper
- Garnish with 2 tsp roasted watermelon seeds.

To turn the recipe into a non-veg meal-

Select a non-veg source like eggs, chicken, beef, mutton, seafood, or any meat of your choice. Season the chosen protein with spices, herbs, marinades, or sauces that align with the flavours of the vegetarian dish.
Ensure that the meat cooks thoroughly.
Adjust the seasoning and flavours of the dish to accommodate the addition of meat. Consider the impact of the meat's flavours on the overall taste of the dish and make any necessary adjustments to ensure a harmonious balance.
Garnish and Serve.

3. *Sprouts Salad*.

Total Average Calories: 100 kcal per serving.
Preparation Time: 12 hours.
Mixing Time: 5 minutes.
Servings: 2 persons.

Ingredients-
- One cup of sprouts.
- One medium size grated carrot.
- One small size finely chopped onion.
- One small size finely chopped tomato.
- 2 stalks coriander, finely chopped.
- ½ of a medium sized cucumber, finely chopped
- 1 tsp lemon juice.
- 2 tsp virgin coconut oil / olive oil.
- Pinch of salt and pepper powder.

How to make Sprouts-
- Choose the type of sprouts you want to make.
- Soak the seeds or grains in boiled water for about 12 hours.
- Drain the water and transfer seeds or grains to a clean cloth and tie it in a tight knot.
- Keep it in a dark place, till it sprouts.

Preparation-
- In a mixing bowl, add sprouts, finely chopped cucumber, onion and tomato, grated carrot and 2 tsp of virgin olive oil or cold-pressed coconut oil.
- Squeeze 1 tsp lemon juice and add pinch of salt and pepper powder. Mix all ingredients. Garnish with coriander leaves.

To turn the recipe into a non-veg meal – *Kindly refer the instructions under the same heading, in the **previous** recipe.*

4. _Sautéed Vegetables Salad_.

Total Average Calories: 500 kcal.
Preparation Time: 10 minutes.
Cooking Time: 15 minutes.
Servings: 1 person.

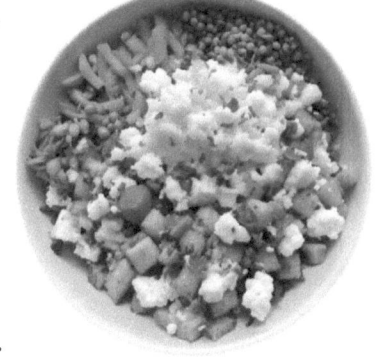

Ingredients-

- 1 bowl green peas.
- 1 onion, finely chopped.
- 50 gm diced paneer.
- 1 tomato, finely chopped.
- 1 carrot, finely chopped.
- 2 beans, finely chopped.
- Half of a coconut grated.
- 1 bunch coriander leaves.
- 2 tsp virgin coconut oil.
- 3 tsp ghee.
- Salt and pepper powder.

Preparation-

- Boil green peas and keep aside.
- Sauté chopped onion, carrot, beans, tomato and peas, in ghee.
- Add coconut oil and sauté coconut gratings and paneer.
- Add salt and pepper powder.
- Garnish with coriander leaves.

To turn the recipe into a non-veg meal-

Select a non-veg source like eggs, chicken, beef, mutton, seafood, or any meat of your choice. Season the chosen protein with spices, herbs, marinades, or sauces that align with the flavours of the vegetarian dish.
Ensure that the meat cooks thoroughly.
Adjust the seasoning and flavours of the dish to accommodate the addition of meat. Consider the impact of the meat's flavours on the overall taste of the dish and make any necessary adjustments to ensure a harmonious balance.
Garnish and Serve.

5. *Chickpea - Avocado Salad*.

Total Average Calories: 133 kcal per serving.
Preparation Time: 15 minutes.
Mixing Time: 10 minutes.
Servings: 3 persons.

Ingredients-
- 1 sliced avocado.
- $1/2$ finely chopped carrot.
- 1 cup (soaked and boiled) chickpea.
- 1 cup finely chopped cucumber.

For yogurt dressing-
- $3/4$ cup curd.
- 1 unseeded green chili.
- 2 stems coriander leaves finely chopped.
- Salt as required.

Preparation-
- Soak the chick peas in enough water and leave it for overnight. Next day morning just strain the water and wash twice in running water. And pressure cook the chick pea by adding the enough salt. Leave for 3 to 4 whistles. Again once cooked strain the water and transfer the chick pea to the bowl. Then add the carrot, cucumber and adjust salt.
- Take other bowl, add the curd and whisk it nicely so that it won't form any lumps, then add the required amount of salt and green chilli along with chopped coriander leaves. Mix well and transfer this yogurt mixture to the chick pea mixture. Mix well!

To turn the recipe into a non-veg meal – *Kindly refer the instructions under the same heading, in the **previous** recipe.*

Healthy Soupy Meals

The following recipes are called "Soupy Meals" because they have the potential in itself to be a one-time meal, without the hassle of having to cook more than one dish, in order to bring a complete meal to the table. But of-course other elements can be included, and enhance the experience of consuming healthy meals.

1. *Carrot Butter Cashew Soup*.

    Total Average Calories: 175 kcal per serving.
    Preparation Time: 7 minutes.
    Cooking Time: 20 minutes.
    Servings: 2 persons.

    Ingredients-

    - 20 cashews.
    - 50 gm butter.
    - 1 onion chopped.
    - Half a bunch coriander leaf.
    - 3 medium sized carrots diced.
    - Salt and pepper.

    Preparation-

    - Sauté cashews, carrots and onion in butter, until browned.
    - Add coriander leaves and boil in pressure cooker with $1\frac{1}{2}$ cups of water.
    - Switch off the heat after 1 whistle.
    - Mix the content in a blender.
    - Add salt and pepper to taste and serve.

    To turn the recipe into a non-veg meal – *Kindly refer the instructions under the same heading, in the* **next** *recipe.*

2. *Spinach Mushroom Soup*.

Total Average Calories: 400 kcal.
Preparation Time: 5 minutes.
Cooking Time: 20 minutes.
Servings: 1 person.

Ingredients-

- 5 leaves of spinach.
- 5 mushrooms, finely chopped.
- 1 onion, finely chopped.
- ½ tsp fennel seeds.
- 50 gm mashed paneer.
- 25 gm butter.
- 20 ml fresh cream.
- Salt and pepper powder.

Preparation-

- Boil spinach with pinch of salt and blend after half cooled.
- Heat butter and sauté the onion for 5 minutes.
- Sauté fennel seeds, chopped mushroom, mashed paneer.
- Add the blended spinach and fresh cream, and let it simmer.
- Garnish with salt and pepper powder.

To turn the recipe into a non-veg meal-

Select a non-veg source like eggs, chicken, beef, mutton, seafood, or any meat of your choice. Season the chosen protein with spices, herbs, marinades, or sauces that align with the flavours of the vegetarian dish.
Ensure that the meat cooks thoroughly.
Adjust the seasoning and flavours of the dish to accommodate the addition of meat. Consider the impact of the meat's flavours on the overall taste of the dish and make any necessary adjustments to ensure a harmonious balance.
Garnish and Serve.

3. *Traditional Herbal "Rasam."*

Total Average Calories: 125 kcal per serving.
Preparation Time: 7 minutes.
Cooking Time: 20 minutes.
Servings: 2 persons.

Ingredients-
- 2 large tomatoes.
- ½ cup split grain.
- ½ tsp black gram.
- 2 tsp cumin seeds.
- 1 tbs chickpeas.
- ½ tsp asafoetida.
- 2 tsp coriander seeds.
- 4 pieces of long pepper (tippali).
- 2 strings of curry leaves and 1 green chilli.
- 1 tbs coconut oil, 1 tsp turmeric, 1 tbs ginger garlic paste.
- 1 tsp mustard seeds, 1 bunch coriander leaves, salt to taste.

Preparation-
- Pressure cook chickpeas with ¼ tsp turmeric and keep aside.
- Sauté chickpeas, coriander seeds, ½ tsp cumin seeds, black pepper, and tippali.
- Remove from flame and grind it with ½ tsp fresh cumin seeds, a string of curry leaves, ginger garlic paste and water to a cake batter consistency.
- Boil tomatoes in 3 cups of water, for 5 mins, with asafoetida.
- Add salt and the ground paste to the boiling water and let it froth for 5 mins. Let it boil for 5-10 mins. Rasam is ready.
- Sauté mustard and the remaining 1 tsp of cumin seeds in oil and drop into the boiling Rasam. Let it simmer for a minute and remove from flame. Garnish with chopped coriander leaves and a string of curry leaves and serve.

To turn the recipe into a non-veg meal – *Kindly refer the instructions under the same heading, in the **previous** recipe.*

4. *Instant Bone Broth*.

Total Average Calories: 140 kcal per serving.
Preparation Time: 10 minutes.
Cooking Time: 1 hour.
Servings: 4 to 6 persons.

Ingredients-

- 1 onion, quartered.
- 4 cloves garlic, smashed.
- 2 tbsp apple cider vinegar.
- 2 carrots, roughly chopped.
- 2 celery stalks, roughly chopped.
- 1 kg mutton, beef or chicken bones (preferably with some meat left on them).
- 1 bay leaf, 1 tsp whole black pepper.
- 1 to 2 sprigs fresh thyme or rosemary (optional).
- 3 to 4 litres of water (enough to cover the bones).
- Salt to taste.

Preparation-

- In a large pressure cooker, add the roasted bones, chopped vegetables, smashed garlic, apple cider vinegar, bay leaf, peppercorns, thyme, and enough water to cover everything.
- Bring the mixture to a boil, then reduce the heat to low, skimming off any foam or impurities that rise to the surface.
- Cover and simmer on medium for 1 hour or 4 to 5 whistles (if opting for pot cooking, let it cook on low flame for 4 to 6 hours or longer if using a slow cooker, stirring occasionally).
- Once the broth is ready, strain out the solids such as bones and vegetables (optional) and return the liquid to the pot.
- Season with salt to taste. Add additional herbs if you like.

Serve the broth hot as a soup or use it in other recipes. You can also customise the soup according to your preference with increased meat or vegetables etc. Enjoy the nourishing collagen rich bone broth!

5. *Steamed Vegetables in Coconut Milk*.

Total Average Calories: 175 kcal per serving.
Preparation Time: 7 minutes.
Cooking Time: 20 minutes.
Servings: 2 persons.

Ingredients-

- 25 gm of ghee.
- 1 cup coconut milk.
- 25 gm of potato, finely chopped.
- 50 gm of cauliflower, finely chopped.
- 50 gm of broccoli, finely chopped.
- Salt and pepper powder.

Preparation-

- Pressure cook the vegetables with salt for 2 whistles.
- Heat ghee in a pan, sauté cauliflower, broccoli and potato for 5 to 10 minutes.
- Add coconut milk and boil for a few minutes on low flame.
- Add salt and pepper powder and mix well.
- Garnish with coriander leaves.

To turn the recipe into a non-veg meal-

Select a non-veg source like eggs, chicken, beef, mutton, seafood, or any meat of your choice. Season the chosen protein with spices, herbs, marinades, or sauces that align with the flavours of the vegetarian dish. Ensure that the meat cooks thoroughly.
Adjust the seasoning and flavours of the dish to accommodate the addition of meat. Consider the impact of the meat's flavours on the overall taste of the dish and make any necessary adjustments to ensure a harmonious balance. Garnish and Serve.

Healthy Sandwiches

1. *Grilled Cheese Sandwich*.

    Total Average Calories: 550 kcal.
    Preparation Time: 5 minutes.
    Cooking Time: 10 minutes.
    Servings: 1 person.

    Ingredients-

    - 2 large eggs.
    - 1 tbsp whole milk.
    - 2 tbsp butter (for grilling).
    - 2 slices cheese (cheddar, mozzarella, or your choice).
    - Whole grain bread or sourdough bread.
    - 1 tbsp butter (for spreading on bread).
    - Salt and pepper powder.

    Preparation-

    - Crack the eggs into a bowl and whisk them until the yolks and whites are fully combined. Add a pinch of salt and pepper. If you like a fluffier texture, you can add a splash of milk or cream (about 1 tbsp).
    - Pour whisked eggs into a preheated skillet and spread evenly. Let the eggs cook undisturbed on medium-low heat. Flip it once it solidifies, and set aside the omelette once cooked.
    - Heat 1 tbsp butter in a skillet over medium heat. Spread butter on one side of bread slice, and place one slice of cheese between the bread slices, buttered side out.
    - Grill the sandwich in the skillet for 2-3 minutes on each side, until golden brown and the cheese is melted.
    - Place the omelette between the slices. Serve warm.

2. *Cuban Roast Sandwich*.

Total Average Calories: 700 kcal.
Preparation Time: 5 minutes.
Cooking Time: 10 minutes.
Servings: 1 person.

Ingredients-

- 2 large eggs.
- 1 slices of Swiss cheese.
- 1 tbsp healthy mayonnaise.
- Whole grain bread or sourdough bread.
- Half cup shredded cheese (mozzarella or cheddar).
- 4 slices roasted chicken (or any meat of your choice).
- 1 tbsp ghee or butter (for grilling).
- Salt and pepper to taste.

Preparation-

- In a bowl, whisk the eggs with shredded cheese, and season it with salt and pepper.
- Preheat an iron skillet. Pour the mixture into it, and close with a lid. Let it cook for about 5 minutes until golden and crispy. Remove the omelette and set aside.
- Heat ghee or butter in a pan over medium heat. Place one slice of bread in the pan, layer with roasted chicken, Swiss cheese, omelette, and mayonnaise.
- Top it with the second slice of bread and grill the sandwich for around 3 minutes on each side, pressing slightly to melt the cheese and crisp the slices of bread.
- Remove from heat, slice, and serve warm.

3. *Lettuce Wrap Sandwich*.

Total Average Calories: 500 kcal.
Preparation Time: 5 minutes.
Cooking Time: 20 minutes.
Servings: 1 person.

Ingredients-

- ¼ avocado, sliced.
- 1 tbsp healthy mayonnaise.
- 2 slices cheese of your choice.
- Whole grain chapati or sourdough rotis.
- 4 large butter lettuce or romaine leaves (or cabbage leaves).
- 2 slices meat (chicken, mutton, or any meat of your choice).
- Optional: Sliced tomatoes, pickles, or other veggies.
- Salt and pepper to taste.

Preparation-

- Wash and dry the lettuce leaves carefully, keeping them intact for wrapping.
- Lay the lettuce leaves flat on top of the roti, overlapping slightly if needed, to make a sturdy wrap.
- Spread a thin layer of mayonnaise or mustard on the leaves.
- Layer the cooked meat, cheese, and avocado slices on top of the lettuce leaves.
- Add optional veggies like tomatoes / pickles for extra flavour.
- Season with salt and pepper, then carefully fold the roti around the fillings like a wrap. Serve immediately, and enjoy your fresh and customizable lettuce wrap sandwich!

4. *Pro-Steak Sandwich*.

Total Average Calories: 550 kcal.
Preparation Time: 10 minutes.
Cooking Time: 20 minutes.
Servings: 1 person.

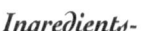

Ingredients-

- 2 large eggs.
- 1 tbsp ghee or butter (for grilling).
- Whole grain or sourdough bread.
- Half cup shredded cheese of your choice.
- 100 gm thinly sliced meat of your choice.
- ½ cup sauerkraut, drained.
- Salt and pepper to taste.

Preparation-

- Crack the eggs into a preheated skillet, add a pinch of salt and pepper and let it cook, closed with a lid, undisturbed on medium-low heat.
- Once the whites solidifies, and yolks are halfway cooked, set aside the *bulls-eye* egg (also called as *one-sides* or *half-boils*).
- Heat ghee or butter in a pan over medium heat and grill slices of bread. Layer the cooked meat, sauerkraut, and shredded cheese on one slice and place the second slice on top.
- Place the cooked egg on the top, or inside the sandwich, as you prefer.
- Let it cool slightly before slicing. Serve warm and enjoy.

5. *Layered Top Sandwich*.

Total Average Calories: 350 kcal per serving.
Preparation Time: 5 minutes.
Cooking Time: 10 minutes.
Servings: 2 persons.

Ingredients-

- 1 tbsp olive oil.
- 1 tbsp butter.
- Whole grain or sourdough bread.
- 200 gm thinly sliced steak or any meat of your choice.
- 1 medium onion, thinly sliced,
- 2 slices of a cheese of your choice.
- Salt and pepper to taste.

Preparation-

- Heat olive oil in a skillet over medium heat. Add the sliced onions and cook for around 4 minutes until caramelized.
- Remove from the pan and set aside.
- In the same skillet, melt butter and add the thinly sliced meat. Season with salt and pepper, and cook for around 4 minutes, stirring occasionally, until meat is cooked to your preference.
- Place cooked onions back into pan with steak and mix well.
- Warm the bread wraps in the pan for a few seconds.
- Lay one slice of cheese on each slice of bread, then add the meat and onion mixture on each slice. Add fresh tomatoes on one side and combine both the slices of bread. You can dress it with mayonnaise or add more toppings like lettuce, pickles or avocadoes, up to your preferences.
- Cut the sandwich through the center, and serve immediately.

Healthy Fillers

1. ## *Sprouts Dosa*.

   Total Average Calories: 250 kcal.
   Preparation Time: 12 hours.
   Cooking Time: 7 minutes.
   Servings: 1 person.

   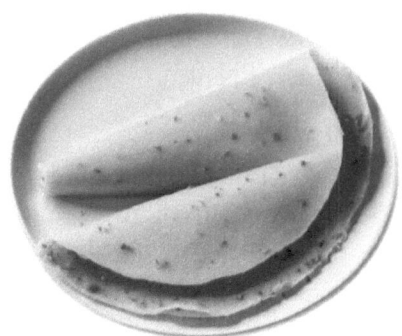

   ### *Ingredients-*
   - 1 cup sprouts.
   - 2 green chillies.
   - 2 cloves garlic.
   - ½ tsp cumin.
   - Ghee and oil for cooking as required.

   ### *For topping-*
   - 1 chopped onion.
   - Cumin seeds.

   ### *How to make Sprouts-*
   - Choose the type of sprouts you want to make.
   - Soak the seeds or grains in boiled water for about 12 hours.
   - Drain the water and transfer seeds or grains to a clean cloth and tie it in a tight knot.
   - Keep it in a dark place, till it sprouts.

   ### *Preparation-*
   - Add sprouts along with rest of the ingredients, and blend to an almost smooth batter. Let it rest for half an hour before making the dosas.
   - When ready to make the dosas, heat a tawa, pour a ladle full of batter, simmer and top with finely chopped onions along with cumin seeds. Flip on the other side and cook on low flame for the onions to get cooked well.
   - Sprinkle little oil and ghee. Serve with chutney, or gravies.

2. *Millet Upma.*

Total Average Calories: 300 kcal.
Preparation Time: 10 minutes.
Cooking Time: 15 minutes.
Servings: 1 person.

Ingredients-

- Groundnut oil.
- 1 potato chopped.
- 1 carrot chopped.
- 1 onion chopped.
- 1 tomato chopped.
- 15 gm green peas.
- 50 gm millets of your choice.
- 3 green chillies, ginger, salt and pepper.

To Garnish-

- Half a coconut grated.
- 20 gm cashew or ground nut.
- 1 tsp ghee.

Preparation-

- In a pan, dry roast the millets for couple minutes on high flame, turn off and keep it aside.
- In the same pan, heat oil and add mustard seeds, urad dal, curry leaves, slit green chillies, cashew nuts, sauté well.
- Add boiled and cooked vegetables, and sauté for couple of minutes. Add 1 cup of water, salt and bring to a boil.
- When the water starts to boil, add the roasted millets and mix well. Let it simmer and cover with lid and cook for a minute. Since the millets are already roasted, it hardly takes time to cook. Garnish and serve.

To turn the recipe into a non-veg meal – *Kindly refer the instructions in any one of the recipes under the same heading.*

3. *Meat Loaf.*

Total Average Calories: 580 kcal per serving.
Preparation Time: 10 minutes.
Cooking Time: 1 hour.
Servings: 4 to 6 persons.

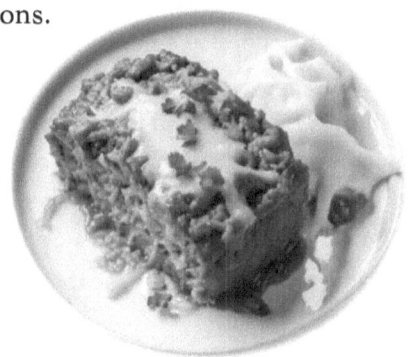

Ingredients-

- 3 large eggs.
- 1/4 cup grated coconut.
- 4 cloves garlic (finely chopped).
- 1 tbsp ginger (finely grated).
- 2 green chili (finely chopped).
- 1 medium onion (finely chopped).
- 700 gm Ground mutton (or meat of your choice, with preferably fatty cuts 7:3)
- 1 tsp cumin powder.
- 1 tsp coriander powder.
- 1 tsp garam masala powder.
- 1/2 tsp red chili powder, 1/4 tsp turmeric powder.
- 2 tbsp fresh cilantro (chopped).
- 3 slices cheese of your choice (optional).
- 3 tbsp ghee or coconut oil (for greasing and basting).
- Salt and pepper to taste.

Preparation-

- In a large mixing bowl, combine the ground meat.
- Add the eggs, grated coconut, garlic, ginger, and green chili.
- Add the onion, cumin powder, coriander powder, garam masala, red chili powder, turmeric powder, salt, and pepper.
- Mix in the chopped cilantro and stir everything until well combined (the mixture should be moist but firm).
- Grease a loaf pan with ghee or coconut oil and transfer the meat mixture into the pan, pressing it down evenly.
- If using, heat 1 tbsp of ghee in a small pan and sauté the cumin seeds and curry leaves until fragrant (1-2 minutes).
- Drizzle this over the meatloaf before baking for additional flavour.
- Place the loaf pan in preheated oven and bake for 1 hour, and the top is browned.
- If you prefer to cook in a pressure cooker, cook for 30 minutes on medium heat, and grill both sides lightly in a fry pan for the brown crust.
- Once done, remove from oven or cooker and let rest for 10 minutes before slicing and serving.

4. *Millet Idli* and *Dosa*.

Total Average Calories: 250 kcal.
Preparation Time: 10 minutes.
Cooking Time: 15 minutes.
Servings: 1 person.

Ingredients-

- 1 cup millets of your choice.
- ½ tsp fenugreek seeds.
- Salt as needed.
- Oil or ghee to grease.

Preparation-

- Take the millet and fenugreek in a bowl.
- Wash well and soak for about 4 hours.
- In a mixer / grinder, grind all the soaked ingredients adding very little water. (If you add too much water and grind to smooth, idlis will turn soft and sticky and be difficult to handle. If required water can add next day while making the dosa or idly)
- If you intend to use the same batter to make both idli and dosa, grind to medium smoothness.
- Transfer to a bowl, add salt and mix well.
- Set aside overnight or for 6 to 10 hrs for fermentation (which drastically reduces the carbohydrate content).
- Mix well before pouring into greased idli moulds or before making dosa .

To make Dosa-

- Heat a tawa, grease with oil, pour a ladle full of batter, spread it in circle, drizzle few drops of oil or ghee over it, cover and cook on medium flame for about 1 to 2 mins.
- Once it's done, the dosas come out easily from the tawa and there won't be any need to flip over and cook.
- Fold and serve the millet dosa accompanied with chutney or sambar or chutney powder of your choice.

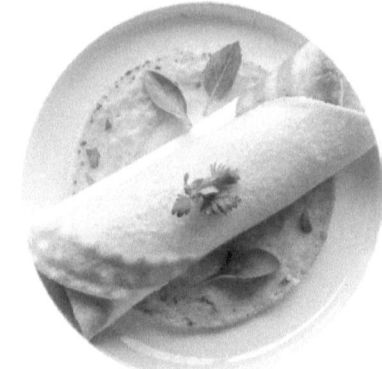

To make Idli-

- Heat water in a steamer, grease idli mold with oil, pour the batter into idli stand and steam for 10 to 12 mins on medium flame.
- Stick a fork or knife in the idli and if it comes clean, then it is cooked well.
- Allow it to cool a bit and remove from mold using a spoon.
- Soft, spongy and healthy millet idlis are ready to serve, with Chutney / Sambar / Chutney Powder or non-veg gravies.

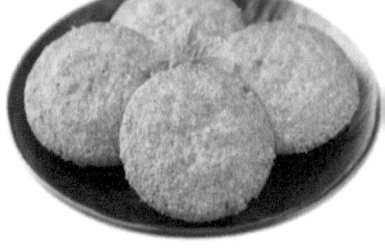

5. *Keto Curd Rice*.

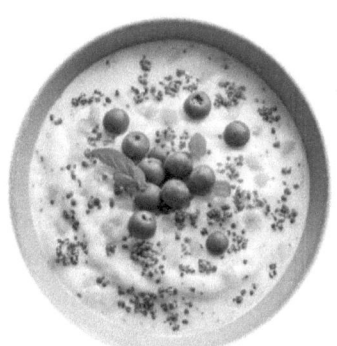

Total Average Calories: 400 kcal.
Preparation Time: 30 minutes.
Cooking Time: 7 minutes.
Servings: 1 person.

Ingredients-

- 100 gm sabja or chia seeds.
- 1 cup curd.
- 50 gm peanuts.
- ½ inch ginger.
- 2 green chillies.
- Coconut oil.
- 5 to 6 curry leaves.
- Half a handful coriander leaves.
- Salt and pepper.

Preparation-

- Soak sabja or chia seeds in double volume of water for 30 minutes or until the seeds soak up the water and have doubled in volume.
- In a pan, fry the peanuts, ginger, chillies and curry leaves in oil for couple minutes on high flame.
- In mixing bowl, add the sabja seeds, curd, salt and mix well.
- Add fried ingredients and coriander leaves to garnish.

❈❈❈❈❈❈❈

I have only shared a few, most simple and easy-to-do recipes, most of which, seem familiar to our traditional foods, in order to convey to you dear reader, that the bare minimum, required for healthy living, can be as simple as tweaking a few ingredients, from our current diet pattern.

These few recipes are more than enough to serve as a guide, for you to start taking baby steps, and once you feel comfortable, you can keep building on these, with more advanced, and extravagant recipes of your choice, that which better suits your palate, and according to what you can afford.

This diet chart and the accompanying recipes have been thoughtfully designed with the financial considerations of middle-class households in mind, who represent a significant portion of the Indian population. While foods like eggs and meat are known for their nutritional benefits, their frequent inclusion may not always be economically feasible for many families.

I do have an arsenal of over the top, exotic recipes, but as the aim of this book is to somehow nudge you towards healthier living, by making everything as simple as possible, and not give you any more excuses to shy away from it, I have chosen to dedicate another book to compile all the advanced recipes and diet charts for you.

So until then…

The End.

Well, not really.
You see, if I were to include every little detail, every fascinating snippet, every twist and turn that I've explored, and learned along the way, this book would never end.
In fact, I'd probably still be writing it ten years from now.
Every day, I discover something new,
and the more I learn, the more I realize
there's always something more to uncover.
So, for the sake of your sanity, and my own, let's just say this is the end...
for now.

But I'm sure there's more to come. In fact, I'm certain of it.
There's always more to be understood and discovered.
Maybe one day I'll release an expanded edition.

For now, though, I'll leave you with this,
The end is just the beginning... and the journey? It's still unfolding.

From the depths of my heart, I wish each and every one of you a life filled with health, happiness, and abundant success.
May your journey be enriched with peace, and fulfilment.

****

SUB-TOPICS

Chapter- 4.1 – Insulin Resistance... 36
Chapter- 5.1 – Free Radicals & Anti-Oxidants (Redox Health)...... 46
Chapter- 7.1 – Good Fat Bad Fat!.. 57
Chapter- 8.1 – Omega-6 Fatty Acids are Good and Bad!............... 72
Chapter- 8.2 – Yummy Deep-Fries are a Mistake....................... 76
Chapter- 13.1 – The Myth of The Leaky Gut............................ 103
Chapter- 16.1 – The Pickle Mechanism................................... 119
Chapter- 17.1 – Glycaemic INDEX vs. Glycaemic LOAD............ 128
Chapter- 18.1 – Autophagy.. 137
Chapter- 20.1 – Is Veganism a Scam?...................................... 170
Chapter- 24.1 – Overweight & Obesity................................... 202
Chapter- 24.2 – Diabetes Mellitus.. 206
Chapter- 24.3 – Type-3 Diabetes or Alzheimer's Disease.............. 208
Chapter- 24.4 – Poly-Cystic Ovarian Syndrome (PCOS) 210
Chapter- 24.5 – Male Infertility... 212
Chapter- 24.6 – Hyper-Triglyceridemia (HTG)......................... 214
Chapter- 24.7 – Non-Alcoholic Fatty Liver Disease (NAFLD)....... 216
Chapter- 24.8 – High Blood Pressure or Hypertension (HTN)...... 219
Chapter- 24.9 – Atherosclerosis (Thickening of Arteries).............. 221
Chapter- 24.10 – Erectile Dysfunction (ED)............................. 223
Chapter- 24.11 – Deep Vein Thrombosis (DVT)....................... 225
Chapter- 24.12 – Varicose Vein.. 227
Chapter- 24.13 – Estrogen Dominance (ED)............................ 229
Chapter- 24.14 – Thyroiditis (Functional)................................ 231
Chapter- 24.15 – Gall-Bladder Stone (Cholelithiasis).................. 234
Chapter- 24.16 – Hyper-uricemia & Gouty Arthritis................... 236
Chapter- 24.17 – Gut Related Disorders.................................. 238
Chapter- 24.18 – Chronic Gastritis... 241
Chapter- 24.19 – Hypo-chlorhydria (Hypo-Acidity).................... 245
Chapter- 24.20 – Hyper-chlorhydria (Hyper-Acidity).................. 251

Chapter- 24.21 – Gastroesophageal reflux disease (GERD)........... 254
Chapter- 24.22 – Migraine & Epilepsy..................................... 258
Chapter- 24.23 – IBS (Irritable Bowel Syndrome)..................... 262
Chapter- 24.24 – Constipation.. 266
Chapter- 24.25 – Diarrhoea.. 269
Chapter- 24.26 – Urinary Tract Infection (UTI)........................ 273
Chapter- 24.27 – Halitosis.. 275
Chapter- 24.28 – IBD (Crohn's Disease & Ulcerative Colitis)......... 277
Chapter- 24.29 – Ankylosing Spondylitis (AS)........................... 279
Chapter- 24.30 – Ig-A nephropathy (Berger's Disease)................ 281
Chapter- 24.31 – Systemic Lupus Erythematosus (SLE).............. 283
Chapter- 24.32 – Rheumatoid Arthritis (RA)............................ 285
Chapter- 24.33 – Immune Thrombocytopenia (ITP)................... 288
Chapter- 24.34 – Thyroiditis (Hashimoto's & Graves')................ 290
Chapter- 24.35 – Multiple Sclerosis (MS)................................. 295
Chapter- 24.36 – Type-1 Diabetes Mellitus (DMT1).................. 299
Chapter- 24.37 – Sjögren's Syndrome....................................... 303
Chapter- 24.38 – Vitiligo.. 305
Chapter- 24.39 – Fibromyalgia.. 307
Chapter- 24.40 – Prostatitis.. 309
Chapter- 24.41 – Myasthenia Gravis (MG).............................. 312
Chapter- 24.42 – Depression... 316
Chapter- 24.43 – Autism Spectrum Disorder (ASD)................... 319
Chapter- 24.44 – Dermatitis & Eczema.................................... 322
Chapter- 24.45 – Psoriasis.. 324
Chapter- 24.46 – Sinusitis... 326
Chapter- 24.47 – Bronchial Asthma (BA)................................. 329
Chapter- 24.48 – Urticaria (Hives)... 331
Chapter- 24.49 – Fissures, Fistula & Haemorrhoids................... 335
Chapter- 24.50 – Pigmentation.. 339
Chapter- 24.51 – Acne... 341

Chapter- 24.52 – Osteo Arthritis (OA).................................... 345
Chapter- 24.53 – Osteopenia & Osteoporosis........................... 348
Chapter- 24.54 – Carpal Tunnel Syndrome (CTS)..................... 350
Chapter- 24.55 – Plantar Fasciitis (PF).................................. 352
Chapter- 24.56 – Frozen Shoulder (Adhesive Capsulitis)............. 354
Chapter- 24.57 – Sciatica.. 356
Chapter- 24.58 – Inter-Vertebral Disc Prolapse (IVDP).............. 358
Chapter- 24.59 – Urinary Incontinence................................... 360
Chapter- 24.60 – Dental Health.. 362
Chapter- 24.61 – Cancer... 368

****

(Major) REFERENCES

- B. D. Chaurasia's Human Anatomy.
- Textbook of Anatomy - Vishram Singh.
- Essentials of Medical Physiology - K Sembulingam.
- Biochemistry - Dr. U. Sathyanarayanan, Dr. U. Chakrapani.
- Ananthanarayan and Paniker's textbook of Microbiology.
- Practical Microbiology - Bharti Arora and D. R. Arora.
- Practical Pathology - Harsh Mohan.
- Textbook of Electrotherapy - Jagmohan Singh.
- Textbook of Orthopaedic Physiotherapy - P. S. Kapoor.
- Davidson's Principles and Practices of Medicine.
- DC Dutta's Textbook of Gynaecology.
- Pharmacology - Karen Whalen.
- Nutrition Diagnosis-Related Care - Escott Stump.
- Preventive and Social Medicine – Rabindra Nath Roy.
- Park's Textbook of Preventive and Social Medicine – K. Park.
- Hatha Yoga Pradipika – Svātmārāma.
- Why Evolution is True – Jerry. A. Coyne.
- Soil Grass & Cancer – Andre Voisin.
- The straight dope on cholesterol by Peter Attia.
- Fish-Rich Diet, Leptin, and Body Mass PMID:12663785.
- Schisgall, Oscar, Eyes on Tomorrow: "The Evolution of Procter & Gamble", J.G. Ferguson Pub Co., Distributed by Doubleday, 1981.
- Pendleton S. "Man's Most Important Food is Fat: The Use of Persuasive Techniques in Procter & Gamble's Public Relations Campaign to Introduce Crisco, 1911-1913," Public Relations Quarterly, March, 1999.
- Mary G. E and Fallon, Sally, *"The Oiling of America."* Wise Traditions, Summer 2001.
- https://www.zeroacre.com/white-papers/seed-oils-as-a-driver-of-heart-disease
- https://www.zeroacre.com/white-papers/how-vegetable-oil-makes-us-fat
- French paradox PMID: 14676260.
- Indian paradox PMID: 9861517.
- Surgical removal of visceral fat reverses hepatic insulin resistance, PMID: 9892227.
- mTOR: from growth signal integration to cancer, diabetes and ageing, PMID: 21157483.
- Insulin regulation of gluconeogenesis, PMID: 28868790.
- Mechanisms of lipotoxicity in NAFLD and clinical implications, PMID: 21629127.

- Role of endoplasmic reticulum stress in the pathogenesis of NAFLD, PMID: 24587654.
- The lysosomal-mitochondrial axis in free fatty acid-induced hepatic lipotoxicity, PMID: 18220271.
- Increased VLDL secretion, hepatic steatosis, and insulin resistance, PMID: 21616678.
- Carbohydrate Sensing Through the Transcription Factor ChREBP, PMID: 31275349.
- Fructose drives de novo lipogenesis affecting metabolic health, PMID: 36753292.
- Structural and functional properties of deep abdominal subcutaneous adipose tissue explain its association with insulin resistance and cardiovascular risk in men, PMID: 24186879.
- Omentin: A Key Player in Glucose Homeostasis, Atheroprotection, & Metabolic Disorders, PMID:38397886.
- https://drcate.com/pufa-project/
- https://pubmed.ncbi.nlm.nih.gov/9844997/
- https://www.sciencedirect.com/science/article/abs/pii/S0891584915000891
- https://www.drberg.com/blog/a-carrot-a-day-keeps-the-doctor-away
- Mushrooms as Future Generation Healthy Foods PMID: 36562045.
- Periodontal Pathogens as Risk Factors of Cardiovascular Diseases, Diabetes, Rheumatoid Arthritis, Cancer, and Chronic Obstructive Pulmonary Disease-Is There Cause for Consideration?, PMID: 31600905.
- Prevotella Copri and Microbiota in Rheumatoid Arthritis, PMID: 31683983.
- The Relationship Between Porphyromonas Gingivalis and Rheumatoid Arthritis PMID: 35923803.
- Molecular Mechanisms of Skatole-Induced Inflammatory Responses in Intestinal Epithelial Cells: Implications for Colorectal Cancer and Inflammatory Bowel Disease, PMID: 39451248.
- The role of short-chain fatty acids in inflammatory skin diseases PMID: 36817115.
- Microbial metabolite p-cresol inhibits gut hormone expression and regulates small intestinal transit in mice, PMID: 37534214.
- Migraine and the trigemino-vascular system, 40 years and counting, PMID: 31160203.
- Calcitonin gene-related peptide (CGRP): role in migraine pathophysiology and therapeutic targeting, PMID:32003253.
- Gut microbiota generation of protein-bound uremic toxins and related metabolites is not altered at different stages of chronic kidney disease, PMID: 32317112.
- Bile Acids Improve Psoriasiform Dermatitis through Inhibition of IL-17A Expression and CCL20-CCR6-Mediated Trafficking of T Cells, PMID: 34808237.

- Junctional adhesion molecule 1 (JAM-1), PMID: 15065765.
- Leaky Gut As a Danger Signal for Autoimmune Diseases, PMID: 28588585.
- Microbial Influences of Mucosal Immunity in Rheumatoid Arthritis, PMID: 33025188.
- Zonulin, regulation of tight junctions, and autoimmune diseases, PMID: 22731712.
- Vitamin A and vitamin D regulate the microbial complexity, barrier function, and the mucosal immune responses to ensure intestinal homeostasis, PMID: 31084433.
- Role of Zinc in Mucosal Health and Disease: A Review of the Literature, PMID: 32572355.
- Artificial Sweeteners Disrupt Tight Junctions and Barrier Function in the Intestinal Epithelium through Activation of the Sweet Taste Receptor, T1R3, PMID: 32580504.
- Association of Long-Term Risk of Respiratory, Allergic, and Infectious Diseases With Removal of Adenoids and Tonsils in Childhood, PMID: 29879264.
- Glucose but Not Fructose Alters the Intestinal Paracellular Permeability and Inflammatory Status in Mice, PMID: 35024040.
- Zinc Deficiency in Men Over 50 and Its Implications in Prostate Disorders, PMID: 32850402.
- Vitamin D suppresses Th17 cytokine production by inducing C/EBP homologous protein (CHOP) expression PMID: 20974859.
- Crosstalk between omega-6 oxylipins and the enteric nervous system: Implications for gut disorders?, PMID:37056732.
- IgA antibodies against Klebsiella and other Gram-negative bacteria in HLA-B27 associated ankylosing spondylitis and acute anterior uveitis, PMID: 8835503.
- Cancer as a Metabolic Disease: On the Origin, Management, and Prevention of Cancer, by Thomas Seyfried
- On the Origin of Cancer Cells by Otto Warburg PMID: 16376957.
- Is cancer a metabolic disease? PMID: 24388298.
- Antitumor efficacy of EDTA co-treatment with cisplatin in tumor-bearing mice. PMID: 33199253.
- Effect of a parenteral ozone-oxygen mixture on the concentration of immuno-globulins (IgA, IgG, IgM), of vitamin A and lysozyme activity in patients with cervical cancer PMID: 3471679.
- Vitamin D signalling pathways in cancer: potential for anticancer therapeutics PMID: 17514235.
- Novel cancer therapy targeting microbiome, PMID: 31492480.

****

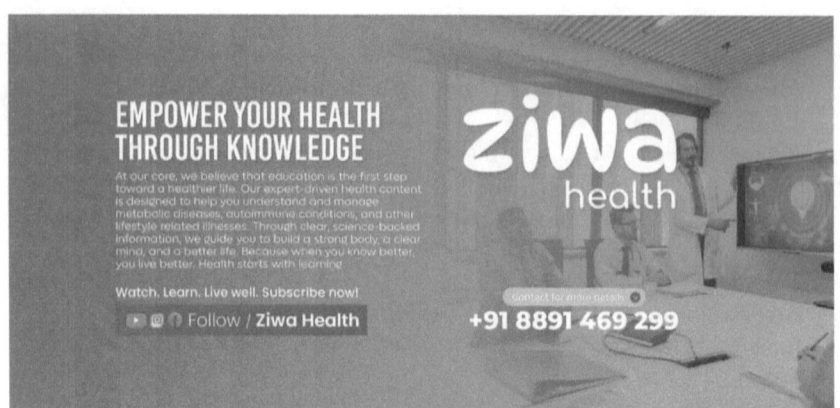

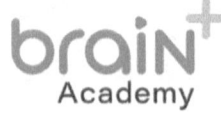

Let's Learn to Read and Write!

Unlock the joy of reading and writing! Age doesn't matter. Learn various languages through personal mentoring from language experts.

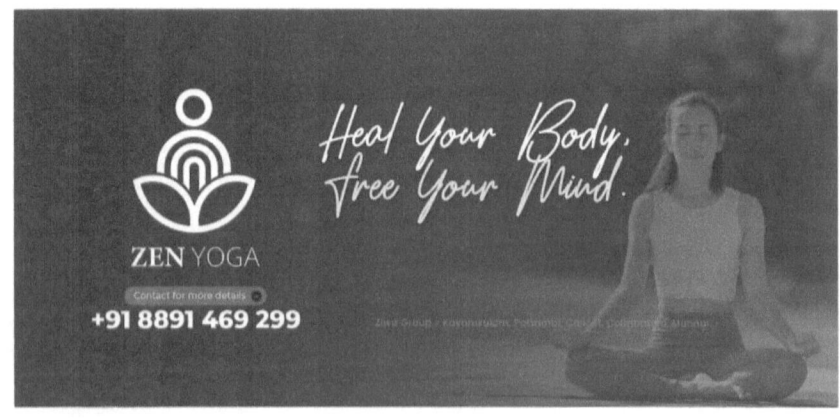

Calm Within Reach

Discover simple and proven supportive strategies to manage mental stress and regain balance, focus, inner peace and emotional well-being in your daily life, with support from psychology experts.

zerene
WELLNESS-HUB

Contact for more details
+91 95440 10087

Health is the Aim
Weight Loss is Bonus

Focus on feeling better, moving with ease, and living with energy. With a mindful approach, you can shed excess weight while keeping your overall well-being at the center. No quick fixes or harsh diets, just balanced habits, nourishing food, and self-care. Lose weight the right way, with care and intention, and let your health shine from the inside out.

ziwa
Doctor Diet

Contact for more details
+91 7025 414 169

Better Choice
Better Life

Treating metabolic diseases, autoimmune conditions, and other lifestyle-related illnesses requires a focus on addressing the root cause. Balanced nutrition, appropriate medications, regular physical activity, and stress management helps enhance the body's resilience, improve mental clarity, and prevent chronic conditions. Embrace a healthy lifestyle that nurtures both body and mind for lasting well-being and vitality.

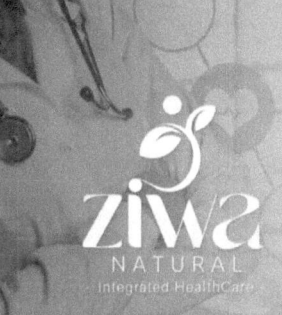

Contact for more details
+91 8891 469 299

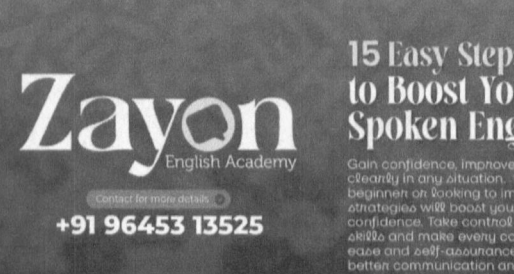
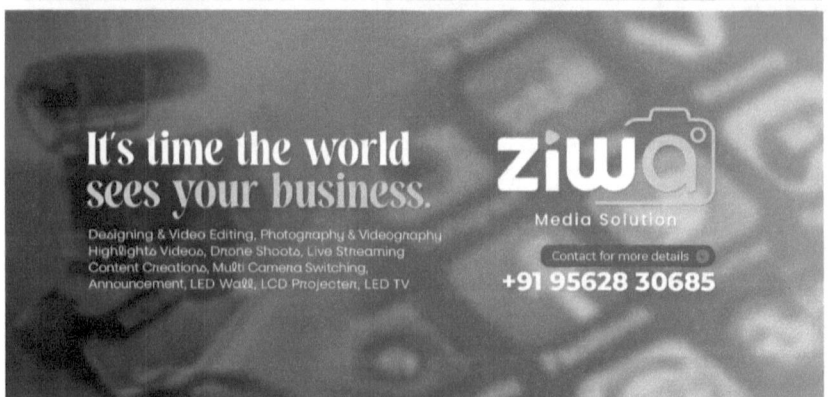

www.ingramcontent.com/pod-product-compliance
Lightning Source LLC
LaVergne TN
LVHW091613070526
838199LV00044B/780